Otologic and Lateral Skull Base Trauma

Otologic and Lateral Skull Base Trauma

Edited by

Elliott D. Kozin, MD
*Department of Otolaryngology,
Massachusetts Eye and Ear, Boston, MA, United States;
Department of Otolaryngology, Harvard Medical School,
Boston, MA, United States*

ELSEVIER

Publisher: Sarah E. Barth
Acquisitions Editor: Jessica L. McCool
Editorial Project Manager: Sam Young
Project Manager: Kiruthika Govindaraju
Cover Designer: Matthew Limbert

3251 Riverport Lane
St. Louis, Missouri 63043

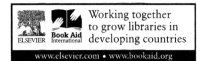

Contents

CHAPTER 16   Management of pediatric otologic trauma 207
Evette A. Ronner, MD and Michael S. Cohen, MD

CHAPTER 17   Pediatric vestibular dysfunction following head injury: Diagnosis and management 217
Graham Cochrane, PhD and Jacob R. Brodsky, MD, FACS, FAAP

List of contributors

Kalil Abdullah, MD, MSc
Department of Neurosurgery, University of Pittsburgh School of Medicine, Pittsburgh, PA, United States; Hillman Comprehensive Cancer Center, University of Pittsburgh Medical Center, Pittsburgh, PA, United States

Reef K. Al-Asad, BA
Department of Otolaryngology, Massachusetts Eye and Ear, Boston, MA, United States

Syeda Maheen Batool
Department of Neurosurgery, Massachusetts General Hospital, Boston, MA, United States

Jacob R. Brodsky, MD, FACS, FAAP
Department of Otolaryngology and Communication Enhancement, Boston Children's Hospital, Boston, MA, United States; Department of Otolaryngology, Harvard Medical School, Boston, MA, United States

Ricky Chae, BA
T.H. Chan School of Medicine, University of Massachusetts Chan Medical School, Worcester, MA, United States; Department of Otolaryngology-Head and Neck Surgery, University of Massachusetts Chan Medical School, Worcester, MA, United States

Divya A. Chari, MD
T.H. Chan School of Medicine, University of Massachusetts Chan Medical School, Worcester, MA, United States; Department of Otolaryngology-Head and Neck Surgery, University of Massachusetts Chan Medical School, Worcester, MA, United States; Department of Otolaryngology-Head and Neck Surgery, Harvard Medical School, Boston, MA, United States; Department of Otolaryngology-Head and Neck Surgery, Massachusetts Eye and Ear, Boston, MA, United States

Graham Cochrane, PhD
University of Alabama, School of Medicine, Birmingham, AL, United States

Michael S. Cohen, MD
Department of Otolaryngology-Head and Neck Surgery, Massachusetts Eye and Ear, Harvard Medical School, Boston, MA, United States

Scott Connors, MD
Department of Neurological Surgery, University of Texas Southwestern Medical Center, Dallas, TX, United States

Matthew Gordon Crowson, MD, MPA, MASc, FRCSC
Department of Otolaryngology-Head and Neck Surgery, Massachusetts Eye and Ear, Boston, MA, United States

Keelin Fallon, BA
Department of Otolaryngology, UMass Memorial Healthcare, UMass Chan Medical School, Worcester, MA, United States

Tomas Garzon-Muvdi, MD, MSc
Department of Neurological Surgery, Emory University, Atlanta, GA, United States

Robert M. Gramer
Department of Neurosurgery, Massachusetts General Hospital, Boston, MA, United States

Seth Herman
California Rehabilitation Institute, Cedars Sinai Medical Center, Los Angeles, CA, United States

Sara Holmes, BA
Department of Otolaryngology, UMass Memorial Healthcare, UMass Chan Medical School, Worcester, MA, United States

Nicole T. Jiam, MD
Department of Otolaryngology-Head and Neck Surgery, Massachusetts Eye and Ear, Harvard Medical School, Boston, MA, United States

Amy F. Juliano, MD
Department of Radiology, Massachusetts Eye and Ear, Harvard Medical School, Boston, MA, United States

David H. Jung, MD, PhD
Department of Otolaryngology-Head and Neck Surgery, Harvard Medical School, Boston, MA, United States; Department of Otolaryngology-Head and Neck Surgery, Massachusetts Eye and Ear, Boston, MA, United States

Leanna W. Katz
Boston University, Boston, MA, United States

Judith S. Kempfle, MD
Department of Otolaryngology, Massachusetts Eye and Ear, Boston, MA, United States

Renata M. Knoll, MD
Department of Otolaryngology, Massachusetts Eye and Ear, Boston, MA, United States; Department of Otolaryngology, Harvard Medical School, Boston, MA, United States

Elliott D. Kozin, MD
Department of Otolaryngology, Massachusetts Eye and Ear, Boston, MA, United States; Department of Otolaryngology, Harvard Medical School, Boston, MA, United States

Daniel J. Lee, MD
Department of Otolaryngology-Head and Neck Surgery, Massachusetts Eye and Ear, Harvard Medical School, Boston, MA, United States

Philip D. Littlefield, MD
Department of Otolaryngology, Sharp Rees-Stealy Medical Group, San Diego, CA, United States

Kathryn C. MacDonald
Wentworth-Douglass Hospital, Dover, NH, United States

Krupa R. Patel, MD
Division of Facial Plastic and Reconstructive Surgery, Department of Otolaryngology-Head and Neck Surgery, Massachusetts Eye and Ear, Harvard Medical School, Boston, MA, United States

Aaron Plitt, MD
Department of Neurological Surgery, University of Texas Southwestern Medical Center, Dallas, TX, United States

Katherine L. Reinshagen
Department of Radiology, Massachusetts Eye and Ear, Harvard Medical School, Boston, MA, United States

Aaron K. Remenschneider, MD, MPH, FACS
Department of Otolaryngology, UMass Memorial Healthcare, UMass Chan Medical School, Worcester, MA, United States; Department of Otolaryngology, Massachusetts Eye and Ear Infirmary, Harvard Medical School, Boston, MA, United States

Evette A. Ronner, MD
Department of Otolaryngology-Head and Neck Surgery, Boston University Medical Center, Boston, MA, United States

Felipe Santos, MD
Department of Otolaryngology-Head and Neck Surgery, Massachusetts Eye and Ear, Harvard Medical School, Boston, MA, United States

David A. Shaye, MD, MPH
Division of Facial Plastic and Reconstructive Surgery, Department of Otolaryngology-Head and Neck Surgery, Massachusetts Eye and Ear, Harvard Medical School, Boston, MA, United States

Yohan Song, MD
Department of Otolaryngology-Head and Neck Surgery, Massachusetts Eye and Ear, Harvard Medical School, Boston, MA, United States

Christopher J. Stapleton
Department of Neurosurgery, Massachusetts General Hospital, Boston, MA, United States

Justin E. Vranic
Department of Neurosurgery, Massachusetts General Hospital, Boston, MA, United States; Department of Radiology, Massachusetts General Hospital, Boston, MA, United States

Matthew J. Wu, MD
Department of Otolaryngology, Massachusetts Eye and Ear, Boston, MA, United States; Department of Otolaryngology-Head and Neck Surgery, Washington University School of Medicine in St Louis, St Louis, MO, United States

Epidemiology of traumatic brain injury and lateral skull base injury in the United States

Matthew J. Wu, MD [1,2], Elliott D. Kozin, MD [1,3]

[1]*Department of Otolaryngology, Massachusetts Eye and Ear, Boston, MA, United States;* [2]*Department of Otolaryngology-Head and Neck Surgery, Washington University School of Medicine in St Louis, St Louis, MO, United States;* [3]*Department of Otolaryngology, Harvard Medical School, Boston, MA, United States*

Overview

Traumatic brain injury (TBI) is a major public health issue globally[1−3] and in the United States.[4−6] The Centers for Disease Control (CDC) defines TBI as an insult (blow or bump to the head) or penetrating head injury affecting the normal function of the brain.[7] TBI can vary in severity, and in the United States, the majority are mild and clinically often described as a "concussion."[8] Recent research over the past decade has demonstrated that there is a growing societal cost[8] involved in the management of the long-term physical and psychosocial sequelae of TBI.[9−11] Following a head injury, trauma may also occur to the lateral skull base, which is an area that includes critical neurovascular structures within the middle and posterior fossae and temporal bone, which, similar to TBI, may greatly affect quality of life.[12] Given the rising incidence of TBI and growing public health concern,[5] understanding the epidemiologic patterns of these types of injuries is important for identifying and managing populations at risk.

Incidence and epidemiology of traumatic brain injury in the United States

Each year in the United States, the overall incidence of TBI is 823.7 per 100,000 people.[5] The overall incidence of TBI can be further subdivided in different settings: 403, 85, and 18 per 100,000 people for emergency department (ED) visits, hospitalizations, and deaths, respectively.[6] Annually, these account for 2.5 million patients who are treated in the ED (87%), hospitalized (11%), or die from their injuries (2%).[13] These annual estimates, however, likely underestimate the true incidence as they do not account for individuals who do not seek medical treatment or receive

Otologic and Lateral Skull Base Trauma. https://doi.org/10.1016/B978-0-323-87482-3.00018-1

care in either an outpatient setting or federal facility (e.g., Veterans Affairs hospital).[13]

Among individuals who experience a TBI in the United States, there are several etiologies that are major contributors to annual ED visits, hospitalizations, and death.[5] The top three most common etiologies resulting in TBI-related ED visits are falls (658,668 individuals; 41%), being struck by or against an object (304,797 individuals; 19%), and being in a motor vehicle traffic accident (232,240; 15%).[5] Among patients who were hospitalized, the leading etiologies resulting in TBI-related hospitalizations are falls (66,291 individuals; 24%) and motor vehicle traffic accidents (53,391 individuals; 19%).[5] Major causes of TBI-related death are motor vehicle traffic accidents (14,795; 29%), self-inflicted/suicide (14,713; 29%), and falls (10,944; 21%).[5]

Sports-related TBI is also a growing area of public health interest.[14] At present, data from the National Electronic Injury Surveillance System—All Injury Program suggest that the majority of TBI-related ED visits are due to contact sports (football and soccer) as well as from basketball, bicycling, and playground activities.[4] Recent studies suggest that within the past two decades, there has been a 62% increase in the treatment of pediatric sports-related TBI[4,5]; this may, however, be driven by public health initiatives to raise awareness for sports-related concussions, such as the CDC's HEADS UP campaign, which prompted more patients to recognize and seek care in the ED following a suspected TBI.[14] A recent study examining a large epidemiologic sample of pediatric patients with TBI suggested that children were more likely to have auditory dysfunction.[15] Further studies are needed to understand how head trauma management in this population can be improved to reduce the known long-term negative developmental sequelae of TBI, such as disrupted cognitive and social performance.[16−18]

Prior studies have highlighted that specific populations are at increased risk for TBI, which include people within certain age groups and males. Individuals who are at the extremes of age ranges (0−4 years, 15−19 years, and ≥75 years) are at increased risk for TBI, leading to an ED visit or hospitalization[13] whereas those ≥75 years old are at greatest risk for TBI-related hospitalizations and death.[13] Determining if a patient suffered a TBI who is in the extremes of age may be challenging as symptoms may be indolent. Children without visible physical injury may present with a delayed onset effects of TBI including poor academic performance and difficulty with social relationships.[16,19] Older adults with past TBI may have their symptoms misattributed to the normal process of aging. As a result, providers should maintain a high clinical suspicion for TBI, especially given the recent epidemiologic shift toward falls being the leading cause of TBI,[5] which are common in the elderly.[20] Additionally, compared with females, males contribute to the majority (59%) of TBI-related medical visits,[13,21] which may be due to males participating in more high-risk activities.

Other patient characteristics associated with elevated risk for TBI include lower socioeconomic status, minority races, and living in rural geographical regions, which are factors that may be interrelated.[22] Comparing insurance status as a surrogate for socioeconomic status, patients who were uninsured were nearly twice as likely to have a TBI compared with those with private insurance.[23] Individuals who are from Black,[24] Hispanic,[24] or American Indian/Alaska Native[25] backgrounds within the United States have greater risk of TBI compared with white individuals. Additionally, those living in rural regions also have increased risk of suffering from a TBI compared with those living in urban settings.[26] Several studies suggest that these populations, in addition to experiencing TBI more frequently than the general population, may also have poorer outcomes.[26] Differences in clinical outcomes may be due to several factors including reduced access to care,[27] delayed presentation,[27,28] and lower likelihood to participate in follow-up care.[29] Future studies are needed to understand how improved resource distribution may reduce rates of TBI in these populations and improve patient outcomes.

Incidence and epidemiology of lateral skull base trauma in the United States

In addition to TBI, lateral skull base trauma is a growing public health concern,[30] but recognition of the lateral skull base as a distinct anatomical area has been fairly recent over the past three decades.[12] The lateral skull base is defined by a combination of two subregions.[12] The first region is the area that extends from the orbit's posterior wall to the petrous temporal bone and formed by the pterygopalatine and infratemporal fossae with the overlying part of the middle cranial fossa, which contains vasculature structures such as the internal carotid artery, and cranial nerves (maxillary and mandibular divisions of the trigeminal nerve, facial, and vestibulocochlear nerves).[12] The second region is primarily composed of the posterior cranial fossa and the posterior segment of the middle cranial fossa, which contains vasculature structures such as the internal jugular vein and cranial nerves (glossopharyngeal, vagus, spinal accessory, and hypoglossal nerves).[12] The following section, however, will focus on primarily temporal bone fractures (TBFs) as robust epidemiologic studies of other areas of the lateral skull base are limited.

Following head injury, the high energy impact may lead to fractures of the skull base and temporal bone. It is estimated that 4%–30% of head injuries lead to skull base fractures and 18%–40% of these result in TBFs[31–34] where the majority of TBFs are unilateral and bilateral TBF occurs in only 4.4%–20% of patients.[34–38] Given the amount of force required to cause a TBF, it is common for trauma to occur to other structures such as the facial nerve or tympanic membrane[36,39] or result in cerebrospinal fluid (CSF) leaks.[36] TBF occurs through three primary mechanisms: motor vehicle accidents (MVAs) (12%–47%), falls (16%–40%), and assaults (10%–37%),[34,39,40] where MVA is currently the most common mechanism of injury,[36] but recent studies suggest that falls are becoming increasingly common.[35] The increased use of automotive safety features such as airbags and seat belts may contribute to the decline in MVA.[35] Risk factors for sustaining a TBF include patient characteristics such as younger age (second to fourth decades) and male gender,[36] which is similar to the risk factors in TBI, and may be due to males participating in risky behavior. Consistent with the severity of injury resulting in TBF, mortality rates following TBF range are high and estimated to be 7.9%—12%.[35,36,41,42]

Historically, TBFs have been classified by the orientation of the fracture line relative to the long axis of the petrous temporal bone as either transverse (perpendicular) or longitudinal (parallel) fractures.[43] Prior studies suggest that using this classification scheme, 70%—90% of TBFs are transverse and 10%—30% of TBFs are longitudinal.[32,34,36,38,40,44] Growing evidence, however, suggests that a significant amount of TBF cannot be discretely organized in these two categories, where most TBFs have a mixed fracture pattern.[34,38] Given the inability for this earlier TBF scheme to prognosticate important clinical information, such as neurotologic deficits,[40] a newer scheme describing involvement of the otic capsule, which is a bony structure that contains the cochlea, vestibule, and semicircular canals, has been increasingly used.[34,36,40,45—47] TBFs using this scheme are categorized as otic capsule-violating (OCV) or otic capsule-sparing (OCS); compared with OCS TBF, OCV TBFs are associated with significantly higher rates of facial nerve paralysis, sensorineural hearing loss, CSF leak, and intracranial complications.[34,36,40,45—47] Since the more recent adoption of the otic capsule classification scheme, the prevalence of OCV appears to occur in 2%—8% of TBF.[32,34—36,44,48] The mechanism of injury that results in OCV TBF is often due to impact of the occipital area toward the foramen magnum, petrous pyramid, and otic capsule. Future studies are needed to assess individuals at risk for experiencing OCV TBF to help improve the diagnosis and management of these injuries.

Healthcare resource utilization due to traumatic brain injury and lateral skull base injury

In addition to being a leading cause of mortality in the United States, TBI and its associated sequelae are associated with significant morbidity.[5] The comorbidities from TBI can greatly affect quality of life by limiting physical function and disturbing cognitive function (e.g., memory, attention) and mood.[5,49,50] The domains that TBI and lateral skull base injury are extensive and can impact both social relationships and the ability to work of those directly injured and for caregivers.[51,52]

In the United States, it is estimated that TBI results in 2.5 million ED visits, inpatient stays, and deaths, and between 3.2 and 5.3 million people have a TBI-related disability.[53—55] Managing TBI acutely and its sequelae places a large financial burden on the healthcare system; the annual expenditure for TBI-related care in the United States is approximately 60 billion dollars.[56] Healthcare-related costs for TBI are composed of several domains: direct medical (acute medical treatment and follow-up), societal (lost productivity due to disability), and rehabilitation (cost due to use of rehabilitation centers).[57] In a study analyzing patients with severe TBI, the majority of expenditures were societal costs followed by direct medical and rehabilitation costs,[57] suggesting that the main cost is opportunity cost due to lost productivity. As a result, areas for reduced healthcare resource utilization related to TBI care should be focused on education, prevention, and targeted treatment protocols. Over the past 40 years, the Brain Trauma Foundation, which is an organization created by the CDC provided evidence-based guidelines for the treatment and monitoring of TBI.[58] Authors who performed a cost–benefit analysis utilizing the Brain Trauma Foundation guidelines noted that if widely adopted, the national cost of TBI-related care could be reduced by 4 billion dollars while decreasing mortality rates.[57] Future studies are needed to identify additional patient-related factors to further lower this societal cost.

Conclusion

TBI and lateral skull base injuries are major public health issues in the United States. Individuals who suffer from these injuries may experience reduced functional status that may affect them socially and cognitively. Economically, TBI and lateral skull base injuries also place a significant burden on the healthcare system. Increased awareness and adoption of evidence-based protocols may help improve clinical outcomes and reduce healthcare resource utilization.

References

1. Hyder AA, Wunderlich CA, Puvanachandra P, Gururaj G, Kobusingye OC. The impact of traumatic brain injuries: a global perspective. *NeuroRehabilitation*. 2007;22(5): 341–353.
2. Roozenbeek B, Maas AI, Menon DK. Changing patterns in the epidemiology of traumatic brain injury. *Nat Rev Neurol*. 2013;9(4):231–236.
3. Taylor CA, Bell JM, Breiding MJ, Xu L. Traumatic brain injury-related emergency department visits, hospitalizations, and deaths—United States, 2007 and 2013. *MMWR Surveill Summ*. 2017;66(9):1–16.
4. Prevention CfDCa. Nonfatal traumatic brain injuries related to sports and recreation activities among persons aged ≤19 years—United States, 2001–2009. *MMWR (Morb Mortal Wkly Rep)*. 2011;60:1337–1342.
5. Prevention CfDCa. *Report to Congress on Traumatic Brain Injury in the United States: Epidemiology and Rehabilitation*. National Center for Injury Prevention and Control; Division of Unintentional Injury Prevention; 2015.
6. Langlois JA, Rutland-Brown W, Thomas KE. *Traumatic Brain Injury in the United States: Emergency Department Visits, Hospitalizations, and Deaths*. Division of Injury and Disability Outcomes and Programs National Center for Injury Prevention and Control Centers for Disease Control and Prevention Department of Health and Human Services; 2004.

7. Marr AL, Coronado VG. *Central Nervous System Injury Surveillance Data Submission Standards—2002*. Centers for Disease Control and Prevention, National Center for Injury Prevention and Control; 2004.

8. Pavlov V, Thompson-Leduc P, Zimmer L, et al. Mild traumatic brain injury in the United States: demographics, brain imaging procedures, health-care utilization and costs. *Brain Inj.* 2019;33(9):1151−1157.

9. Howell DR, O'Brien MJ, Beasley MA, Mannix RC, Meehan 3rd WP. Initial somatic symptoms are associated with prolonged symptom duration following concussion in adolescents. *Acta Paediatr.* 2016;105(9):e426−e432.

10. Kontos AP, Elbin RJ, Schatz P, et al. A revised factor structure for the post-concussion symptom scale: baseline and postconcussion factors. *Am J Sports Med.* 2012;40(10):2375−2384.

11. DeKosky ST, Ikonomovic MD, Gandy S. Traumatic brain injury: football, warfare, and long-term effects. *Minn Med.* 2010;93(12):46−47.

12. Irish JC, Gullane PJ, Gentili F, et al. Tumors of the skull base: outcome and survival analysis of 77 cases. *Head Neck.* 1994;16(1):3−10.

13. Faul M, Xu L, Wald MM, Coronado VG. *Traumatic Brain Injury in the United States; Emergency Department Visits, Hospitalizations, and Deaths, 2002−2006*. Centers for Disease Control and Prevention, National Center for Injury Prevention and Control; 2010.

14. Sarmiento K, Hoffman R, Dmitrovsky Z, Lee R. A 10-year review of the Centers for Disease Control and Prevention's Heads Up initiatives: bringing concussion awareness to the forefront. *J Saf Res.* 2014;50:143−147.

15. Kozin ED, Knoll RM, Bhattacharyya N. Association of pediatric hearing loss and head injury in a population-based study. *Otolaryngol Head Neck Surg.* 2021;165(3):455−457.

16. Ewing-Cobbs L, Prasad MR, Kramer L, et al. Late intellectual and academic outcomes following traumatic brain injury sustained during early childhood. *J Neurosurg.* 2006;105(suppl 4):287−296.

17. Yeates KO, Swift E, Taylor HG, et al. Short- and long-term social outcomes following pediatric traumatic brain injury. *J Int Neuropsychol Soc.* 2004;10(3):412−426.

18. Schwartz L, Taylor HG, Drotar D, Yeates KO, Wade SL, Stancin T. Long-term behavior problems following pediatric traumatic brain injury: prevalence, predictors, and correlates. *J Pediatr Psychol.* 2003;28(4):251−263.

19. Gerrard-Morris A, Taylor HG, Yeates KO, et al. Cognitive development after traumatic brain injury in young children. *J Int Neuropsychol Soc.* 2010;16(1):157−168.

20. Berry SD, Miller RR. Falls: epidemiology, pathophysiology, and relationship to fracture. *Curr Osteoporos Rep.* 2008;6(4):149−154.

21. Schneider ALC, Wang D, Ling G, Gottesman RF, Selvin E. Prevalence of self-reported head injury in the United States. *N Engl J Med.* 2018;379(12):1176−1178.

22. Bruns Jr J, Hauser WA. The epidemiology of traumatic brain injury: a review. *Epilepsia.* 2003;44(s10):2−10.

23. Selassie AW, Pickelsimer EE, Frazier Jr L, Ferguson PL. The effect of insurance status, race, and gender on ED disposition of persons with traumatic brain injury. *Am J Emerg Med.* 2004;22(6):465−473.

24. Schiraldi M, Patil CG, Mukherjee D, et al. Effect of insurance and racial disparities on outcomes in traumatic brain injury. *J Neurol Surg A Cent Eur Neurosurg.* 2015;76(3):224−232.

25. Adekoya N, Thurman DJ, White DD, Webb KW. Surveillance for traumatic brain injury deaths—United States, 1989—1998. *MMWR Surveill Summ.* 2002;51(10):1—14.

26. Brown JB, Kheng M, Carney NA, Rubiano AM, Puyana JC. Geographical disparity and traumatic brain injury in America: rural areas suffer poorer outcomes. *J Neurosci Rural Pract.* 2019;10(1):10—15.

27. Jarman MP, Castillo RC, Carlini AR, Kodadek LM, Haider AH. Rural risk: geographic disparities in trauma mortality. *Surgery.* 2016;160(6):1551—1559.

28. Carr BG, Bowman AJ, Wolff CS, et al. Disparities in access to trauma care in the United States: a population-based analysis. *Injury.* 2017;48(2):332—338.

29. Graves JM, Mackelprang JL, Moore M, et al. Rural-urban disparities in health care costs and health service utilization following pediatric mild traumatic brain injury. *Health Serv Res.* 2019;54(2):337—345.

30. Feldman JS, Farnoosh S, Kellman RM, Tatum 3rd SA. Skull base trauma: clinical considerations in evaluation and diagnosis and review of management techniques and surgical approaches. *Semin Plast Surg.* 2017;31(4):177—188.

31. Cannon CR, Jahrsdoerfer RA. Temporal bone fractures. Review of 90 cases. *Arch Otolaryngol.* 1983;109(5):285—288.

32. Nosan DK, Benecke Jr JE, Murr AH. Current perspective on temporal bone trauma. *Otolaryngol Head Neck Surg.* 1997;117(1):67—71.

33. Alvi A, Bereliani A. Acute intracranial complications of temporal bone trauma. *Otolaryngol Head Neck Surg.* 1998;119(6):609—613.

34. Dahiya R, Keller JD, Litofsky NS, Bankey PE, Bonassar LJ, Megerian CA. Temporal bone fractures: otic capsule sparing versus otic capsule violating clinical and radiographic considerations. *J Trauma.* 1999;47(6):1079—1083.

35. Schubl SD, Klein TR, Robitsek RJ, et al. Temporal bone fracture: evaluation in the era of modern computed tomography. *Injury.* 2016;47(9):1893—1897.

36. Brodie HA, Thompson TC. Management of complications from 820 temporal bone fractures. *Am J Otol.* 1997;18(2):188—197.

37. Cvorovic L, Jovanovic MB, Markovic M, Milutinovic Z, Strbac M. Management of complication from temporal bone fractures. *Eur Arch Otorhinolaryngol.* 2012;269(2):399—403.

38. Ghorayeb BY, Yeakley JW. Temporal bone fractures: longitudinal or oblique? The case for oblique temporal bone fractures. *Laryngoscope.* 1992;102(2):129—134.

39. Johnson F, Semaan MT, Megerian CA. Temporal bone fracture: evaluation and management in the modern era. *Otolaryngol Clin North Am.* 2008;41(3):597—618, x.

40. Ishman SL, Friedland DR. Temporal bone fractures: traditional classification and clinical relevance. *Laryngoscope.* 2004;114(10):1734—1741.

41. Goodwin Jr WJ. Temporal bone fractures. *Otolaryngol Clin North Am.* 1983;16(3):651—659.

42. Yeakley JW. Temporal bone fractures. *Curr Probl Diagn Radiol.* 1999;28(3):65—98.

43. Gurdjian ES, Lissner HR. Deformation of the skull in head injury; a study with the stress-coat technique. *Surg Gynecol Obstet.* 1945;81:679—687.

44. Aguilar 3rd EA, Yeakley JW, Ghorayeb BY, Hauser M, Cabrera J, Jahrsdoerfer RA. High resolution CT scan of temporal bone fractures: association of facial nerve paralysis with temporal bone fractures. *Head Neck Surg.* 1987;9(3):162—166.

45. Little SC, Kesser BW. Radiographic classification of temporal bone fractures: clinical predictability using a new system. *Arch Otolaryngol Head Neck Surg.* 2006;132(12):1300—1304.

46. Fisch U. Facial paralysis in fractures of the petrous bone. *Laryngoscope*. 1974;84(12): 2141−2154.

47. Vrabec JT. Otic capsule fracture with preservation of hearing and delayed-onset facial paralysis. *Int J Pediatr Otorhinolaryngol*. 2001;58(2):173−177.

48. Saraiya PV, Aygun N. Temporal bone fractures. *Emerg Radiol*. 2009;16(4):255−265.

49. Riggio S. Traumatic brain injury and its neurobehavioral sequelae. *Psychiatr Clin North Am*. 2010;33(4):807−819.

50. Walker WC, Pickett TC. Motor impairment after severe traumatic brain injury: a longitudinal multicenter study. *J Rehabil Res Dev*. 2007;44(7):975−982.

51. Aitken ME, McCarthy ML, Slomine BS, et al. Family burden after traumatic brain injury in children. *Pediatrics*. 2009;123(1):199−206.

52. Wade SL, Carey J, Wolfe CR. The efficacy of an online cognitive-behavioral family intervention in improving child behavior and social competence following pediatric brain injury. *Rehabil Psychol*. 2006;51(3):179−189.

53. Selassie AW, Zaloshnja E, Langlois JA, Miller T, Jones P, Steiner C. Incidence of long-term disability following traumatic brain injury hospitalization, United States, 2003. *J Head Trauma Rehabil*. 2008;23(2):123−131.

54. Thurman DJ, Alverson C, Dunn KA, Guerrero J, Sniezek JE. Traumatic brain injury in the United States: a public health perspective. *J Head Trauma Rehabil*. 1999;14(6): 602−615.

55. Zaloshnja E, Miller T, Langlois JA, Selassie AW. Prevalence of long-term disability from traumatic brain injury in the civilian population of the United States, 2005. *J Head Trauma Rehabil*. 2008;23(6):394−400.

56. Finkelstein EA, Corso PS, Miller TR. *The Incidence and Economic Burden of Injuries in the United States*. New York: Oxford University Press; 2006.

57. Faul M, Wald MM, Rutland-Brown W, Sullivent EE, Sattin RW. Using a cost-benefit analysis to estimate outcomes of a clinical treatment guideline: testing the Brain Trauma Foundation guidelines for the treatment of severe traumatic brain injury. *J Trauma*. 2007; 63(6):1271−1278.

58. Carney N, Totten AM, O'Reilly C, et al. Guidelines for the management of severe traumatic brain injury, fourth edition. *Neurosurgery*. 2017;80(1):6−15.

Imaging of the temporal bone following otologic and lateral skull base trauma

Katherine L. Reinshagen

Department of Radiology, Massachusetts Eye and Ear, Harvard Medical School, Boston, MA, United States

Introduction

Extent and severity of injury in the setting of otologic and lateral skull base trauma are readily detected noninvasively by imaging. Due to its speed and excellent spatial resolution, multidetector CT (MDCT) remains the primary modality of choice in the acute traumatic setting to delineate temporal bone trauma. Detection of subtle fractures and involvement of the otic capsule, carotid canal, and facial nerve canal can be readily assessed with MDCT. MDCT is also considered the primary imaging method of choice due to its ability to visualize the intracranial structures and exclude an acute intracranial hemorrhage or additional signs of intracranial trauma such as cerebral edema or infarct. Depending on the severity of the trauma or clinical suspicion of skull base involvement, CT angiogram (CTA) can also be acquired to assess the internal carotid artery or dural venous system.

In the nonacute setting, MDCT or cone beam CT (CBCT) can also be used to provide excellent delineation of the middle ear anatomy. Magnetic resonance imaging (MRI) may also be used to assess for subtle changes in the labyrinth, including intralabyrinthine hemorrhage or postinflammatory changes from labyrinthitis. In addition, MRI can help to characterize persistent soft tissue abnormalities in the temporal bone, in particular, to assess for a site of cerebrospinal fluid (CSF) leak or possible meningoencephalocele.

Multidetector CT

MDCT provides fast, high spatial resolution images (0.5—0.6 mm), which can be readily reconstructed in multiple planes. Reconstructed images of the temporal bone in an axial plane parallel to the lateral/horizontal semicircular canal, coronal images 90 degrees from the axial reformatted images, Pöschl reformats perpendicular to the long axis of the temporal bone, and Stenvers reformats parallel to the long axis of the temporal bone can help to assess for signs of trauma. In addition, MDCT images can provide soft tissue window images, which are critical to assess for signs of intracranial trauma, such as intraparenchymal, subarachnoid, subdural or epidural hemorrhage, cerebral edema, infarct, mass effect, or midline shift. When a patient arrives in an acute trauma or demonstrates unstable or concerning clinical symptoms, MDCT is the best modality to exclude more severe sequelae of trauma and is the safest modality due to its speed.

CT angiography (CTA) can be added to an MDCT temporal bone protocol to assess for injury to the internal carotid arteries or dural venous sinuses based on clinical indication or concern for significant skull base trauma. CTA can be timed in the early arterial and delayed venous phases to better delineate the type of vascular injury. With faster MDCT units becoming more readily available, these images can be acquired alongside dedicated chest, abdomen, and pelvis images to further assess the entire degree of bodily trauma.

Cone beam CT

In the nonacute setting, CBCT can provide excellent delineation of temporal bone anatomy. However, due to its slower speed of acquisition, it typically requires patient cooperation to perform without substantial motion artifact. As a result, this modality is best used in adult patients who are alert and cooperative. Some CBCT units require a sitting position and may be further limited due to height restrictions, limiting its use in some pediatric settings. CBCT also does not provide adequate soft tissue characterization[1] and should be avoided when there is concern for intracranial disease or an extracranial soft tissue abnormality.

Magnetic resonance imaging

MRI should be reserved for the nonacute traumatic setting when the patient has stabilized and the patient has been carefully screened for any MRI safety considerations, such as implants or foreign bodies. MRI is preferred for better delineation of the soft tissue structures, intracranial anatomy, and fluid within the labyrinth. MRI can be acquired at 1.5 or 3 T magnetic field strengths. High-resolution (2–3 mm slice thickness), small field-of-view images of the temporal bone are necessary to provide adequate information. In addition, a cisternographic sequence that is heavily T2-weighted with 0.5–0.6 mm slice thickness is very helpful for assessing the fluid signal within the inner ear structures. Phase-corrected/sensitive inversion recovery MR images in the coronal and/or sagittal plane are also helpful additions to assess for sites of meningoencephalocele. Intravenous gadolinium can be considered particularly when assessing for labyrinthitis.

Temporal bone fractures

Temporal bone fractures can be classified in two main classifications, in relation to the axis of the temporal bone (longitudinal, transverse, or mixed)[2] or in relation to its involvement of the otic capsule (otic capsule sparing or otic capsule violating) or petrous involvement. Longitudinal fractures as defined as along the long axis of the temporal bone are more common accounting for approximately 70%—90% of temporal bone fractures.[3,4] These longitudinal fractures are more likely to be associated with injury to the ossicular chain resulting in conductive hearing loss. Transverse fractures, along the short axis of the temporal bone, are less common and are associated with damage to the inner ear structures resulting in sensorineural hearing loss. Unfortunately, the exact orientation of a fracture can be in the practical sense challenging to classify and may be oblique or mixed.[5] As a result, this classification scheme does not tend to correlate well with patient outcomes.[5–7] Thus, the otic capsule violating or sparing terminology is often preferred as it has been better correlated with clinical outcomes in relation to facial nerve injury and sensorineural hearing loss.[7,8] Otic capsule sparing fractures or nonpetrous fractures as defined by Ishman et al. (Figs. 2.1 and 2.2) are associated with more middle ear abnormalities and can result in conductive hearing loss,[6] while otic capsule violating fractures tend to involve inner ear structures resulting in higher incidences of sensorineural hearing loss, as well as injury to the facial nerve, carotid canal, and tegmen resulting in vascular injury and CSF leaks, respectively (Fig. 2.3).[6–9] Temporal bone fractures can often be seen long after the initial injury due to the slow healing of the temporal bone and otic capsule (Fig. 2.1).

Ossicular chain injury can be readily detected by both MDCT and CBCT. Dislocation of the ossicles is most frequently seen with direct fractures of the ossicles considered rare.[10] Incudostapedial and incudomalleal dislocations are the most frequently seen ossicular chain injuries.[10] In incudostapedial dislocation, a gap between the distal incus and the stapes superstructure can be seen, although may be subtle. Incudomalleal dislocation can be best appreciated in the axial plane as separation of the head of the malleus from the body of the incus, resulting in an "ice cream" falling off the "ice cream cone" appearance (Fig. 2.1). Frank dislocation of the stapes can also be detected by CT (Fig. 2.4). Lateral to medial trauma can result in displacement of the stapes into the vestibule and can result in perilymphatic fistula (Fig. 2.5). Complete dislocation of the malleus and incus can also occur, resulting in free-floating ossicles in the middle ear.

Intracranial hemorrhage

Given the relative high force required to cause fractures of the temporal bone, associated intracranial hemorrhage must always be excluded. MDCT is the imaging modality of choice in the acute setting to exclude acute intracranial hemorrhage.

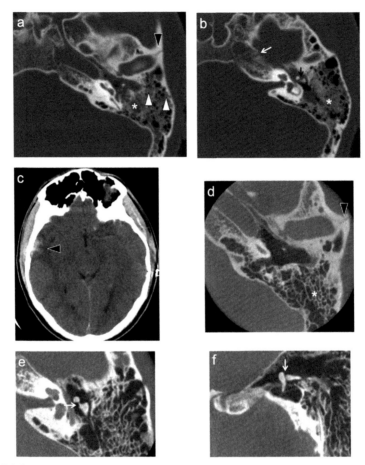

FIGURE 2.1

(A and B) Axial MDCT of the temporal bone demonstrates an otic capsule sparing fracture lines through the lateral temporal bone extending to the mandibular fossa (*black arrowhead*) and mastoid air cells (*white arrowheads*) with opacification in the mastoid (asterisk) and middle ear. A fracture line is seen extending into the petrous apex extending near the carotid canal (*white arrow*). There is widening of the incudomalleal articulation with a classic "ice cream off the ice cream cone" appearance (*black arrow*). (C) Soft tissue windows of the MDCT of the brain demonstrates a hemorrhagic contusion in the contralateral right temporal lobe (*black arrowhead*), consistent with a contrecoup type injury. (D–F) CBCT of the temporal bone 6 months after initial injury demonstrates persistent, slightly fainter fracture lines (*black arrowhead*) consistent with interval healing. There has been near complete resolution of the mastoid opacification (asterisk). There is persistent widening of the incudomalleal articulation (*white arrow*) shown in axial plane (E) and Stenvers plane (F).

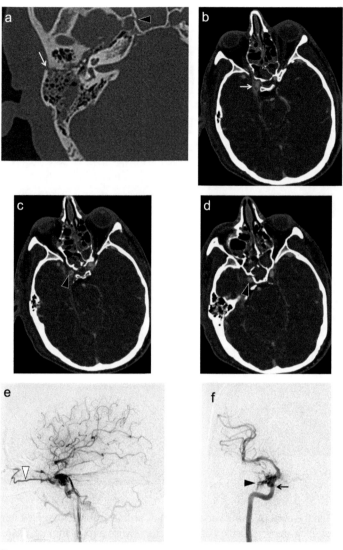

FIGURE 2.2

(A) Axial MDCT images of the right temporal bone demonstrate a displaced comminuted otic capsule sparing fracture of the mastoid (*white arrow*) with a mildly displaced fracture line extending into the petrous carotid canal (*black arrowhead*). (B–D) Due to the extent of injury through the petrous right carotid canal, dedicated CT angiogram was performed. There is early asymmetric contrast filling of the right cavernous sinus (*white arrow*) with a dissection flap and irregularity of the right internal carotid artery (*black arrowhead*), concerning for arterial dissection and traumatic direct carotid-cavernous fistula. (E and F) Conventional cerebral angiogram in the lateral (F) and AP (G) projections following selective injection into the right internal carotid artery demonstrates early venous filling of the superior ophthalmic vein (*white arrowhead*), cavernous sinus (*black arrowhead*), and pseuodoaneurysm of the right internal carotid artery (*black arrow*).

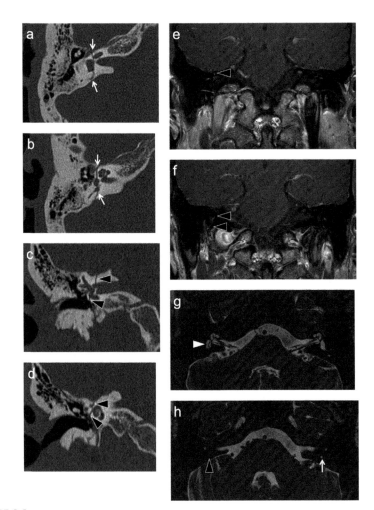

FIGURE 2.3

(A–D) MDCT in the axial (A and B) and coronal (C and D) planes of the right temporal bone demonstrating an otic capsule violating fracture (*white arrows*) through the cochlea, vestibule, posterior semicircular canal, and anterior/first genu and labyrinthine segment of the facial nerve (D, *upper black arrowhead*). (E and F) Postcontrast coronal T1-weighted MR images demonstrate an enhancing fracture line corresponding with the coronal MDCT images involving the labyrinthine segment of the right facial nerve canal and vestibule. (G and H) Axial heavily T2-weighted cisternographic MR images demonstrate abnormal linear signal void extending through the vestibule with diminished fluid signal in the vestibule, and absent fluid signal in the posterior limb of the right superior semicircular canal (*black arrowhead*), likely sequelae of posttraumatic labyrinthitis. The normal fluid signal in the posterior limb of the left superior semicircular canal is shown (*white arrow*).

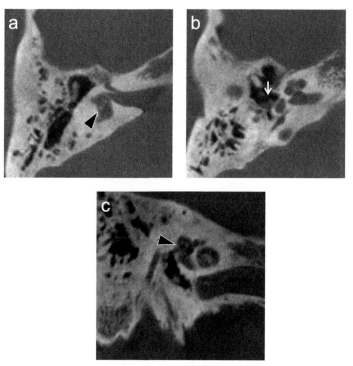

FIGURE 2.4

(A and B) Axial CBCT of the right temporal bone demonstrates displacement of the right stapes into the vestibule (*black arrowhead*) and a large gap between the distal incus and stapes superstructure (*white arrow*), consistent with stapes dislocation. (C) Oblique multiplanar reconstruction view from the CBCT of the right temporal bone demonstrates the entire stapes in the vestibule (*black arrowhead*).

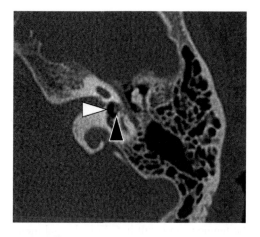

FIGURE 2.5

Axial MDCT image of the left temporal bone demonstrates a displaced stapes (*black arrowhead*) into the vestibule with air in the vestibule (*white arrowhead*), consistent with traumatic displacement of the stapes and perilymphatic fistula.

In patients with associated clinical signs to suggest a severe skull base injury, CT angiogram of the head and neck can also be performed at the same time to assess for vascular injury. Coup and contrecoup type injuries with parenchymal hemorrhage in the brain can be demonstrated and result in surrounding cerebral edema (Fig. 2.1). In addition, epidural hematomas are particularly worrisome with severe clinical consequences. These can be detected as lentiform-shaped hemorrhages in the extraaxial space between the calvaria and dura. Subdural hemorrhages and subarachnoid hemorrhages can also be seen in the acute traumatic setting and should be excluded, usually by CT.

Vascular injury

Carotid canal involvement is particularly worrisome in the setting of skull base trauma (Fig. 2.2). Carotid canal fractures are accompanied by a high incidence of carotid injury, leading to pseudoaneurysm, dissection, occlusion, arteriovenous or carotid cavernous fistula, or in very rare cases, transection.[11]

Venous injury can occur with fracture involvement of the sigmoid groove or jugular fossa. Venous thrombosis within the sigmoid sinus or jugular vein can be an associated complication. On noncontrast CT, this can sometimes be detected as subtle hyperdensity within the dural venous sinus.[12] On delayed venous-phased images, a filling defect within the dural venous sinus is suggestive of thrombosis.[12]

In the setting of a known fracture through the carotid canal or along a venous sinus, CT angiogram is recommended and provides the timeliest and least invasive method to assess for vascular injury. CT angiogram can be timed for both arterial and venous phases. If there is an equivocal or treatable finding, patients can then go to catheter angiogram for both diagnostic confirmation and treatment.

Facial nerve injury

Facial nerve injury is a serious complication of temporal bone trauma. Fractures can occur through the facial nerve canal in various locations. Injury to the facial nerve can result from direct transection, contusion, or compression from a bony spicule. CT plays an important role in preoperative imaging to assess for fracture lines extending through the facial nerve canal (Fig. 2.3), suggesting possible injury to the facial nerve itself, or to assess for a compressive cause for facial nerve injury, such as a bony spicule.

Tegmen defects and cerebrospinal fluid leaks

Tegmen defects are a possible complication from temporal bone trauma. Fractures extending through the tegmen can result in CSF leaks and meningoencephaloceles. Initial imaging with CT can be helpful to visualize the tegmen defect.

High-resolution CT has a reported sensitivity ranging from 60% to 93% in active skull base CSF leaks.[13–15] MR is complementary by allowing assessment of the neighboring soft tissue. Inversion recovery sequences can be used to distinguish meningoencephaloceles from otherwise nonspecific soft tissue opacification on CT (Fig. 2.6). If a CSF leak is suspected, and a source is not obviously visible, then further imaging with cisternographic imaging can be considered.[13] These techniques include CT cisternogram, which requires injection of intrathecal contrast via lumbar puncture, MR cisternography, which can be performed with or without intrathecal contrast, or nuclear medicine imaging, which also requires intrathecal administration of radioactive tracer (Tc-99m DTPA or In-111 DTPA) via lumbar puncture. Radionuclide tracer can be seen transgressing the tegmen in the temporal bone, although spatial resolution from nuclear medicine studies is somewhat poor.

Intralabyrinthine hemorrhage

Intralabyrinthine hemorrhage is best appreciated on MR[16] and can vary substantially in signal characteristics depending on the age of the hemorrhage. This is due to the presence of oxy- and deoxy- or met-hemoglobin within the area of hemorrhage.[17]

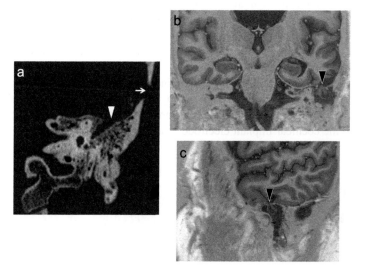

FIGURE 2.6

(A) Coronal MDCT image of the left temporal bone demonstrates a large widened fracture line extending through the squamous portion of temporal bone (*white arrow*) and extending through the tegmen mastoideum (*white arrowhead*). (B and C) Corresponding MRI with inversion recovery images in the coronal (B) and sagittal (C) planes demonstrates a large meningoencephalocele from the inferior left temporal lobe extending through the widened tegmen defect (*black arrowhead*).

There are 5 stages of hemorrhage: hyperacute (less than 1 day), acute (1−3 days), early subacute (3−7 days), late subacute (7−28 days), and chronic (older than 28 days). In the hyperacute phase, hemorrhage is typically isointense on both T1-weighted and T2-weighted images to fluid, making this stage the most challenging to detect. In the acute phase, hemorrhage will begin to become hypointense on T2-weighted images while isointense to fluid on T1-weighted images. In the early subacute phase, hemorrhage will become hyperintense on T1-weighted images and dark on T2-weighted images. In the late subacute phase, hemorrhage will become hyperintense on both T1- and T2-weighted images. In the chronic phase, hemorrhage will be both low signal on T1- and T2-weighted images. Fig. 2.7 shows an example of intralabyrinthine hemorrhage in the subacute phase.

Labyrinthitis ossificans

Labyrinthitis ossificans following otic capsule violating fractures is a concerning feature and has important clinical consequences. The combination of CT and MR is particularly helpful for determining the stage of labyrinthitis ossificans. In the early fibrous stage, CT will not demonstrate ossification in the labyrinth; however, MR with a heavily T2-weighted cisternographic sequence will demonstrate absence of fluid signal in the affected areas.[18] On postcontrast T1-weighted images, the labyrinth will demonstrate enhancement, suggesting labyrinthitis. Over time, these findings will evolve as the labyrinth begins to ossify. In the ossified stage, MDCT or CBCT readily demonstrates ossification within the affected labyrinth. On MR, this will remain hypointense on the heavily T2-weighted cisternographic sequence (Fig. 2.3). Imaging in the early stage of labyrinthitis ossificans is crucial to providing timely treatment. In the ossified stage of labyrinthitis, treatment with cochlear implantation becomes particularly challenging and may result in kinking or incomplete rotation of the cochlear implant electrode array.

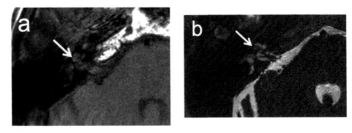

FIGURE 2.7

(A) Axial precontrast T1-weighted image demonstrates intrinsic T1 shortening (hyperintensity) in the right cochlea (*white arrow*). (B) Corresponding axial heavily T2-weighted cisternographic sequence demonstrates diminished fluid signal in the corresponding areas. In the setting of prior trauma, this likely represents sequelae of subacute intralabyrinthine hemorrhage.

Perilymphatic fistula

Imaging findings of perilymphatic fistula may be subtle, and often the clinical history is helpful. While highly specific, air in the labyrinth is best detected by MDCT[19]; however, perilymphatic fistula particularly due to a small leak or focus of damage at the round window and oval window may be subtle including only nonspecific soft tissue along the round window niche and adjacent to the oval window. In the setting of a displaced stapes into the vestibule resulting in perilymphatic fistula, CT is the modality of choice for detecting the displaced stapes[20] (Fig. 2.5).

Conclusion

Imaging in the setting of otologic and lateral skull base trauma is particularly important to detect the severity and extent of traumatic injury. In the acute setting, MDCT is the primary modality of choice due to its speed, excellent delineation of bony anatomy, and detection of vascular and intracranial injury. MRI and CBCT can be used when the patient is more cooperative and stabilized to detect sequelae of otologic and lateral skull base trauma.

References

1. Miracle AC, Mukherji SK. Conebeam CT of the head and neck, part 1: physical principles. *AJNR Am J Neuroradiol.* 2009;30:1088–1095.
2. Ulrich K. Verletzungen des Gehörorganes bei Schädelbasisfrakturen. *Acta Otolaryngol Stockh, Suppl VI.* 1926:1–50.
3. Tos M. Course of and sequelae to 248 petrosal fractures. *Acta Otolaryngol.* 1973;75: 353–354.
4. Nosan DK, Benecke Jr JE, Murr AH. Current perspective on temporal bone trauma. *Otolaryngol Head Neck Surg.* 1997;117(1):67–71.
5. Ghorayeb BY, Yeakley JW. Temporal bone fractures: longitudinal or oblique? The case for oblique temporal bone fractures. *Laryngoscope.* 1992;102(2):129–134.
6. Ishman SL, Friedland DR. Temporal bone fractures: traditional classification and clinical relevance. *Laryngoscope.* 2004;114(10):1734–1741.
7. Dahiya R, Keller JD, Litofsky NS, et al. Temporal bone fractures: otic capsule sparing versus otic capsule violating clinical and radiographic considerations. *J Trauma.* 1999; 47(6):1079–1083.
8. Little SC, Kesser BW. Radiographic classification of temporal bone fractures: clinical predictability using a new system. *Arch Otolaryngol Head Neck Surg.* 2006;132(12): 1300–1304.
9. Diaz RC, Cervenka B, Brodie HA. Treatment of temporal bone fractures. *J Neurol Surg B Skull Base.* 2016;77(5):419–429.
10. Meriot P, Veillon F, Garcia JF, et al. CT appearances of ossicular injuries. *Radiographics.* 1997;17(6):1445–1454.

11. McKinney A, Ott F, Short J, et al. Angiographic frequency of blunt cerebrovascular injury in patients with carotid canal or vertebral foramen fractures on multidetector CT. *Eur J Radiol.* 2007;62(3):385−393.

12. Poon CS, Chang JK, Swarnkar A, et al. Radiologic diagnosis of cerebral venous thrombosis: pictorial review. *AJR Am J Roentgenol.* 2007;189(suppl 6):S64−S75.

13. Stone JA, Castillo M, Neelon B, et al. Evaluation of CSF leaks: high-resolution CT compared with contrast-enhanced CT and radionuclide cisternography. *AJNR Am J Neuroradiol.* 1999;20(4):706−712.

14. LaFata V, McLean N, Wise SK, et al. CSF leaks: correlation of high-resolution CT and multiplanar reformations with intraoperative endoscopic findings. *AJNR Am J Neuroradiol.* 2008;29(3):536−541.

15. Shetty PG, Shroff MM, Sahani DV, Kirtane MV. Evaluation of high-resolution CT and MR cisternography in the diagnosis of cerebrospinal fluid fistula. *AJNR Am J Neuroradiol.* 1998;19(4):633−639.

16. Mark AS, Seltzer S, Harnsberger HR. Sensorineural hearing loss: more than meets the eye? *AJNR Am J Neuroradiol.* 1993;14(1):37−45.

17. Bradley W. MR appearance of hemorrhage in the brain. *Radiology.* 1993;189(1):15−26.

18. Juliano AF, Ginat DT, Moonis G. Imaging review of the temporal bone: part I. anatomy and inflammatory and neoplastic processes. *Radiology.* 2013;269(1):17−33.

19. Mafee MF, Valvassori GE, Kumar A, et al. Pneumolabyrinth: a new radiologic sign for fracture of the stapes footplate. *Am J Otol.* 1984;5(5):374−375.

20. Hatano A, Rikitake M, Komori M, et al. Traumatic perilymphatic fistula with the luxation of the stapes into the vestibule. *Auris Nasus Larynx.* 2009;36(4):474−478.

Surgical management of auricular trauma

3

Krupa R. Patel, MD, David A. Shaye, MD, MPH

Division of Facial Plastic and Reconstructive Surgery, Department of Otolaryngology-Head and Neck Surgery, Massachusetts Eye and Ear, Harvard Medical School, Boston, MA, United States

Auricular anatomy

Mastery of auricular anatomy is a prerequisite for achieving successful reconstruction. The majority of the auricle is composed of an intricate cartilaginous framework with an overlying taut skin envelope, creating distinct topographical landmarks (Fig. 3.1). The lobule lacks underlying cartilage and is made up of thin skin overlying fibrofatty tissue. Between the cartilage and skin along the posterior surface of the auricle exists a minimal amount of intervening adipose tissue, which is absent on the anterior surface of the auricle.[1] The rich vascular supply to the auricle is derived from two branches of the external carotid artery: the superficial temporal artery and the posterior auricular artery. Venous drainage occurs via the superficial

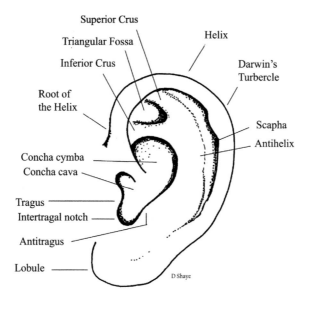

FIGURE 3.1

The topographical landmarks of the auricle.

Otologic and Lateral Skull Base Trauma. https://doi.org/10.1016/B978-0-323-87482-3.00014-4

temporal, posterior auricular, and retromandibular veins into the external and internal jugular veins.[2]

The average height and width of the adult auricle is 5–6 cm and 3–4 cm, respectively. In the Frankfort horizontal plane, the root of the adult helix is 6–7 cm posterior to the lateral canthus. The superior and inferior most points of the auricle align with the superior orbital rim and subnasale, respectively. The longitudinal axis of the auricle is inclined 15–20 degrees off the true vertical axis. The auriculocephalic angle, defined as the protrusion of the auricle from the scalp, is between 25 and 35°. The ear protrudes from the postauricular skin approximately 1.5–2 cm.[3–5] Despite these established anthropomorphic standards for the ideal ear, auricular reconstruction is best modeled on the patient's contralateral ear to ensure symmetry and facial harmony.

Primary survey

Primary survey of the auricular injury should include assessment of the size, location and depth of the defect, viability of any avulsed segments and adjacent tissue, and patient goals based on comorbidities and trauma burden. A complete head and neck examination should be performed with special attention to evaluation of the tympanic membrane, presence of cerebrospinal fluid otorrhea, temporal bone fractures, facial nerve function, and external auditory canal (EAC) edema and lacerations. For lacerations extending into the EAC, a wick is placed to prevent canal stenosis, and otic drops are initiated until wick removal. All auricular injuries in the acute setting should be copiously irrigated and debrided of foreign bodies and visibly necrotic tissue. Tetanus and rabies vaccines should be administered if necessary.[5] Topical antibiotic ointment is applied to all lacerations and open wounds. With regard to systemic prophylactic antibiotic therapy, superficial lacerations with intact perichondrium can be covered with a first-generation oral cephalosporin. For wounds with exposed cartilage in adults, oral fluoroquinolones are recommended to reduce the risk of auricular chondritis.

Principles of auricular reconstruction

The primary goal of auricular reconstruction is to restore the function of the auricle to converge, amplify, and transmit sound to the middle ear. The secondary, more formidable goal is to recreate the complex topographic landmarks and three-dimensional structure of the auricle and to maintain symmetry in its position, protrusion, height, and width when compared to the contralateral ear. For minor skin lacerations with intact perichondrium, the wound can often be closed primarily. If cartilage is exposed, the framework is reestablished either by primary repair or with use of cartilage grafts, with the most common donor sites being the conchal bowl, septum, and autologous rib. Any exposed or grafted cartilage must be covered with vascularized tissue. A multilayered, composite closure is performed with use of cartilage grafts, local advancement flaps, and skin grafts. Bolsters are applied to prevent hematoma or seroma formation and resultant auricular deformity.

Minor auricular trauma

Auricular hematoma

Auricular hematomas (Fig. 3.2) result from accumulation of blood in the subperichondrial plane ultimately forming a dense, fibrin clot.[3] A delay in clot evacuation can lead to an unsightly cauliflower ear deformity.[6] Auricular hematomas are drained via a small, dependent incision down to cartilage overlying the area of fluctuance and hidden within a concavity of the lateral auricle. Dental roll or xeroform bolsters are contoured and secured to the anterior and posterior surface of the auricle via through-and-through large, nonabsorbable monofilament sutures in a quilting fashion to obliterate potential dead space and to prevent reaccumulation of the hematoma.

Auricular lacerations

Auricular lacerations should be repaired with a layered primary closure within the first 24 hours of injury to prevent infection, cartilage devascularization, scar contracture and an unfavorable aesthetic outcome. The site of injury should first be copiously irrigated of debris. A regional peripheral nerve block will facilitate primary

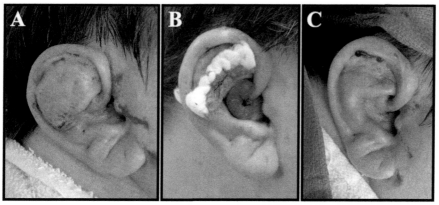

FIGURE 3.2

(A) Auricular hematoma, (B) placement of a dental roll after incision and drainage and (C) subsequent appearance of the auricle.

repair without the anatomical distortion associated with direct infiltration. Local anesthetic is infiltrated just inferior to the lobule to block the great auricular nerve and posterosuperiorly within the auriculocephalic sulcus to block the auriculotemporal branch of the mandibular division of the trigeminal nerve (V3). Nonviable tissue should then be debrided prior to performing a layered closure. If there is no cartilage exposure, a simple skin closure with minimal tension and wound edge eversion should be performed using fast-absorbing plain gut or nylon sutures. If there is cartilage exposure or involvement, 4-0 or 5-0 long-lasting absorbable monofilament suture should be used to reapproximate the cartilage framework. Extra care should be taken during repair if the laceration involves the helical rim, where slight imperfections in cartilage reapproximation can result in a noticeable soft tissue step-off deformity. A bolster dressing should be applied for relatively large and complex lacerations to prevent auricular hematoma formation.

Lobule tears

Due to the round, smooth contour of the ear lobe, repair of lobule tears can present a significant reconstructive challenge. To prevent notching of the inferior border of the ear lobe, lobule tears can be repaired with a small Z-plasty such that the resultant scar lies parallel to the inferior border of the ear lobe.[7] Given that the lobule is composed of thin skin and subcutaneous tissue with lack of rigid structural support, lobule tears with substantial skin loss can result in significant contraction and lobule deformity. A small cartilage graft harvested from the conchal bowl or septum can therefore be placed in a subcutaneous pocket to reduce contraction.[8,9] A full-thickness skin graft (FTSG) or vascularized local flap can be placed over the cartilage graft if additional skin coverage is needed.

Classification of auricular trauma: depth of defect
Skin defects and auricular burns

Superficial skin defects of concave auricular surfaces with intact perichondrium and cartilage framework can heal by secondary intention with diligent wound care. Larger, lateral skin defects left to heal by secondary intention, however, can contract and cause forward-folding of the auricle. FTSGs can be harvested from the pre- or postauricular skin for a close color match. FTSGs intended for the ear should be thinned aggressively before placement to optimize graft survival and to accentuate the underlying auricular contour.[3] Fast-absorbing gut suture is used to tack down the edges of the FTSG, and quilting sutures can be added along natural lines of concavity.

Due to its superolateral position on the cranium, the auricle is also highly susceptible to thermal injury. Early debridement of burns is crucial for preventing irreversible cartilage damage and deformity.[10] Based on the depth and size of the burn injury and viability of adjacent tissue, options for repair include healing by secondary intention with meticulous wound care, FTSG coverage, and postauricular advancement flaps.

Perichondrium defects

Superficial defects involving both skin and perichondrium with resultant cartilage exposure will not support skin graft survival. Small, 2-mm fenestrations through the exposed cartilage can be created to accelerate the growth of granulation tissue and to promote neovascularization.[11] Subsequent delayed repair of the defect can be performed with a FTSG placed overlying the vascularized bed of granulation tissue overlying the cartilage. If perichondrium defects are present in a location that is not vital to the auricular framework, such as the conchal bowl or scaphoid fossa, the exposed cartilage can be excised and a FTSG can then be placed within the defect. The blood supply for the FTSG will be derived from the opposing perichondrium or subcutaneous tissue. A better aesthetic outcome can be achieved for particular skin and perichondrium defects—such as those located along the sharp contour of the helical rim—with conversion to a composite defect via excision of the underlying cartilage.[12]

Composite defects

Composite defects of the auricle—those that involve skin, perichondrium and cartilage—can be repaired via conversion of the defect to a wedge or star excision (Fig. 3.3). Small composite defects of the middle third of the helical rim can be closed via wedge resection.[13] A triangular full thickness wedge is excised such that the base encompasses the rim defect and the apex lies within the conchal bowl. No more than 1 cm of the conchal rim should be excised to maintain the overall proportions of the auricle. The defect is closed primarily in layers with a staggered closure of the cartilage and skin, referred to as "tongue and groove" fashion.[14] A star resection should be utilized for larger composite defects of the middle third of the helical rim in cases where a traditional wedge resection would cause unsightly distortion. A traditional wedge is first drawn to encompass the defect. Two smaller triangles are then added with their axis oriented parallel to the antihelix. The composite defect is thereby repaired primarily via chondrocutaneous advancement of the adjacent tissue. The entirety of the auricle is slightly reduced in size via the star resection technique while maintaining normal proportions for the individual subunits.[12,14]

Composite defects of the helix that are 2.5 cm or less can be repaired with adjacent soft tissue via the aforementioned chondrocutaneous advancement (Fig. 3.4)

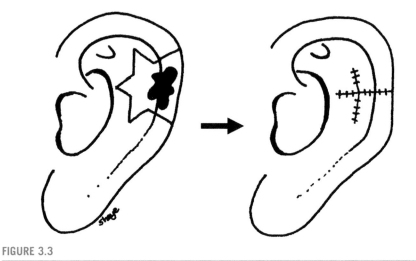

FIGURE 3.3

Star excision of a helical rim defect.

techniques. For defects larger than 2.5 cm, additional tissue is often required in the form of a combination of skin grafts, local fasciocutaneous flaps and cartilage grafts. Skin and soft tissue coverage can be achieved utilizing a variety of reconstructive techniques including a FTSG, postauricular advancement flap (Fig. 3.5) or temporoparietal fascia flap.[15] Options for cartilage grafts include septal cartilage, ipsilateral or contralateral conchal bowl cartilage and autologous costal cartilage.

Classification of auricular trauma: extent of avulsion
Partial and segmental avulsions

Partial avulsions of the auricle should be reattached expeditiously in a multilayered fashion. A primary direct repair can be performed for partial avulsions with a wide pedicle. Even most near-total avulsions of the auricle with a narrow pedicle survive due to the rich vascular supply of the external ear. If the blood supply is tenuous or a direct repair of a partial avulsion fails, a postauricular advancement flap based on the postauricular artery can be used to cover the exposed regions on the auricle. As described above, chondrocutaneous advancement flaps can be used to repair partial avulsions of the helical rim.

Avulsed auricular segments have variable results after reattachment as composite grafts. There are several reports of avulsed auricular segments surviving after reattachment.[16–18] The avulsed segment should be wrapped in a saline-soaked gauze and submerged in a 4°C ice bath after the injury and preceding surgical replantation, which should be performed as soon as possible.[19] Alternatively, one may employ Mladick's pocket principle, which involves deepithelializing and fenestrating the

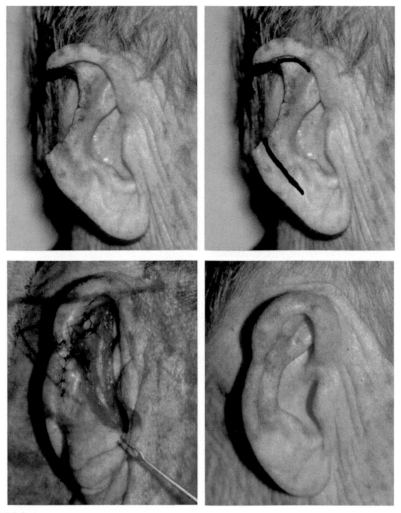

FIGURE 3.4

Helical rim advancement flaps.

avulsed segment first and then burying the denuded cartilage in a postauricular sub-cutaneous pocket. Two to four weeks later, the buried cartilage and overlying post-auricular tissue is raised and contoured in a second stage procedure, and the postauricular pocket is closed primarily.[11,20] Modifications of this technique involve leaving the lateral epidermis in place after exteriorizing the buried cartilage and placing a skin graft over the medial surface. Of note, there are reports of cartilage resorption, weakness and poor auricular definition with use of the pocket

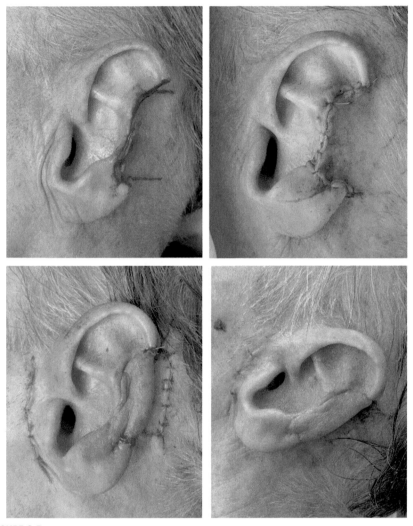

FIGURE 3.5

Postauricular advancement flap, contralateral conchal cartilage graft and full-thickness preauricular skin graft for repair of a composite defect.

technique.[14] Attempts at reattachment have the advantage of potential significant cosmetic benefit if the avulsed segment survives. However, if the likelihood of survival of the avulsed segment is low based on a tenuous, narrow pedicle, one may consider denuding and banking the cartilage for use in future reconstruction rather than attempting reattachment.

Total auricular avulsions

In cases of total auricular avulsion, the availability and viability of the avulsed auricle, amount of time elapsed since the injury and the clinical stability of the patient should be taken into consideration.[19] In the acute setting, microvascular reattachment should be considered if the avulsed auricle has been properly preserved, ischemia time is short and potential suitable vessels are identified under magnification.[3,19] Microvascular reattachment should be performed as soon as possible, but there are case reports of microvascular reattachment being successful after up to 33 hours of ischemia time.[21] If suitable vessels are identified in the avulsed auricle, primary anastomosis to the superficial temporal or posterior auricular artery with potential use of vein grafts can be attempted. According to prior reports in the literature, microvascular anastomosis of total auricular avulsions has been performed with mixed success.[22,23]

If microvascular reattachment fails, there are several options for total auricular reconstruction, including auricular prostheses and techniques involving autologous costal cartilage—the principles of the latter mirror those of microtia repair.[24] Auricular reconstruction with autologous rib grafts is one of the most challenging endeavors undertaken by facial plastic surgeons. The technique necessitates multiple staged procedures including harvest of autologous costal cartilage, meticulous carving of a cartilaginous framework, coverage of the cartilage with FTSG and local advancement flaps, elevation and contouring of the neo-auricle and creation of a lobule and tragus (Fig. 3.6). Even a meticulously crafted cartilage framework through a series of multiple reconstructive surgeries can result in highly variable aesthetic outcomes. However, in comparison to auricular prostheses, reconstruction with autologous costal cartilage offers the advantage of permanent attachment and a natural feel.

Auricular prostheses

For patients who are of advanced age, are unable to tolerate multiple reconstructive procedures, lack viable adjacent tissue or have previously undergone failed reconstructive surgery, an auricular prosthesis remains a practical and relatively low-risk alternative to total auricular reconstruction. Prostheses boast unmatched exquisite detail of the auricle's topographic anatomy and excellent color match and symmetry and therefore offer an outstanding aesthetic result. An auricular prothesis is anchored via a variety of attachment techniques including eyeglasses, head straps, adhesives and surgically implanted posts with osseointegration.[25,26] Overall, auricular prostheses offer an excellent practical alternative to surgery for near-total and complete traumatic avulsions of the auricle.

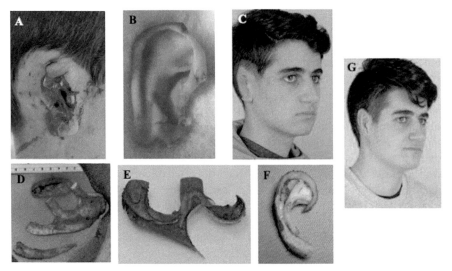

FIGURE 3.6

Autologous costal cartilage graft for near-total auricular reconstruction. (A) Wound at time of dog bite injury. (B) Severed ear at time of injury. (C) Healed auricular defect. (D) Costal cartilage harvest. (E) Template for carving of cartilage framework. (F) Neo-auricle cartilage framework. (G) Postoperative auricle appearance after costal cartilage reconstruction.

Conclusion

The protuberant and lateral anatomical position of the auricle aids its function in converging and transmitting sound while simultaneously endangering it to trauma. A variety of repair techniques can be employed based on the size, location and depth of the auricular defect, the viability of avulsed segments and the adjacent tissue and patient goals. Complex, extensive injuries often require multiple staged procedures and harvesting of cartilage grafts to obtain an aesthetically pleasing result. The intricate three-dimensional structure and topography of the auricle make its reconstruction one of the most challenging and rewarding endeavors undertaken by facial plastic surgeons.

References

1. Netter F. Head and neck. In: Colacino S, ed. *Atlas of Human Anatomy.* 2 ed. East Hanover, NJ: Novartis; 1997:17−18.
2. Zilinsky I, Erdmann D, Weissman O, et al. Reevaluation of the arterial blood supply of the auricle. *J Anat.* 2017;230(2):315−324.

3. Shaye DA, Sykes JM. Reconstruction of the acquired auricular deformity. *Oper Tech Otolaryngol*. 2010:47−52.

4. Tolleth H. Artistic anatomy, dimensions, and proportions of the external ear. *Clin Plast Surg*. 1978;5(3):337−345.

5. Wong K, Wong A, Rousso JJ. Reconstructive options for auricular trauma. *Facial Plast Surg*. 2021;37(4):510−515.

6. Patel BC, Skidmore K, Hutchison J, Hatcher JD. *Cauliflower Ear*. Treasure Island (FL): StatPearls; 2021.

7. Gajiwala K. Repair of the split earlobe using a half Z-plasty. *Plast Reconstr Surg*. 1998; 101(3):855−856.

8. Buonaccorsi S, Terenzi V, Pellacchia V, Indrizzi E, Fini G. Reconstruction of an acquired subtotal ear defect with autogenous septal cartilage graft. *Plast Reconstr Surg*. 2007; 119(6):1960−1961.

9. Sharma RK, Basu A, Parashar A, Makkar SS. Cartilage graft for strengthening repair of torn ear lobes: concept or conjecture? *J Plast Reconstr Aesthetic Surg*. 2010;63(12): e846−e847.

10. Ebrahimi A, Kazemi A, Rasouli HR, Kazemi M, Kalantar Motamedi MH. Reconstructive surgery of auricular defects: an overview. *Trauma Mon*. 2015;20(4):e28202.

11. Park SS, Hood RJ. Auricular reconstruction. *Otolaryngol Clin*. 2001;34(4):713−738. v-vi.

12. Shonka Jr DC, Park SS. Ear defects. *Facial Plast Surg Clin North Am*. 2009;17(3): 429−443.

13. Al-Shaham A. Helical advancement: pearls and pitfalls. *Can J Plast Surg*. 2012;20(2): e28−e31.

14. Cook TA, Miller PJ. Auricular reconstruction. *Facial Plast Surg*. 1995;11(4):319−329.

15. Kurbonov U, Davlatov A, Janobilova S, Kurbanov Z, Mirshahi M. The use of temporo-parietal fascia flap for surgical treatment of traumatic auricle defects. *Plast Reconstr Surg Glob Open*. 2018;6(5):e1741.

16. Garcia-Murray E, Adan-Rivas O, Salcido-Calzadilla H. Delayed, bilateral, non-microvascular ear replantation after violent amputation. *J Plast Reconstr Aesthetic Surg*. 2009;62(6):824−829.

17. Gifford Jr GH. Replantation of severed part of an ear. *Plast Reconstr Surg*. 1972;49(2): 202−203.

18. Salyapongse A, Maun LP, Suthunyarat P. Successful replantation of a totally severed ear. *Plast Reconstr Surg*. 1979;64(5):706−707.

19. Lavasani L, Leventhal D, Constantinides M, Krein H. Management of acute soft tissue injury to the auricle. *Facial Plast Surg*. 2010;26(6):445−450.

20. Mladick RA, Horton CE, Adamson JE, Cohen BI. The pocket principle: a new technique for the reattachment of a severed ear part. *Plast Reconstr Surg*. 1971;48(3):219−223.

21. Shelley OP, Villafane O, Watson SB. Successful partial ear replantation after prolonged ischaemia time. *Br J Plast Surg*. 2000;53(1):76−77.

22. Brent B. Reconstruction of the auricle. In: McCarthy J, ed. *Plastic Surgery*. *3*. Philadelphia, PA: Saunders; 1990:2131−2146.

23. Gailey AD, Farquhar D, Clark JM, Shockley WW. Auricular avulsion injuries and reattachment techniques: a systematic review. *Laryngoscope Investig Otolaryngol*. 2020; 5(3):381−389.

24. Baluch N, Nagata S, Park C, et al. Auricular reconstruction for microtia: a review of available methods. *Plast Surg (Oakv)*. 2014;22(1):39−43.

25. Giot JP, Labbe D, Soubeyrand E, et al. Prosthetic reconstruction of the auricle: indications, techniques, and results. *Semin Plast Surg*. 2011;25(4):265−272.

26. Tanner PB, Mobley SR. External auricular and facial prosthetics: a collaborative effort of the reconstructive surgeon and anaplastologist. *Facial Plast Surg Clin North Am*. 2006; 14(2):137−145. vi-vii.

Physiology of acoustic blast injury

Reef K. Al-Asad, BA, Judith S. Kempfle, MD

Department of Otolaryngology, Massachusetts Eye and Ear, Boston, MA, United States

Introduction

Damage to the ear is the most common organ injury after exposure to blast overpressure (BOP).[1] A blast injury occurs due to a rapid overpressurization force to the body. The middle and inner ear are particularly sensitive to sudden pressure changes and are therefore very susceptible to blast injuries. Blast injury to the ear may be caused by the detonation of high-order explosives (e.g., dynamite, nitroglycerine) that produce a supersonic, overpressurization shock wave, or by nonexplosive sudden pressure changes in the external auditory canal (EAC), such as a slap to the side of the head.[2] These mechanisms generally cause a rapid increase in pressure within the EAC and can lead to a variety of middle and inner ear injuries.[2] Patients with otologic damage after BOP often present with tympanic membrane rupture.[1] Additional signs and symptoms may include ossicular chain dislocation, conductive, mixed or sensorineural heading loss, tinnitus, and dizziness/vertigo.[1,3] While it is not uncommon for tympanic membrane perforations and conductive hearing loss to improve spontaneously, a subset of patients continues to experience transient or permanent high-frequency sensorineural hearing loss (SNHL), suggestive of additional inner ear damage.[4] In this chapter, we examine the anatomy and physiology of the ear as it relates to blast injury.

Background: normal anatomy and physiology of the ear

Sound waves travel along the EAC to reach the tympanic membrane (TM), which separates the external ear from the pneumatized middle ear (Fig. 4.1A). The tympanic membrane can be divided into four quadrants and is comprised of the pars tensa and the pars flaccida. The pars tensa, which makes up the majority of the drum, consists of three distinct layers—a lateral epithelial layer, a fibrous middle layer, and an inner mucosal layer. The pars flaccida, located superiorly between the anterior and posterior malleolar ligaments, lacks the fibrous layer and is as such less resistant to pressure changes.[5] The middle ear contains the ossicular chain, specifically the three ossicles, malleus, incus, and stapes. The malleus attaches to the tympanic membrane and medially connects with the incus via the incudomalleolar

Otologic and Lateral Skull Base Trauma. https://doi.org/10.1016/B978-0-323-87482-3.00001-6

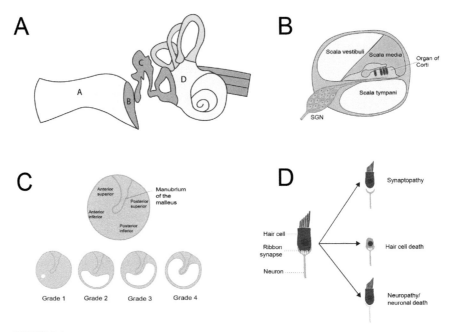

FIGURE 4.1

Otologic blast injury. (A) Overview of the ear with (A) external ear canal (*yellow*), middle ear structures (*purple*), including (B) the tympanic membrane and (C) the ossicular chain; (D) inner ear (*turquoise*), vestibular apparatus (*green*), internal auditory canal with cochleovestibular nerve (*red*). (B) Cross section of the membranous cochlear structures. Three-channel compartment including the scala tympani, vestibuli, and the scala media, which harbors the organ of Corti with the sensory hair cells connected to primary auditory neurons, so called spiral ganglion neurons. (C) Normal tympanic membrane with four anatomical quadrants. Traumatic membrane perforations are graded 1−4 after blast injury depending on size. (D) Sensorineural damage to the inner ear can be divided in loss of sensory hair cells, loss of spiral ganglion neurons, and loss of synapses.

joint. The incus interacts with the stapes through the incudostapedial joint, and the stapes footplate provides direct communication with the inner ear via the oval window (Fig. 4.1A). The ossicular chain acts as a lever, causing relative medial displacement of the stapes footplate at the oval window. The middle ear matches the lower impedance of sound waves in the air to the higher impedance fluid in the cochlea. This amplifying function has been described as middle ear gain, and the impedance matching is essential for the efficiency of air conduction.[6] The vibratory area of the tympanic membrane is about 20 times greater than the area of the stapes footplate. This area ratio together with the mechanical lever effect especially from the malleus and incus achieves a middle ear gain of roughly 25−35 dB. Damage to the middle ear conductive pathway impairs the efficiency of sound conduction and consecutively can lead to conductive hearing loss.[6,7]

In the inner ear, transmitted sounds propagate as frequency-dependent travel waves through inner ear fluids along the turns of the cochlea, moving the basilar membrane and with it the organ of Corti (OC)[8] (Fig. 4.1B). The cochlea is organized in tonotopic fashion, with high frequencies located at the base, and low frequencies located at the apex. Different frequencies result in a distinct peak of a traveling sound wave along the basilar membrane. Its movement creates localized shearing forces along the OC, which, through subsequent steps, initiate the process of mechanotransduction: Mechanical energy of the traveling wave is transformed into electrochemical energy at the apical surface of the inner hair cells within the OC.[9] Stereocilia bundle movement leads to opening of ion channels, potassium influx, and subsequent depolarization of hair cells. Neurotransmitter release from ribbon synapses at the basal portion of inner hair cells stimulates bipolar afferent spiral ganglion neurons. An action potential is generated, and the signal is transmitted along the central auditory pathway in a tonotopic organization. Outer hair cells (OHCs) serve to amplify and tune the cochlear traveling wave through an additional active motile process.[9]

Overview: types of blast explosions and blast injuries to the ear

Detonation of high-order explosives generally causes a supersonic blast wave, resulting in a large increase in pressure as the wave propagates outward from the explosion core.[10] This is followed by the blast wind, which is a rapid decrease in pressure that pulls objects back toward the core of the explosion.[11] This stands in contrast to low-order explosives, which produce subsonic waves without associated blast waves.[11] The use of improvised explosive devices (IEDs) has increased with mounting frequency of terror attacks, and these devices may be a high order, low order, or a mix of both types of explosives, which makes the prediction of injury patterns challenging.[12–14]

Of note, the pathophysiology of explosive blasts is distinct from nonexplosive blast injury to the ear: nonexplosive blast injury is relatively common, with similar symptoms as explosive blast injury, but is caused by sudden sealing of the EAC with associated increased pressure in the EAC (such as a slap or punch to the ear, e.g., in sports accidents), and frequently leads to rupture of the tympanic membrane.[2]

Blast injury can be categorized into four groups: primary, secondary, tertiary, and quaternary blast injuries. Primary blast injury (PBI) affects organs that contain gas or air, such as the lungs and the ear. This type of injury is due to extreme and fast changes in pressure caused by the blast wave. Therefore, this type of injury is unique to high-order explosives. Otologic damage is the most common outcome for survivors of blast injury,[14] with the majority of survivors suffering from tympanic membrane perforations (TMPs).[15] Given its unique anatomy, the tympanic membrane can be perforated at pressure changes as small as 5 psi,[4] making it particularly sensitive to PBI. Other possible outcomes of PBI to the ear include dizziness, hearing loss, and ossicular chain injury or dislocation.[16,17] Hearing loss after BOP can be conductive, sensorineural, or mixed.[18] Conductive hearing loss refers to mechanical damage and impaired sound transmission to the inner ear, as seen with TMP or ossicular chain dysfunction. SNHL affects structures of the inner ear and is generally irreversible.

Secondary blast injuries (SBIs) are caused by rapid movement of items in the air due to the blast wind, which may cause blunt or penetrating injuries to an individual.[1] Resulting injuries to the ear may occur along the outer ear, including damage to the pinna and in the EAC.[17] Similar to PBI, traumatic perforation of the tympanic membrane and ossicular chain dislocation can occur with SBI.[17] Blast wind carrying contaminating particles in the air may lead to infections by depositing them in the ear canal and middle ear. SBI can be protected against by body armor and ear protection; it is therefore more likely to occur in civilian settings than military settings. Tertiary blast injury refers to injury sustained from displacement of the body and may lead to head trauma, which has been linked to hearing loss and/or tinnitus.[1] Hearing loss after traumatic brain injury (TBI) without evidence of skull fractures has been documented and linked to brainstem injury and contusions involving the auditory regions in the brain.[19] Auditory and vestibular symptoms resulting from concussions can last 6 months or longer after blast injury.[20] Quaternary blast injury refers to other types of sustained injuries not aforementioned, from burns to post-traumatic stress disorder.[1]

This chapter mainly focuses on research advances related to the physiology of PBI.

Blast injury to the tympanic membrane

The tympanic membrane (TM) is highly sensitive to pressure changes and is commonly ruptured during exposure to blast overpressure. Injuries caused by BOP lead to severe deformation of the TM as well as the ossicular chain, causing significant structural damage.[14] Ear protection can lower the maximum pressure caused by the blast,[21] but body armor and head protection cannot prevent PBI.[1] Closer proximity to the explosion core increases chances of TMP, but this is additionally influenced by head positioning—a position perpendicular to the blast wave or a frontal blast wave has a higher likelihood of causing TMP than parallel orientation.[4,21] Four grades mark the degree of TMP related to blast injury. Grade 1 includes linear tears or pinpoint defects within the drum, grade 2 includes smaller perforations with defects up to 50% of the drum, grade 3 marks defects of >50% up to 75%, and grade 4 is reserved for total drum defects (Fig. 4.1C).[4,21]

The pars tensa of the drum is most commonly affected, and central perforations outweigh perforations in marginal locations, due to higher vulnerability to disproportionate overpressurization.[22] Spontaneous TMP recovery is possible, but positive outcomes vary widely. The size, shape, location, and often irregular margins of traumatic perforations play a significant role in the lower numbers of spontaneous recovery.[17,23] Generally, larger perforations after blast injury are less likely to heal, as are more centrally located perforations, whereas inferior perforations were the most likely to heal.[21,24]

Multiple mathematical models, animal studies, and studies of human temporal bones have attempted to better understand the underlying changes of mechanical TM properties and damage to its microstructure after BOP.[25] The middle layer of the TM is unique in that it is comprised of radially and circumferentially aligned collagen fibers. This layer significantly influences the elasticity or stiffness of the TM.

Its mechanical properties change based on the level of strain, and changes in TM stiffness in response to an applied force are measured by Young's modulus.[25] In a recent human temporal bone study, cadaveric tympanic membrane strip samples first underwent multiple blasts to create an injury pattern before the TMs were exposed to sound stimulation. Mechanical TM stiffness had decreased significantly, and the Young Modulus was found to be reduced by more than 50%. This reduction was frequency specific in that it affected mainly high-frequency sound conduction, and the residual stiffness corresponded to the degree of injury of the TM.[25] Electron microscopy of the TM after BOP revealed corresponding damage and fractures of both radial and circumferential TM fibers.[25]

Similar results were found in animal studies, where chinchilla tympanic membranes were exposed to BOP levels below the TM rupture threshold. Mechanical properties of the TM were analyzed with a microfringe projection system and characterized using a finite element method (FEM) model. Young's modulus after blast was found to have decreased by more than 50%. This demonstrated that even in TMs that did not rupture after exposure to BOP, there is deformation due to the high strain rate with damage to the collagen fiber layer, softening the TM.[26] When a similar method was used in human cadaveric temporal bones, Young's modulus decreased by up to 20% after multiple blasts.[27] A TM rupture dose−response risk assessment based on the FEM model predicted the probability of injury to the TM dependent on TM displacement, velocity, and acceleration. Assuming that TMP is associated with purely mechanical, structural damage after traumatic blast loading,[22] the fast running algorithm allowed for prediction of possible moderate and severe TM ruptures.

A similar model was employed again in a follow-up study, where the influence of blast wave direction on probability of TMP was further analyzed. Blast wave exposure to the front of the face was more likely to cause rupture of the TM compared with other directions, due to comparably higher changes in maximum stress within the TM.[28]

A novel method using laser Doppler vibrometers (LDVs) was able to successfully assess motion of the TM during BOP.[29] TM motion in cadaveric temporal bones was recorded in response to BOP of 35 kPa, and LDVs reliably measured TM displacement and velocity to provide data on blast wave transduction through the middle ear.[29]

Traumatic TMPs related to explosions have a much lower spontaneous healing rate compared with other traumatic TMPs, even at lower perforation grades, and improved understanding of the pathophysiology, as well as prediction of the injury pattern could significantly aid to determine when and which surgical intervention is needed.[4,17,22,25]

Blast injury to the ossicular chain

PBI to the middle ear in general resulted in conductive hearing loss with impaired sound conduction into the inner ear. In patients exposed to BOP, ossicular injury requiring ossiculoplasty varied anywhere from 10% to 20%.[23] Ossicular damage was frequently associated with TMP, and, as the nature of the blast wave tends to invert the edges of the tympanic membrane, increased risk of middle ear cholesteatoma.[15,23] The incidence of middle ear damage also positively correlated with higher levels of blast overexposure.[18] While the TM has been fairly well studied in various model systems, less is known about the biomechanics of the ossicles during BOP. Damage in the form of dislocation of the ossicular chain or fractures has been clinically described, but the underlying pathophysiology remains elusive.

Recent biomechanical measurements, however, have been able to shed light on overall blast energy transmission through the middle ear.[14,30,31] High-intensity sound from BOP changes middle ear transfer function, and with it the amount of energy that is being transmitted into the cochlea.[28,32,33] Using the previously described approach with LDVs, Jiang et al. measured the displacement of the stapes footplate (SFP) during BOP in a cadaveric human temporal bone study. SFP far exceeded normal movements and ranged from 41.2 to 126.5 µm when a stimulus level of 187 dB was applied. Interestingly, placement of hearing protection devices such as ear plugs reduced movement and displacement of the SFP, indicating a preventative effect during blast exposure.[34]

Blast injury to the inner ear

Blast-induced SNHL with associated tinnitus and vertigo has been well documented as a direct consequence of blast overpressure in military and civilian settings, but the underlying pathophysiology is distinct from the purely mechanical damage seen in the middle ear.[22,35] In cases of inner ear hearing loss, the symptoms can be temporary, and hearing loss presents as temporary threshold shift (TTS) which resolves over time; or, depending on the injury pattern, symptoms and threshold shift may be permanent (PTS).[18,22,35] SNHL is considered irreversible and associated with permanent macroscopic or microscopic damage to auditory structures within the inner ear.[14,36]

Recovery of hearing after initial threshold shift is not uncommon after blast injury.[30,33] In patients with SNHL, high-frequency SNHL appeared to be the most common pattern.[18,26,30] Next to TTS or PTS, tinnitus was one of the most common audiological complaints after blast injury and presented immediately after the injury in the majority of cases, rather than over time.[4,30,35,37] Tinnitus and hyperacusis also remained as symptoms despite recovery of hearing thresholds, with lasting increased sensitivity to noise and hearing difficulties in noisy environments. This was attributed to possible "hidden hearing loss."[4] Hidden hearing loss has recently been described as a new form of SNHL, a cochlear synaptopathy associated with isolated ribbon synapse loss and without visible threshold shift[38–40] (Fig. 4.1D).

In analogy to studies on conductive hearing loss and BOP, computational, cadaveric, and animal studies have been serving as models to investigate SNHL related to traumatic inner ear damage after blast injury.

Previous data indicated that SNHL after high intensity sounds or a blast wave may be a result of enhanced energy transmission through the middle ear via the TM and ossicular chain.[32–34]

This was supported by modeling of a blast wave moving from the external ear to the cochlea, which demonstrated increased displacement of the tympanic membrane and the ossicular chain, and which translated into exaggerated movement and displacement of the stapes footplate during BOP, subsequently leading to significantly increased cochlear pressures and basilar membrane at a level conducive to irreversible structural damage to the inner ear.[41]

An additional study confirmed that SNHL and PTS in mice after BOP were directly related to the blast wave and not associated with concurrent TMP.[14] Lower-pressure blast waves produced elevated auditory brainstem evoked responses (ABRs) and distortion product otoacoustic emission (DPOAE) thresholds on day 0. DPOAEs function as a measure of cochlear hair cell function. ABR thresholds at frequencies lower than 30 kHz recovered completely, while those above 30 kHz did not. DPOAE-elevated thresholds did not recover. Higher pressure blast correlated with larger threshold elevation in ABR and reduced threshold recovery. Cochleas lacked outer hair cells in the blast-exposed, high-frequency regions in up to 40%, and spiral ganglion neurons were increasingly reduced with higher-pressure blast waves. Despite this, the overall morphology of the cochlea was not changed.[14]

When using a blast stimulator on mice for either single or triple blast wave exposure to the inner ear, animals experienced the previously described TMP, as well as ABR threshold elevations of 50–65 dB 1 day after exposure.[42] Single blast animals partially recovered low-frequency thresholds after 1 month, but triple blast exposed mice never showed measurable recovery. DPOAE thresholds were undetectable across all frequencies in both groups up to 1 week after the blast, but partially recovered in the majority of single-blast mice after 6 months. This clearly indicates a dose dependency between SNHL, cochlear damage, and severity of BOP. This was supported by histological analysis, which found significant loss of OHC in basal and middle turns in triple blasted mice.[42] IHC and spiral ganglion numbers were unchanged between control, single, and triple blasted mice, but presynaptic portions of ribbon synapses were reduced in middle and apical cochlear regions of triple-blasted mice and in the middle cochlear region of single-blasted mice, suggesting additional beginning synaptopathy.[42]

To better identify histologic and molecular changes associated with BOP, another study utilized an advanced blast simulator to create inner ear damage in a rat model.[43] Associated TMP was observed after blast exposure, which healed completely by 4 weeks. Presence of inner ear hemorrhage at day 1 and 7 correlated

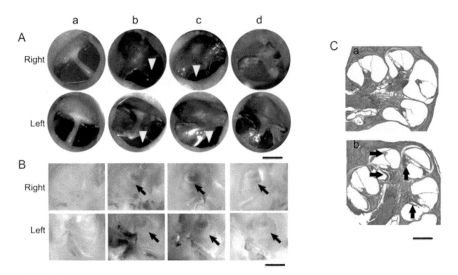

FIGURE 4.2

Damage to the ear after BOP in rats. (A) Right and left TMs before (a) and at 1 (b), 7 (c), and 28 (d) days after BOP. Middle ear hemorrhage, perforation, and malleus scarring are present (*yellow arrowheads*). Scale bar represents 1 mm. (B) Right and left views of the cochlea within the bony labyrinth demonstrate hemolabyrinth (*arrow*). Scale bar represents 1 mm. (C) Paraffin-embedded cochlear cross sections (H&E stain) of control (a) and 7 days after damage (b). Erythrocytes (*black arrows*) can be seen within the scala tympani and vestibuli. Scale bar represents 100 μm.

Reprinted [adapted] from Wang Y, Urioste RT, Wei Y, et al. Blast-induced hearing impairment in rats is associated with structural and molecular changes of the inner ear. Sci Rep. June 30, 2020;10(1):10652. https://doi. org/10.1038/s41598-020-67389-5.

with absent DPOAEs. DPOAEs slightly recovered by 1 month, but remained elevated compared with baseline (Fig. 4.2). ABR thresholds were elevated across all frequencies, in addition to significant reduction and increased latency of ABR wave 1 amplitude, a measure of the distal portion of the spiral ganglion nerves (SGN). Thresholds partially improved, but only in the lower frequencies. RNA sequencing (RNASeq) of inner ear tissue demonstrated differentially expressed genes in the cochlea 1 day (acute) and 1 month (chronic) after blast exposure, underlining additional subcellular changes related to altered transcriptional regulation and activation of immune response within the inner ear. During the acute phase, 1 day after blast exposure, gene upregulation was found in pathways related to cation channel activity, nervous system development, and neurotransmitter release, among others. One month after blast injury, positively regulated pathways involved cell—cell junction, protein binding, and antigen processing and presentation.[43]

To understand the effect of blast waves on the inner ear and SNHL alone, without associated middle ear transfer component, laser-induced shock waves (LISWs) were used to recapitulate low-, middle-, and high-energy blast exposure to the inner ear in a rat model.[36] Immediately after exposure, rats in the middle- and high-energy groups showed significant threshold changes in ABRs, which persisted for 1 month after exposure, while the low-energy group did not exhibit threshold elevation. DPOAEs only demonstrated threshold changes in the high-energy group up to 1 month after exposure at higher frequencies. Additional measurements of wave 1 and 2 signals in the ABR, which reflect responses from the distal and proximal segments of the spiral ganglion nerve, were permanently reduced in the low-energy group up to 1 month after exposure, despite normal DPOAEs, suggesting neural damage across all groups.[36] No gross morphological damage of the tympanic membrane, the middle, or the inner ear was observed. Microscopic exam showed intact outer and inner hair cells (OHCs and IHCs) but revealed a significant loss of HC synaptic ribbon synapses in middle- and high-energy groups across all frequencies (Fig. 4.3).

One month after exposure to high-energy waves, overall SGN numbers had declined and remaining cell bodies in the high-frequency regions had atrophied. Loss of up to 50% of synaptic ribbons in severe cases only produced a small threshold shift. In the low- and middle-energy groups, an ABR threshold was elevated to 30 dB at 16 kHz. Electron microscopy revealed damages to the surface structures of OHCs that had not readily been visible in light microscopy. Deformed stereocilia in the outer row of OHCs correlated with the ABR threshold changes seen in high- and mid-energy groups.[36]

The relationship of synaptopathy and TMP in blast injury is controversial, but has become increasingly important to explain tinnitus and hyperacusis after acoustic trauma. Hickman et al. hypothesized that a perforation during multiple blasts could mitigate transmission into the cochlea and therefore have a protective role against sensorineural damage and synapse loss to the chinchilla inner ear.[44] In contrast to this, a recent study in mice found auditory dysfunction in peripheral and central structures after BOP, independent of TMP.[45] The degree of peripheral synaptopathy, however, was increased in animals without TMP. One day after BOP, ABR thresholds were elevated in all animals that were exposed to a blast, and animals with concurrent TMP demonstrated higher thresholds than animals without TMP. However, after 2 months, and spontaneous healing of TM, thresholds of TMP+ and TMP− animals were similar, albeit still higher compared with control animals. TMP+ ears maintained elevated DPOAE thresholds throughout, suggesting that, apart from a conductive component, additional OHC damage was present. In animals that demonstrated cochlear dysfunction on ABR after BOP, ears were assessed for hair cell and neuron survival. Hair cell and neuron numbers were preserved in all groups independent of TMP. Stereocilia disruption on OHC was present in all blast-induced mice with or without TMP, likely explaining the threshold shifts seen in ABR and DPOAEs after BOP. Interestingly, animals without concurrent TMP showed significantly more reduction in peripheral cochlear synapse numbers.[45] This was in contrast to animals with TMP, which demonstrated preserved peripheral synapse counts. At the level of the brainstem, in the cochlear

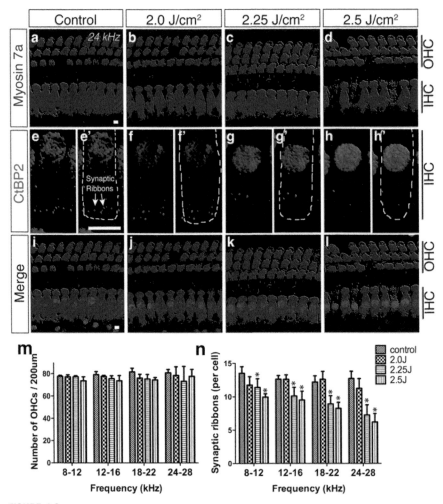

FIGURE 4.3

Organ of Corti changes in response to LISW. (A—L) Confocal microscopy of hair cells. (A—D) 3 rows of OHCs and 1 row of IHC, labeled with hair cell marker myosin 7A (*blue*) in response to increasing LISW. (E—H) CtBP2 labels presynaptic portion of IHC synaptic ribbons (*red*); *dotted line* contours IHCs; anti-CtBP2 also stains the IHC nuclei. Merged images (I—L) at 24 kHz demonstrate maintained hair cell numbers. (M, N) The number of OHCs (M) and IHC synaptic ribbons (N) 1 month after LISW exposure (n = 5 in each group). Despite increased ABR threshold shifts in the 2.25 and 2.5 J/cm^2 groups (C, D), OHC number did not change 1 month after LISW (M) compared with control (A). Synaptic ribbon numbers in IHC decreased with increasing LISW energy levels (E—H, N). Asterisks indicate significant differences ($P < .05$). Scale bar represents 5 μm.

Reprinted [adapted] from Niwa K, Mizutari K, Matsui T, et al. Pathophysiology of the inner ear after blast injury caused by laser-induced shock wave. Sci Rep. August 17, 2016;6:31754. https://doi.org/10.1038/srep31754.

nucleus, the number of synapses was reduced after blast injury, but did not significantly differ between TMP+ and TMP− groups, suggesting that TMP did not influence damage of the central auditory pathway.[45]

In summary, current research has advanced considerably and led to better understanding of the underlying pathophysiology of acoustic blast injury. This research, however, is limited by the nature of BOP—prospective human clinical trials are unethical, and human studies have to rely on retrospective analysis of injury patterns or cadaveric human temporal bone studies. While animal studies and computational models help to elucidate the biomechanical, cellular, and molecular changes related to BOP in the ear, more future work is necessary to ultimately improve prevention and treatment options for patients with acoustic blast injury.

References

1. Mathews ZR, Koyfman A. Blast injuries. *J Emerg Med.* 2015;49:573−587.
2. Berger G, Finkelstein Y, Harell M. Non-explosive blast injury of the ear. *J Laryngol Otol.* 1994;108:395−398.
3. Brown MA, Ji XD, Gan RZ. 3D finite element modeling of blast wave transmission from the external ear to cochlea. *Ann Biomed Eng.* 2021;49:757−768.
4. Remenschneider AK, Lookabaugh S, Aliphas A, et al. Otologic outcomes after blast injury: the Boston Marathon experience. *Otol Neurotol.* 2014;35:1825−1834.
5. Lim DJ. Structure and function of the tympanic membrane: a review. *Acta Otorhinolaryngol Belg.* 1995;49:101−115.
6. Merchant SN, Ravicz ME, Puria S, et al. Analysis of middle ear mechanics and application to diseased and reconstructed ears. *Am J Otol.* 1997;18:139−154.
7. Merchant SN, Ravicz ME, Rosowski JJ. Acoustic input impedance of the stapes and cochlea in human temporal bones. *Hear Res.* 1996;97:30−45.
8. Robles L, Ruggero MA. Mechanics of the mammalian cochlea. *Physiol Rev.* 2001;81:1305−1352.
9. Caprara GA, Peng AW. Mechanotransduction in mammalian sensory hair cells. *Mol Cell Neurosci.* 2022;120:103706.
10. Cernak I. Blast injuries and blast-induced neurotrauma: overview of pathophysiology and experimental knowledge models and findings. In: Kobeissy FH, ed. *Brain Neurotrauma: Molecular, Neuropsychological, and Rehabilitation Aspects.* 2015. Boca Raton (FL).
11. Singh AK, Ditkofsky NG, York JD, et al. Blast injuries: from improvised explosive device blasts to the Boston Marathon bombing. *Radiographics.* 2016;36:295−307.
12. Harrison CD, Bebarta VS, Grant GA. Tympanic membrane perforation after combat blast exposure in Iraq: a poor biomarker of primary blast injury. *J Trauma.* 2009;67:210−211.
13. Wightman JM, Gladish SL. Explosions and blast injuries. *Ann Emerg Med.* 2001;37:664−678.
14. Cho SI, Gao SS, Xia A, et al. Mechanisms of hearing loss after blast injury to the ear. *PLoS One.* 2013;8:e67618.
15. Yeh DD, Schecter WP. Primary blast injuries—an updated concise review. *World J Surg.* 2012;36:966−972.

16. Shah A, Ayala M, Capra G, Fox D, Hoffer M. Otologic assessment of blast and nonblast injury in returning Middle East-deployed service members. *Laryngoscope*. 2014;124: 272–277.
17. Aslier M, Aslier NGY. Analysis of otologic injuries due to blast trauma by handmade explosives. *Turk Arch Otorhinolaryngol*. 2017;55:64–68.
18. Darley DS, Kellman RM. Otologic considerations of blast injury. *Disaster Med Public Health Prep*. 2010;4:145–152.
19. Chen JX, Lindeborg M, Herman SD, et al. Systematic review of hearing loss after traumatic brain injury without associated temporal bone fracture. *Am J Otolaryngol*. 2018; 39:338–344.
20. Fausti SA, Wilmington DJ, Gallun FJ, Myers PJ, Henry JA. Auditory and vestibular dysfunction associated with blast-related traumatic brain injury. *J Rehabil Res Dev*. 2009;46:797–810.
21. Ritenour AE, Baskin TW. Primary blast injury: update on diagnosis and treatment. *Crit Care Med*. 2008;36:S311–S317.
22. Iyoho AE, Ho K, Chan P. The development of a tympanic membrane model and probabilistic dose-response risk assessment of rupture because of blast. *Mil Med*. 2020;185: 234–242.
23. Keller M, Sload R, Wilson J, Greene H, Han P, Wise S. Tympanoplasty following blast injury. *Otolaryngol Head Neck Surg*. 2017;157:1025–1033.
24. Kronenberg J, Ben-Shoshan J, Modan M, Leventon G. Blast injury and cholesteatoma. *Am J Otol*. 1988;9:127–130.
25. Engles WG, Wang X, Gan RZ. Dynamic properties of human tympanic membrane after exposure to blast waves. *Ann Biomed Eng*. 2017;45:2383–2394.
26. Liang J, Yokell ZA, Nakmaili DU, Gan RZ, Lu H. The effect of blast overpressure on the mechanical properties of a chinchilla tympanic membrane. *Hear Res*. 2017;354:48–55.
27. Liang J, Smith KD, Gan RZ, Lu H. The effect of blast overpressure on the mechanical properties of the human tympanic membrane. *J Mech Behav Biomed Mater*. 2019;100: 103368.
28. Gan RZ, Leckness K, Nakmali D, Ji XD. Biomechanical measurement and modeling of human eardrum injury in relation to blast wave direction. *Mil Med*. 2018;183:245–251.
29. Jiang S, Smith K, Gan RZ. Dual-laser measurement and finite element modeling of human tympanic membrane motion under blast exposure. *Hear Res*. 2019;378:43–52.
30. Dougherty AL, MacGregor AJ, Han PP, Viirre E, Heltemes KJ, Galarneau MR. Blast-related ear injuries among U.S. military personnel. *J Rehabil Res Dev*. 2013;50: 893–904.
31. Patterson Jr JH, Hamernik RP. Blast overpressure induced structural and functional changes in the auditory system. *Toxicology*. 1997;121:29–40.
32. Greene NT, Alhussaini MA, Easter JR, Argo TF, Walilko T, Tollin DJ. Intracochlear pressure measurements during acoustic shock wave exposure. *Hear Res*. 2018;365: 149–164.
33. Peacock J, Al Hussaini M, Greene NT, Tollin DJ. Intracochlear pressure in response to high intensity, low frequency sounds in chinchilla. *Hear Res*. 2018;367:213–222.
34. Jiang S, Dai C, Gan RZ. Dual-laser measurement of human stapes footplate motion under blast exposure. *Hear Res*. 2021;403:108177.
35. Joseph AR, AuD, Horton JL, et al. Development of a comprehensive blast-related auditory injury database (BRAID). *J Rehabil Res Dev*. 2016;53:295–306.

36. Niwa K, Mizutari K, Matsui T, et al. Pathophysiology of the inner ear after blast injury caused by laser-induced shock wave. *Sci Rep*. 2016;6:31754.
37. Cave KM, Cornish EM, Chandler DW. Blast injury of the ear: clinical update from the global war on terror. *Mil Med*. 2007;172:726−730.
38. Plack CJ, Barker D, Prendergast G. Perceptual consequences of "hidden" hearing loss. *Trends Hear*. 2014;18.
39. Schaette R, McAlpine D. Tinnitus with a normal audiogram: physiological evidence for hidden hearing loss and computational model. *J Neurosci*. 2011;31:13452−13457.
40. Kujawa SG, Liberman MC. Adding insult to injury: cochlear nerve degeneration after "temporary" noise-induced hearing loss. *J Neurosci*. 2009;29:14077−14085.
41. Brown MA, Bradshaw JJ, Gan RZ. Three-dimensional finite element modeling of blast wave transmission from the external ear to a spiral cochlea. *J Biomech Eng*. 2022:144.
42. Mao B, Wang Y, Balasubramanian T, et al. Assessment of auditory and vestibular damage in a mouse model after single and triple blast exposures. *Hear Res*. 2021;407: 108292.
43. Wang Y, Urioste RT, Wei Y, et al. Blast-induced hearing impairment in rats is associated with structural and molecular changes of the inner ear. *Sci Rep*. 2020;10:10652.
44. Hickman TT, Smalt C, Bobrow J, Quatieri T, Liberman MC. Blast-induced cochlear synaptopathy in chinchillas. *Sci Rep*. 2018;8:10740.
45. Kurioka T, Mizutari K, Satoh Y, Shiotani A. Correlation of blast-induced tympanic membrane perforation with peripheral cochlear synaptopathy. *J Neurotrauma*. 2022; 9(13−14):999−1009.

Acute and chronic management of otologic blast injury

Nicole T. Jiam, MD [1], Philip D. Littlefield, MD [2], Daniel J. Lee, MD [1]

[1]*Department of Otolaryngology-Head and Neck Surgery, Massachusetts Eye and Ear, Harvard Medical School, Boston, MA, United States;* [2]*Department of Otolaryngology, Sharp Rees-Stealy Medical Group, San Diego, CA, United States*

Introduction

In 2005, the Department of Veterans Affairs awarded more than $1 billion for otologic-related disabilities—the majority of which were due to impulse noise exposures and blast injuries.[1] The ear is the body's most sensitive pressure transducer, and as a result, otologic complaints are common after blasts.[2] Fortunately, blast trauma is a rare occurrence in the United States. As a result, much of the civilian literature is drawn from the Boston Marathon bombings,[3] Afghanistan War,[4] and Iraq War.[5] Unique to blast-related otologic trauma, acute management is often dictated by the tactical situation at hand and by the severity of other injuries. In this chapter, we will review evaluation and management patients exposed to otologic blast injuries based on military and civilian experiences as well as animal studies (Table 5.1).

Otologic blast injuries

Aural soft tissue trauma

Facial and neck injuries are common in warfare as these areas are incompletely protected by body armor and helmets.[6–8] Even worse, civilians caught in war zones or terrorist attacks usually have no protection. Acute ear management is highly dependent on the severity of other nonotologic injuries, local resources, the nearest facility with surgical capabilities, and if the patient can be evacuated from the site of injury. History taking is usually abbreviated in this setting, and otologic injuries will not have priority compared with more emergent injuries. For example, the incidence of emergent surgeries and perioperative mortality rates were higher in Iraq than in Afghanistan, and as a result, US soldiers and civilians were less likely to be cared for by head and neck surgeons in Iraq.[9]

During the initial trauma evaluation, a thorough examination of the pinna and surrounding soft tissue should be performed. Profusely bleeding soft tissue injuries

Table 5.1 Common otologic injuries after blast trauma.

Otologic injuries:
Soft tissue injuries
Auricular laceration
Auricular hematoma
Temporal bone fractures
External ear injuries
External auditory canal lacerations
Tympanic membrane
Middle ear injuries
Ossicular chain discontinuity/fracture
Inner ear injuries
Cochlea
Sensorineural hearing loss
Tinnitus
Vestibular system
Vestibular organ damage
Benign paroxysmal positional vertigo
Postconcussive migraines/vestibular migraines
Semicircular canal dehiscence

should be addressed, and initial surgery should be limited to primary closure and soft tissue coverage of exposed bone.[9] Mastoid ecchymosis (otherwise known as Battle's sign) may be indicative of a skull base fracture and brain trauma. This usually takes at least one day to appear, so examination of the postauricular region should not be overlooked after the initial trauma evaluation.

The external auditory canal should be evaluated for any soft tissue lacerations and tympanic membrane perforations. If an otoscope or microscope is not available, a headlight, loupes, and nasal speculum may be used instead. This is often necessary even in the hospital since most initial exams are at the bedside. Many such patients, however, have other injuries that require acute management in the operating room. It often is possible to perform an operative microscope exam under anesthesia simultaneously, if not interfering with the other surgeons, and they usually are accommodating. During this time, remove as much foreign material (e.g., metal fragments, wood, dirt, pebbles) as possible. Saline irrigation may be used to clear blood and foreign debris.

Tympanic membrane perforation

If a tympanic membrane perforation is present, then unfurl the remnants to avoid cholesteatoma formation. These remnants can also be supported with absorbable foam or a paper patch, but this is not the time to attempt a formal tympanoplasty. Apply an ototopical fluoroquinolone if there is a moist or contaminated perforation or soft tissue injury to the external auditory canal. Topical aminoglycosides should be avoided since they may be ototoxic and risk sensorineural hearing loss and vestibulopathy.[10] There is no need for topical antibiotics with a clean and dry perforation as this may delay healing.[11] However, many of these patients also have acute sensorineural hearing loss, for which middle ear delivery of steroids (e.g., dexamethasone) may be indicated, although this too may influence closure of the tympanic membrane perforation.[12]

The detonation of one pound of trinitrotoluene (TNT) at a 15-feet distance is approximately 180 dB SPL.[13] Blast pressures greater than five pounds per square inch (34.5 kPa) above atmosphere can rupture the tympanic membrane.[14] A murine study that examined tympanic membrane perforation following exposure to 30 or 63 kPa blast waves reported significant and unanimous tympanic membrane damage at 63 kPa (mean perforation size of $57.8 \pm 3.5\%$ ($n = 5$) of the total surface area).[15] Smaller perforations (mean perforation size of $5.9 \pm 1.7\%$ of the total surface area) were observed in some animals exposed to the 30 kPa blast level. Tympanic membrane perforations are common after explosions and have been reported to be present in 5%−90% of explosion-wounded patients.[3,16,17] Proximity to the blast and significant nonotologic injuries have been reported to be positive predictors of tympanic membrane perforation.

Spontaneous tympanic membrane perforation closure occurs in 38%−82% of patients[18−21], particularly with smaller perforations (<50% of the tympanic membrane). Surgical intervention via tympanoplasty may be necessary for persistent perforations, especially when there is conductive hearing loss and/or persistent otorrhea. These perforations should be given sufficient time to heal spontaneously, and it is possible for even large perforations to heal, or at least partially. Six weeks of observation is typical but can be extended if subsequent visits show that the perforation is getting smaller. These patients often need to wait this long anyway as they are being treated for other injuries, and some patients with multiple amputations have had upward of 40 surgeries. Tympanoplasty should be delayed as anesthesia induction and intubations risk displacing grafts in the middle ear. Also, many of these patients are on anticoagulants, and this should be taken into consideration. The success rates of tympanoplasties (∼82%-85%) for blast-related perforations are lower than non−blast-related perforations due to the size of the perforation (e.g., total or near-total), ossicular displacement, and inflammatory responses to foreign material[22−24], and this is despite normal eustachian tube function.

The same tympanoplasty techniques that are used for chronic ear surgery are applicable to blast-induced perforations. These perforations tend to be large so simple transcanal fascia underlays are usually insufficient. More advanced techniques such as lateral grafting, anterior tab pull-through, and the over—under technique are usually necessary.[23,24] Whatever technique is used, it is important to inspect the tympanum for implanted epithelium and cholesteatomas[23,25]; endoscopes are useful adjuncts for examining the hidden recesses of the middle ear (retrotympanum, protympanum, etc.). It is also important to inspect for ossicular discontinuity and perilymphatic fistulas.[24] Ossiculoplasty is usually best performed at a second stage given the concerns of cholesteatoma with keratin implantation following implosion injury.

Sensorineural hearing loss

Hearing loss and tinnitus often follow blast injuries to the ear. For example, among 36,917 Afghanistan and Iraq war veterans that underwent traumatic brain injury evaluations, 65.7% reported subjective auditory impairments.[26]

Impulse noise (such as from rifles or supersonic blast waves from explosions) is more damaging than sustained noise exposure, as cochlear injury is both mechanical and biochemical.[27] Blasts cause stereociliary bundle disruption that results in immediate outer hair dysfunction.[28] It used to be thought that noise damage was limited to within the cochlea. This is the most immediate result, but it is now known that the damage is more extensive and progressive and can eventually cause auditory nerve degeneration. For example, in vivo cochlear imaging of mice exposed to blast waves revealed endolymphatic hydrops, hair cell loss, and cochlear synaptopathy.[29] Another histological animal study demonstrated a loss of outer hair cells within the basal turn of the cochlea, decreased spiral ganglion neurons, and diminished afferent nerve synapses 1 week and 3 months after blast injury.[30] These progressive effects are contrary to the traditional thinking that noise-induced hearing loss only occurs at the time of the injury. Furthermore, recent clinical data show that this is not just limited to the lab; noise-induced sensorineural hearing loss from military service accelerates what otherwise looks like normal hearing loss from aging.[31,32]

Blasts may also cause temporary hearing threshold shifts without permanent hair cell damage, and yet there may be hearing damage despite this apparent audiometric recovery. This is because significant synaptic and neuronal loss may have occurred. Studies in chinchillas have revealed 20%—45% ribbon synapse loss in the mid and basal cochlea after blasts of 160—175 dB sound pressure levels.[33] This phenomenon is called hidden hearing loss, and blast victims with hidden hearing loss often report hyperacusis and difficulty with speech-in-noise despite normal audiometric thresholds.

Timely audiometric evaluations are important to quantify and establish an objective verification of hearing loss. Unfortunately, audiometry often is not available in a combat theater, but treatment should not be delayed and should be initiated if there is a clinical suspicion of a sensorineural hearing loss. Even at Walter Reed Army

Medical Center (2007–12), most initial audiograms were performed at the bedside and with background noise because it was impractical (or impossible) to transport polytrauma patients into a sound-proof booth. As usual, a Weber tuning fork exam is helpful to confirm a low-frequency sensorineural hearing loss, but one should be aware that it does not rule out higher-frequency hearing losses. Noise-induced hearing loss typically causes decreased high-frequency hearing sensitivity and an audiometric "noise" notch at 4000 Hz due to the transfer function of the ear.[34] Blast-induced hearing losses not only affect these frequencies the most but also tend to involve the low- to mid-frequency thresholds with a flatter audiogram pattern.[35] The presence of a tympanic membrane perforation should increase suspicion and empiric treatment of sensorineural hearing loss; a study conducted at the Walter Reed National Military Medical Center reported an incidence of sensorineural hearing loss of 36% in patients with blast-induced tympanic membrane perforations that required tympanoplasty.[23] The strongest predictor of severe or profound hearing loss is the presence of ossicular chain discontinuity.[35] Even when there is intact tympanic membrane, empiric steroid treatment should be considered if there is new-onset tinnitus or subjective hearing loss.

Steroids are the mainstay treatment for acute acoustic trauma.[36,37] Steroids may be otoprotective by scavenging oxygen free radicals and inhibiting lipid peroxidation.[38] Animal studies have demonstrated a strong, acute otoprotective effect from topical steroids after impulse noise exposure or drill trauma.[39–42] When sensorineural hearing loss is suspected, it is important to initiate high-dose oral steroids (e.g., 60 mg prednisone daily for 14 days, followed by a taper) or weekly intratympanic steroid injections (e.g., 0.4 mL of dexamethasone 10 mg/mL). This strategy mirrors the management of sudden sensorineural hearing loss. As such, American Academy of Otolaryngology—Head and Neck Surgery Clinical Practice Guideline recommends initiating steroids in patients with sudden sensorineural hearing loss within 2 weeks of symptom onset.[43] Intratympanic steroid therapy can be offered to patients with incomplete recovery from sensorineural hearing loss 2–6 weeks after the onset of their symptoms. There is no evidence to suggest corticosteroid delivered intratympanically is more beneficial than systemic treatment in the case of moderate-to-severe idiopathic sudden sensorineural hearing loss,[22] but this so far has not been studied for noise-induced hearing loss. Regardless, oral steroids may be more logistically feasible to administer in a combat environment. On the other hand, systemic steroids may hinder wound healing among polytrauma patients, so intratympanic steroids are sometimes a better option in a multidisciplinary setting.

Other compounds that have been studied in laboratory animals exposed to acoustic trauma include acetyl-L-carnitine and *N*-acetylcysteine (NAC)[44–46], 2,4-disulfonyl α-phenyl tertiary butyl nitrone,[47] astragaloside IV,[48] leupeptin49; Src-protein kinase inhibitors,[50] AM-111,[51] caroverine,[52] and magnesium.[53] However, none of these have come into common use, and at present, they should only be considered adjuncts to steroids rather than replacements.

Noise injury has been shown to increase calcium levels in hair cells and stimulate reactive oxygen species production,[18,54] resulting in the activation of cell death pathways.[55] Accordingly, antioxidants have been studied as therapeutics to reduce reactive oxygen species levels in the hair cells after acoustic trauma. Eleven military officers who received oral NAC after an indoor shooting session received a small protective effect in hearing thresholds compared to controls.[56] Unlike some of the other compounds, NAC is often available in military pharmacies because it is the antidote for acetaminophen overdose, and also a common respiratory therapy treatment. Given the low risk-to-benefit ratio of steroids and NAC, there should be a low threshold for initiation NAC with steroids after a blast injury.[57–59]

Auditory hair cells may be more sensitive to further insults after a blast injury. Therefore, ear protection and minimization of hazardous noise exposure is critical. Any hearing loss should be followed up in the long term with annual audiograms and an otolaryngologist as needed. Many blast-injured patients require hearing aids, but there are cases that have ultimately required cochlear implants due to the severity of sensorineural hearing loss.

Hair cell repair is critical for auditory function. Thus, hair cell regeneration and viral gene therapy have been an active source of investigation for sensorineural hearing loss.[60] In Zebrafish, epigenetic factors LSD1 and HDAC seem to be required for hair cell regeneration.[61,62] However, hair cells in mature mammals do not regenerate, and paths of regeneration may be different than from those of development. As a result, morphologic and transcriptome profiles may differ across species and maturity; there has been no effect of HDAC inhibitors on Atoh1-mediated conversion in the adult mouse cochleae.[62] Posttranscriptional regulation (e.g., micro-RNA-induced gene silence) may play a role in hair cell development and regeneration, especially the miRNA 183 family[63–65], miRNA 124,[66] and let7.[67] Mizutari et al. found that introducing Notch inhibitor LY411575 in vivo in noise-damaged mouse cochleae activated Atoh1 and induced new hair cell formation with an 8-decibel hearing improvement.[68] However, this finding was shown in neonatal mice and not in adult mammals.[69] Combination therapies targeting multiple factors and epigenetic pathways hold promise for hair cell regeneration in mature mammalian cochleae following noise-induced sensorineural hearing loss.

Secondary effects of sensorineural hearing loss include tinnitus. Blast-induced tinnitus is common among veterans; approximately 49% of patients with blast-related injuries from war report tinnitus, as compared with a prevalence of 10%–15% within the normal population.[17] The degree of severity can be influenced by stress, anxiety, and depression[70]—which are common mental health disorders in the veteran and military population.[25,71] As a result, blast-exposed veterans may suffer greatly from the effects of tinnitus.

Currently, there is no cure or clinically recommended drug or device treatment for tinnitus. Sound-based therapy and cognitive behavioral therapy are mainstay management strategies to reduce the potentiation of tinnitus signal.[72] Animal models have been widely used for pharmaceutical treatment research for tinnitus. Unfortunately, successful pharmacologic treatments in animal models (e.g., memantine, esketamine, AUT00063) have failed to share the same level of efficacy in humans.[73–75] Studies adopting a bimodal neuromodulation approach toward tinnitus have reported a significant reduction in tinnitus symptom severity.[76–79] Cochlear implants have also been shown to reduce tinnitus, particularly in those with a fluctuating type of tinnitus, greater tinnitus handicap, and shorter duration of tinnitus prior to implantation.[80] In recent years, technological innovation has spurred the development of digital smart therapy platforms for personalized tinnitus modulation.[81]

Vestibular injuries

Vestibular dysfunction is a frequent complaint among blast-exposed service members and civilians.[82,83] The most direct cause is labyrinthine concussion, which is thought to be acute damage to the vestibular organs from a pressure wave within the intralabyrinthine fluids.[84,85] Presenting symptoms are typical of an acute unilateral vestibulopathy and include vertigo, nausea, vomiting, and spontaneous nystagmus, all of which may be exacerbated with head movements. Murine studies have observed histological changes to the vestibular organs after blasts[86]; there was a significant loss of stereocilia in the cristae ampullaris and the macule after exposure to a 63-kPa peak blast wave (akin to an improved explosive device [IED] injury).[15] As with any acute vestibular injury, these symptoms typically improve over weeks to months through vestibular compensation. Physical therapy may help blast-exposed patients with peripheral vestibular injuries, particularly older adults who may have difficulties with vestibular compensation due to age-related declines in neuroplasticity.[87]

Explosions were the most common cause of traumatic brain injuries (TBIs) among military service members in the recent Middle East wars, accounting for approximately 80% of cases.[88] Consequently, many patients with blast injuries have a mix of central and peripheral vestibular dysfunction, such as postconcussive syndrome combined with a labyrinthine injury. These can be difficult to separate from one another clinically although there are sometimes localizing signs. For example, a pure upbeat positional nystagmus cannot be explained by peripheral causes alone, but this is often seen (using videonystagmography goggles) after a mild TBI.[89] Patients with pure upbeat positional nystagmus after a trauma therefore should be screened for TBI (assuming no nicotine, which also causes an upbeat nystagmus). This is also true for other central findings that may be seen during a bedside exam or during videonystagmography. These include pure torsional nystagmus, direction-changing nystagmus, poor fixation suppression of nystagmus, overshoots with saccades, and dysconjugate eye movements.

Posttraumatic headaches and postconcussive migraines are highly prevalent among this patient population.[90] Even in cases of mild head trauma, disequilibrium was reported to persist for at least 2 or more years in approximately 18% of TBI patients.[91] Any blast victim with symptoms of disequilibrium of moderate or severe intensity lasting 5 min to 72 h should be screened for the Bárány Society and International Headache Society's diagnostic criteria for definitive or probable vestibular migraines.[92] Vestibular migraine management often includes avoidance of triggers, dietary and behavioral modifications, sleep hygiene, over-the-counter supplementation, and/or antimigraine medications.[93]

Benign paroxysmal positional vertigo (BPPV) is also common after ear and head traumas.[94,95] It is therefore important to evaluate any patient with dizziness after head trauma with Dix-Hallpike maneuvers, assuming no neck injuries (and then cervical vertigo is another possibility). Personal experience suggests Dix-Hallpike maneuvers should be performed even if the symptoms do not sound like classic BPPV, as it is not unusual to see a positive response (with the typical upbeat and geotropic torsional nystagmus) in trauma patients with atypical symptoms.

Patients that report autophony after blast exposure should undergo a temporal bone CT scan and vestibular evoked myogenic potential testing to evaluate for superior semicircular canal dehiscence syndrome. It is not unusual for superior semicircular canal dehiscence to become symptomatic after head traumas.[96] For example, there is a case report on a 26-year-old service member who was near two IED blasts during his deployment, and then had new onset of oscillopsia and vertigo in response to loud and low-pitch sounds.[97] The hypothesized etiology was pressure-induced mobilization of (presumably thin) bone overlaying the superior semicircular canal. Surgical plugging of such a dehiscence is no different than with nontrauma cases, but the perioperative management may be more complicated by comorbidities such as TBI and migraine.

Perilymphatic fistula is another cause of hearing loss and vestibular dysfunction. However, the authors have only one surgically confirmed case (and several negative explorations) from the Walter Reed and Boston Marathon bombing experiences, so this is possible but seems to be uncommon. Many of these patients require prolonged bedrest, so perhaps breaches of the otic capsule heal without causing subsequent symptoms.

Vestibular screening should be conducted even if a blast-exposed individual appears relatively unscathed.[98] For example, a study evaluating 100 patients after blast injury or exposure demonstrated that individuals without severe extremity injuries were more likely to suffer from imbalance and vertigo than those with severe extremity injuries.[99] However, this is in part explained by the higher prevalence of TBI in the latter group. Also, symptoms often take time to manifest and may go unnoticed while these patients are confined to hospital beds or light activities. Furthermore, autonomic deconditioning is another consequence of prolonged bedrest, so it is common for these patients to be lightheaded with standing or incur cervicogenic dizziness once they start to resume more routine activities.[100] This can result in referrals for suspected vestibular dysfunction. It fortunately tends to resolve spontaneously, but this can take time.

Conclusion

Otologic injuries are common after blast trauma. Acute management of otologic injuries among the military personnel and civilians is influenced by the combat terrain and proximity to facilities with surgical capabilities and specialty care. Blast-exposed patients are likely to suffer from long-term effects of hearing loss, tinnitus, tympanic membrane perforations, and dizziness—and should be followed by an otolaryngologist for chronic care and management.

References

1. Chandler D. Blast-related ear injury in current U.S. Military operations: role of audiology on the interdisciplinary team. *ASHA Leader.* 2006;11:8−9+29.
2. Esquivel CR, Parker M, Curtis K, et al. Aural blast injury/acoustic trauma and hearing loss. *Mil Med.* 2018;183(suppl_2):78−82.
3. Remenschneider AK, Lookabaugh S, Aliphas A, et al. Otologic outcomes after blast injury: the Boston Marathon experience. *Otol Neurotol.* 2014;35(10):1825−1834.
4. Swan AA, Nelson JT, Swiger B, et al. Prevalence of hearing loss and tinnitus in Iraq and Afghanistan veterans: a chronic effects of neurotrauma consortium study. *Hear Res.* 2017;349:4−12.
5. Shah A, Ayala M, Capra G, Fox D, Hoffer M. Otologic assessment of blast and nonblast injury in returning Middle East-deployed service members. *Laryngoscope.* 2014;124(1):272−277.
6. Breeze J, Gibbons AJ, Shieff C, Banfield G, Bryant DG, Midwinter MJ. Combat-related craniofacial and cervical injuries: a 5-year review from the British military. *J Trauma.* 2011;71(1):108−113.
7. Kelly JF, Ritenour AE, McLaughlin DF, et al. Injury severity and causes of death from operation Iraqi freedom and operation enduring freedom: 2003-2004 versus 2006. *J Trauma.* 2008;64(2 Suppl):S21−S26. discussion S6-7.
8. Holcomb JB, McMullin NR, Pearse L, et al. Causes of death in U.S. special operations forces in the global war on terrorism: 2001−2004. *Ann Surg.* 2007;245(6):986−991.
9. Brennan J. Head and neck trauma in Iraq and Afghanistan: different war, different surgery, lessons learned. *Laryngoscope.* 2013;123(10):2411−2417.
10. Winterstein AG, Liu W, Xu D, Antonelli PJ. Sensorineural hearing loss associated with neomycin eardrops and nonintact tympanic membranes. *Otolaryngol Head Neck Surg.* 2013;148(2):277−283.
11. Dirain CO, Kosko B, Antonelli PJ. Effects of common ear drops on tympanic membrane healing in rats. *Otolaryngol Head Neck Surg.* 2018;158(5):917−922.
12. Antonelli PJ, Winterstein AG, Schultz GS. Topical dexamethasone and tympanic membrane perforation healing in otitis media: a short-term study. *Otol Neurotol.* 2010;31(3):519−523.

13. Agency) EUSEP. *Technical Fact Sheet—2,4,6-Trinitrotoluene (TNT)*. Office of Solid Waste and Emergency Response (5106P); 2014. EPA 505-F-14-009:1-8.

14. Jensen JH, Bonding P. Experimental pressure induced rupture of the tympanic membrane in man. *Acta Otolaryngol*. 1993;113(1):62−67.

15. Lien S, Dickman JD. Vestibular injury after low-intensity blast exposure. *Front Neurol*. 2018;9:297.

16. Ritenour AE, Wickley A, Ritenour JS, et al. Tympanic membrane perforation and hearing loss from blast overpressure in Operation Enduring Freedom and Operation Iraqi Freedom wounded. *J Trauma*. 2008;64(2 Suppl):S174−S178. discussion S8.

17. Cave KM, Cornish EM, Chandler DW. Blast injury of the ear: clinical update from the global war on terror. *Mil Med*. 2007;172(7):726−730.

18. Peng TI, Jou MJ. Oxidative stress caused by mitochondrial calcium overload. *Ann N Y Acad Sci*. 2010;1201:183−188.

19. Kronenberg J, Ben-Shoshan J, Wolf M. Perforated tympanic membrane after blast injury. *Am J Otol*. 1993;14(1):92−94.

20. Miller IS, McGahey D, Law K. The otologic consequences of the Omagh bomb disaster. *Otolaryngol Head Neck Surg*. 2002;126(2):127−128.

21. Kerr AG, Byrne JE. Concussive effects of bomb blast on the ear. *J Laryngol Otol*. 1975; 89(2):131−143.

22. Mirian C, Ovesen T. Intratympanic vs systemic corticosteroids in first-line treatment of idiopathic sudden sensorineural hearing loss: a systematic review and meta-analysis. *JAMA Otolaryngol Head Neck Surg*. 2020;146(5):421−428.

23. Sridhara SK, Rivera A, Littlefield P. Tympanoplasty for blast-induced perforations: the Walter Reed experience. *Otolaryngol Head Neck Surg*. 2013;148(1):103−107.

24. Song SA, Sridhara SK, Littlefield PD. Tympanoplasty outcomes for blast-induced perforations from Iraq and Afghanistan. *Otolaryngol Head Neck Surg*. 2017;156(2): 353−359.

25. Finnegan A, Randles R. Prevalence of common mental health disorders in military veterans: using primary healthcare data. *BMJ Mil Health*. 2022:e002045.

26. Lew HL, Pogoda TK, Baker E, et al. Prevalence of dual sensory impairment and its association with traumatic brain injury and blast exposure in OEF/OIF veterans. *J Head Trauma Rehabil*. 2011;26(6):489−496.

27. Clifford RE, Rogers RA. Impulse noise: theoretical solutions to the quandary of cochlear protection. *Ann Otol Rhinol Laryngol*. 2009;118(6):417−427.

28. Niwa K, Mizutari K, Matsui T, et al. Pathophysiology of the inner ear after blast injury caused by laser-induced shock wave. *Sci Rep*. 2016;6:31754.

29. Kim J, Xia A, Grillet N, Applegate BE, Oghalai JS. Osmotic stabilization prevents cochlear synaptopathy after blast trauma. *Proc Natl Acad Sci USA*. 2018;115(21): E4853−E4860.

30. Cho SI, Gao SS, Xia A, et al. Mechanisms of hearing loss after blast injury to the ear. *PLoS One*. 2013;8(7):e67618.

31. Xiong M, Yang C, Lai H, Wang J. Impulse noise exposure in early adulthood accelerates age-related hearing loss. *Eur Arch Oto-Rhino-Laryngol*. 2014;271(6):1351−1354.

32. Moore BCJ. The effect of exposure to noise during military service on the subsequent progression of hearing loss. *Int J Environ Res Publ Health*. 2021;18(5).

33. Hickman TT, Smalt C, Bobrow J, Quatieri T, Liberman MC. Blast-induced cochlear synaptopathy in chinchillas. *Sci Rep*. 2018;8(1):10740.

34. McBride DI, Williams S. Audiometric notch as a sign of noise induced hearing loss. *Occup Environ Med.* 2001;58(1):46−51.

35. Littlefield PD, Brungart DS. Long-term sensorineural hearing loss in patients with blast-induced tympanic membrane perforations. *Ear Hear.* 2020;41(1):165−172.

36. Ahmed MM, Allard RJ, Esquivel CR. Noise-induced hearing loss treatment: systematic review and meta-analysis. *Mil Med.* 2021;187(5−6):e661−e666.

37. Zhou Y, Zheng G, Zheng H, Zhou R, Zhu X, Zhang Q. Primary observation of early transtympanic steroid injection in patients with delayed treatment of noise-induced hearing loss. *Audiol Neuro Otol.* 2013;18(2):89−94.

38. Hall ED. The neuroprotective pharmacology of methylprednisolone. *J Neurosurg.* 1992; 76(1):13−22.

39. Zhou Y, Zheng H, Shen X, Zhang Q, Yang M. Intratympanic administration of methyl-prednisolone reduces impact of experimental intensive impulse noise trauma on hearing. *Acta Otolaryngol.* 2009;129(6):602−607.

40. Chi FL, Yang MQ, Zhou YD, Wang B. Therapeutic efficacy of topical application of dexamethasone to the round window niche after acoustic trauma caused by intensive impulse noise in Guinea pigs. *J Laryngol Otol.* 2011;125(7):673−685.

41. El-Hennawi DM, El-Deen MH, Abou-Halawa AS, Nadeem HS, Ahmed MR. Efficacy of intratympanic methylprednisolone acetate in treatment of drill-induced sensorineural hearing loss in Guinea pigs. *J Laryngol Otol.* 2005;119(1):2−7.

42. Sendowski I, Abaamrane L, Raffin F, Cros A, Clarencon D. Therapeutic efficacy of intra-cochlear administration of methylprednisolone after acoustic trauma caused by gunshot noise in Guinea pigs. *Hear Res.* 2006;221(1−2):119−127.

43. Chandrasekhar SS, Tsai Do BS, Schwartz SR, et al. Clinical Practice guideline: sudden hearing loss (update). *Otolaryngology-Head Neck Surg (Tokyo).* 2019;161(1_suppl): S1−S45.

44. Duan M, Qiu J, Laurell G, Olofsson A, Counter SA, Borg E. Dose and time-dependent protection of the antioxidant N-L-acetylcysteine against impulse noise trauma. *Hear Res.* 2004;192(1−2):1−9.

45. Kopke R, Bielefeld E, Liu J, et al. Prevention of impulse noise-induced hearing loss with antioxidants. *Acta Otolaryngol.* 2005;125(3):235−243.

46. Bielefeld EC, Kopke RD, Jackson RL, Coleman JK, Liu J, Henderson D. Noise protection with N-acetyl-l-cysteine (NAC) using a variety of noise exposures, NAC doses, and routes of administration. *Acta Otolaryngol.* 2007;127(9):914−919.

47. Ewert DL, Lu J, Li W, Du X, Floyd R, Kopke R. Antioxidant treatment reduces blast-induced cochlear damage and hearing loss. *Hear Res.* 2012;285(1−2):29−39.

48. Xiong M, Lai H, He Q, Wang J. Astragaloside IV attenuates impulse noise-induced trauma in Guinea pig. *Acta Otolaryngol.* 2011;131(8):809−816.

49. Gavriel H, Shulman A, Stracher A, Sohmer H. Leupeptin reduces impulse noise induced hearing loss. *J Occup Med Toxicol.* 2011;6:38.

50. Bielefeld EC, Hangauer D, Henderson D. Protection from impulse noise-induced hearing loss with novel Src-protein tyrosine kinase inhibitors. *Neurosci Res.* 2011;71(4): 348−354.

51. Coleman JK, Littlesunday C, Jackson R, Meyer T. AM-111 protects against permanent hearing loss from impulse noise trauma. *Hear Res.* 2007;226(1−2):70−78.

52. Duan M, Chen Z, Qiu J, et al. Low-dose, long-term caroverine administration attenuates impulse noise-induced hearing loss in the rat. *Acta Otolaryngol.* 2006;126(11): 1140−1147.

53. Abaamrane L, Raffin F, Gal M, Avan P, Sendowski I. Long-term administration of magnesium after acoustic trauma caused by gunshot noise in Guinea pigs. *Hear Res.* 2009; 247(2):137—145.

54. Böttger EC, Schacht J. The mitochondrion: a perpetrator of acquired hearing loss. *Hear Res.* 2013;303:12—19.

55. Henderson D, Bielefeld EC, Harris KC, Hu BH. The role of oxidative stress in noise-induced hearing loss. *Ear Hear.* 2006;27(1):1—19.

56. Lindblad AC, Rosenhall U, Olofsson A, Hagerman B. The efficacy of N-acetylcysteine to protect the human cochlea from subclinical hearing loss caused by impulse noise: a controlled trial. *Noise Health.* 2011;13(55):392—401.

57. Chen SL, Ho CY, Chin SC. Effects of oral N-acetylcysteine combined with oral prednisolone on idiopathic sudden sensorineural hearing loss. *Medicine (Baltim).* 2022; 101(26):e29792.

58. Bai X, Chen S, Xu K, et al. N-acetylcysteine combined with dexamethasone treatment improves sudden sensorineural hearing loss and attenuates hair cell death caused by ROS stress. *Front Cell Dev Biol.* 2021;9:659486.

59. Angeli SI, Abi-Hachem RN, Vivero RJ, Telischi FT, Machado JJ. L-N-Acetylcysteine treatment is associated with improved hearing outcome in sudden idiopathic sensorineural hearing loss. *Acta Otolaryngol.* 2012;132(4):369—376.

60. Wagner EL, Shin JB. Mechanisms of hair cell damage and repair. *Trends Neurosci.* 2019;42(6):414—424.

61. He Y, Cai C, Tang D, Sun S, Li H. Effect of histone deacetylase inhibitors trichostatin A and valproic acid on hair cell regeneration in zebrafish lateral line neuromasts. *Front Cell Neurosci.* 2014;8:382.

62. He Y, Tang D, Cai C, Chai R, Li H. LSD1 is required for hair cell regeneration in zebrafish. *Mol Neurobiol.* 2016;53(4):2421—2434.

63. Ebeid M, Sripal P, Pecka J, Beisel KW, Kwan K, Soukup GA. Transcriptome-wide comparison of the impact of Atoh1 and miR-183 family on pluripotent stem cells and multipotent otic progenitor cells. *PLoS One.* 2017;12(7):e0180855.

64. Li H, Kloosterman W, Fekete DM. MicroRNA-183 family members regulate sensorineural fates in the inner ear. *J Neurosci.* 2010;30(9):3254—3263.

65. Weston MD, Pierce ML, Jensen-Smith HC, et al. MicroRNA-183 family expression in hair cell development and requirement of microRNAs for hair cell maintenance and survival. *Dev Dynam.* 2011;240(4):808—819.

66. Huyghe A, Van den Ackerveken P, Sacheli R, et al. MicroRNA-124 regulates cell specification in the cochlea through modulation of sfrp4/5. *Cell Rep.* 2015;13(1):31—42.

67. Golden EJ, Benito-Gonzalez A, Doetzlhofer A. The RNA-binding protein LIN28B regulates developmental timing in the mammalian cochlea. *Proc Natl Acad Sci U S A.* 2015;112(29):E3864—E3873.

68. Mizutari K, Fujioka M, Hosoya M, et al. Notch inhibition induces cochlear hair cell regeneration and recovery of hearing after acoustic trauma. *Neuron.* 2013;77(1):58—69.

69. Maass JC, Gu R, Basch ML, et al. Changes in the regulation of the Notch signaling pathway are temporally correlated with regenerative failure in the mouse cochlea. *Front Cell Neurosci.* 2015;9:110.

70. Kleinstäuber M, Weise C. Psychosocial variables that predict chronic and disabling tinnitus: a systematic review. *Curr Top Behav Neurosci.* 2021;51:361—380.

71. Inoue C, Shawler E, Jordan CH, Jackson CA. *Veteran and Military Mental Health Issues*. Treasure Island (FL): StatPearls; 2022. StatPearls Publishing Copyright © 2022, StatPearls Publishing LLC.

72. Searchfield GD, Durai M, Linford T. A state-of-the-art review: personalization of tinnitus sound therapy. *Front Psychol*. 2017;8:1599.

73. Figueiredo RR, Langguth B, Mello de Oliveira P, Aparecida de Azevedo A. Tinnitus treatment with memantine. *Otolaryngol Head Neck Surg*. 2008;138(4):492−496.

74. Bing D, Lee SC, Campanelli D, et al. Cochlear NMDA receptors as a therapeutic target of noise-induced tinnitus. *Cell Physiol Biochem*. 2015;35(5):1905−1923.

75. Hall DA, Ray J, Watson J, et al. A balanced randomised placebo controlled blinded phase IIa multi-centre study to investigate the efficacy and safety of AUT00063 versus placebo in subjective tinnitus: the QUIET-1 trial. *Hear Res*. 2019;377:153−166.

76. Marks KL, Martel DT, Wu C, et al. Auditory-somatosensory bimodal stimulation desynchronizes brain circuitry to reduce tinnitus in Guinea pigs and humans. *Sci Transl Med*. 2018;10(422).

77. Markovitz CD, Smith BT, Gloeckner CD, Lim HH. Investigating a new neuromodulation treatment for brain disorders using synchronized activation of multimodal pathways. *Sci Rep*. 2015;5:9462.

78. Hamilton C, D'Arcy S, Pearlmutter BA, Crispino G, Lalor EC, Conlon BJ. An investigation of feasibility and safety of Bi-modal stimulation for the treatment of tinnitus: an open-label pilot study. *Neuromodul Technol Neural Interface*. 2016;19(8):832−837.

79. Conlon B, Langguth B, Hamilton C, et al. Bimodal neuromodulation combining sound and tongue stimulation reduces tinnitus symptoms in a large randomized clinical study. *Sci Transl Med*. 2020;12(564):eabb2830.

80. Kloostra FJJ, Verbist J, Hofman R, Free RH, Arnold R, van Dijk P. A prospective study of the effect of cochlear implantation on tinnitus. *Audiol Neurotol*. 2018;23(6):356−363.

81. Searchfield GD, Sanders PJ, Doborjeh Z, et al. A state-of-art review of digital technologies for the next generation of tinnitus therapeutics. *Front Digit Health*. 2021;3:724370.

82. Scherer MR, Schubert MC. Traumatic brain injury and vestibular pathology as a comorbidity after blast exposure. *Phys Ther*. 2009;89(9):980−992.

83. Hoffer ME, Balaban C, Gottshall K, Balough BJ, Maddox MR, Penta JR. Blast exposure: vestibular consequences and associated characteristics. *Otol Neurotol*. 2010;31(2):232−236.

84. Davies RA, Luxon LM. Dizziness following head injury: a neuro-otological study. *J Neurol*. 1995;242(4):222−230.

85. Bartholomew RA, Lubner RJ, Knoll RM, et al. Labyrinthine concussion: historic otopathologic antecedents of a challenging diagnosis. *Laryngoscope Investig Otolaryngol*. 2020;5(2):267−277.

86. Schuknecht HF, Neff WD, Perlman HB. An experimental study of auditory damage following blows to the head. *Ann Otol Rhinol Laryngol*. 1951;60(2):273−289.

87. Allum JHJ, Scheltinga A, Honegger F. The effect of peripheral vestibular recovery on improvements in vestibulo-ocular reflexes and balance control after acute unilateral peripheral vestibular loss. *Otol Neurotol*. 2017;38(10):e531−e538.

88. Eskridge SL, Macera CA, Galarneau MR, et al. Injuries from combat explosions in Iraq: injury type, location, and severity. *Injury*. 2012;43(10):1678−1682.

89. Littlefield PD, Pinto RL, Burrows HL, Brungart DS. The vestibular effects of repeated low-level blasts. *J Neurotrauma.* 2016;33(1):71–81.
90. Dikmen S, Machamer J, Fann JR, Temkin NR. Rates of symptom reporting following traumatic brain injury. *J Int Neuropsychol Soc.* 2010;16(3):401–411.
91. Cartlidge NE. Post-concussional syndrome. *Scot Med J.* 1978;23(1):103.
92. Lempert T, Olesen J, Furman J, et al. Vestibular migraine: diagnostic criteria. *J Vestib Res.* 2012;22(4):167–172.
93. Bisdorff AR. Management of vestibular migraine. *Ther Adv Neurol Disord.* 2011;4(3): 183–191.
94. Fausti SA, Wilmington DJ, Gallun FJ, Myers PJ, Henry JA. Auditory and vestibular dysfunction associated with blast-related traumatic brain injury. *J Rehabil Res Dev.* 2009;46(6):797–810.
95. Shupak A, Doweck I, Nachtigal D, Spitzer O, Gordon CR. Vestibular and audiometric consequences of blast injury to the ear. *Arch Otolaryngol Head Neck Surg.* 1993; 119(12):1362–1367.
96. McCrary HC, Babajanian E, Patel N, et al. Superior semicircular canal dehiscence syndrome following head trauma: a multi-institutional review. *Laryngoscope.* 2021; 131(11):E2810–e8.
97. Mehlenbacher A, Capehart B, Bass D, Burke JR. Sound induced vertigo: superior canal dehiscence resulting from blast exposure. *Arch Phys Med Rehabil.* 2012;93(4): 723–724.
98. Scherer MR, Burrows H, Pinto R, et al. Evidence of central and peripheral vestibular pathology in blast-related traumatic brain injury. *Otol Neurotol.* 2011;32(4):571–580.
99. Johnson CM, Perez CF, Hoffer ME. The implications of physical injury on otovestibular and cognitive symptomatology following blast exposure. *Otolaryngol Head Neck Surg.* 2014;150(3):437–440.
100. Jiam NT, Murphy OC, Gold DR, et al. Nonvestibular dizziness. *Otolaryngol Clin.* 2021; 54(5):999–1013.

Conductive hearing loss after head injury: diagnosis and management

Sara Holmes, BA [1]**, Keelin Fallon, BA** [1]**,**
Aaron K. Remenschneider, MD, MPH, FACS [1,2]

[1]*Department of Otolaryngology, UMass Memorial Healthcare, UMass Chan Medical School, Worcester, MA, United States;* [2]*Department of Otolaryngology, Massachusetts Eye and Ear Infirmary, Harvard Medical School, Boston, MA, United States*

Introduction

Head injury is a major source of disability and mortality worldwide. The CDC reports that in 2017 there were 224,000 head injury-related hospitalizations in the United States.[1] Unintentional falls accounted for nearly 50% of these hospitalizations, motor vehicle crashes 25%, and strikes by an object, intentional self-harm, and assault accounted for the remaining 25% (CDC, Traumatic Brain Injury). Head injury may result in a variety of mild-to-severe neurologic deficits and can impair an individual's ability to communicate normally. Auditory dysfunction can frequently occur as a consequence of head injury and requires a thorough evaluation to localize the problem and permit appropriate rehabilitation.[2]

Conductive hearing loss is a common type of auditory dysfunction that may occur following head injury. Often overlooked in the initial trauma assessment, head injury patients may present with conductive hearing loss in a delayed fashion.[3] Conductive hearing loss may be transient from fluid or blood in the ear canal or middle ear. High-impact head trauma may result in temporal bone fractures that can damage the external auditory canal or middle ear structures[4] and result in persistent conductive hearing loss. In the absence of temporal bone fractures, a small subset of head injury patients has also been shown to sustain conductive hearing loss.[5] Close follow-up of patients with conductive hearing loss following head trauma is necessary to understand persistent external and middle ear issues and manage hearing loss appropriately.[6]

Evaluation

The severity of head injury typically dictates the location of initial consultation and the resources available for patient evaluation. In cases of severe head trauma, patients may be either incapable or impaired in their ability to participate with clinical history, examination, and audiologic evaluation. The clinician must prioritize patient stabilization, and as such, otologic evaluation may be only rudimentary or may be necessarily delayed. Mild cases of head injury may be primarily evaluated in the oto-laryngologists' clinic if the sole complaint is hearing loss. Evaluation of conductive hearing loss following head trauma typically includes a history, physical exam, and audiometry. In some cases, imaging of the temporal bones is also necessary.

History

If the patient is awake and alert, a complete auditory history and examination should be performed at the bedside or in the outpatient clinic. Important aspects of the history include the nature and timing of the head injury, whether the trauma was blunt or penetrating and any direct injury to the ear or temporal bone. Complaints of hearing loss, ear pain, otorrhea, tinnitus, imbalance, nausea, dizziness, vertigo, facial weakness, rhinorrhea, and other neurologic changes should be assessed. In patients with hearing loss, the time course and any transience or gradual improvement should be documented.

Physical examination

In settings of severe head trauma, the priority must be patient stabilization, including airway management, and assessment of breathing, hemorrhage, neurological status, and additional exposures.[7] Patients with significant injury sustained during head trauma may have spinal precautions in place, and the spine should be evaluated and stabilized prior to manipulation of the head.[8] When the patient is deemed hemo-dynamically stable, an otologic examination can occur. Performed by an otolaryn-gologist, the evaluation should include a focused head and neck exam including detailed otomicroscopic exam, bedside hearing evaluations, and subsequent referral for additional testing, when appropriate.

For patients with severe head trauma, the initial otologic exam may occur at the bedside in the emergency department or intensive care unit, and patients may have limited ability to participate. In settings of less severe head trauma, the otologic exam may occur in an otolaryngologists' clinic, with the patient typically able to participate more actively.

A full head and neck examination should be performed to assess for sequelae of head injury. After ensuring the patient is stable, a detailed otologic exam is completed. Examination begins with a thorough inspection of the external auricle looking for any signs of trauma, such as swelling, lacerations, erythema, and discharge from the external auditory canal. If otorrhea is present, the onset, quality, color, and volume should be documented (Fig. 6.1). A cerebral spinal fluid (CSF) leak may mix with blood from the middle ear or ear canal; thus, a large persistent volume leak from the ear should raise suspicion for a CSF leak. A sample should be collected to check for the presence of beta-2 transferrin. Given the typical long time frame for test results to return, a "'halo sign" may be assessed at the bedside.

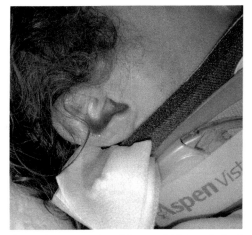

FIGURE 6.1 Cerebrospinal fluid otorrhea in a 34-year-old female following blunt head trauma.

Here, a drop of fluid may be placed on tissue paper and examined for signs of a ring of clear fluid around a drop of blood, indicating the presence of CSF.[9]

Every effort should be made to clear the external auditory canal to permit an examination of the tympanic membrane (TM). If the TM is intact, pneumatic otoscopy may be used to determine TM mobility. Immobility of TM on pneumatic otoscopy, air/fluid levels, and dullness of landmarks may suggest middle ear effusion or hemotympanum. Hemotympanum (and a conductive hearing loss) may be the only sign the patient has a temporal bone fracture and should prompt a high-resolution CT scan of the temporal bones (Fig. 6.2). If there is a visible perforation in the TM, assessment of size, location and any epithelial debris within the middle ear should be noted. Relative location of the ossicular chain should also be documented.

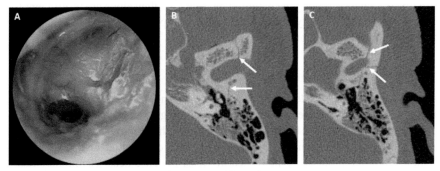

FIGURE 6.2 Hemotympanum following temporal bone fracture.

(A) Endoscopic view showing blood behind the tympanic membrane indicative of hemotympanum. (B, C) Axial images from high-resolution computed tomography showing transverse and oblique fractures of the left temporal bone in a 53-year-old man.

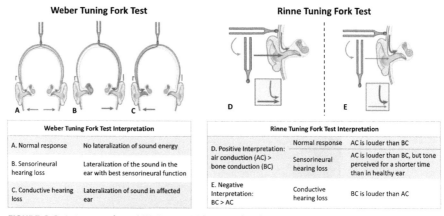

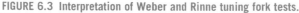

Weber Tuning Fork Test Interpretation	
A. Normal response	No lateralization of sound energy
B. Sensorineural hearing loss	Lateralization of the sound in the ear with best sensorineural function
C. Conductive hearing loss	Lateralization of sound in affected ear

Rinne Tuning Fork Test Interpretation		
	Normal response	AC is louder than BC
D. Positive Interpretation: air conduction (AC) > bone conduction (BC)	Sensorineural hearing loss	AC is louder than BC, but tone perceived for a shorter time than in healthy ear
E. Negative Interpretation: BC > AC	Conductive hearing loss	BC is louder than AC

FIGURE 6.3 Interpretation of Weber and Rinne tuning fork tests.

Weber and Rinne tests can help distinguish between types of hearing loss. Air conduction testing measures the integrity of the entire hearing apparatus from external ear to auditory cortex. Bone conduction testing measures the integrity of the sensorineural structures (cochlear, cochlear nerve, brainstem nuclei, and relays to the auditory cortex).

Hearing evaluation including tuning fork tests and bedside speech reception thresholds should be performed to determine the type and severity of hearing loss. The Weber and Rinne tests can be performed as an early assessment of hearing loss (Fig. 6.3). Both tests can be performed at the bedside typically with a 512-Hz tuning fork. A Weber test is suggestive of conductive hearing loss if the fork is heard loudest in the affected ear. A negative Rinne test is suggestive of a conductive hearing loss of at least 30 dB at 512 Hz if bone conduction is heard louder than air conduction. Interpretation of full Weber and Rinne test results may be found in Fig. 6.3. Whispered word tests can also screen for a drop in speech intelligibility, which may suggest a sensorineural hearing loss. While tuning fork and whispered word tests can be a first step in determining the nature of hearing loss, they alone are insufficient for diagnosis of hearing loss type and severity. Ideally, patients should be referred for behavioral pure tone audiometry.

Audiological evaluation

Threshold audiogram—Alert, responsive patients should be tested via pure tone audiometry to further assess for conductive hearing loss. Ideally, testing is performed in a sound-treated booth, although bedside threshold and speech testing is also possible in some centers. Both air and bone conduction testing should be completed to determine the type of hearing loss. Because head trauma may result in conductive hearing loss from a variety of sources, the degree and frequency dependence of the air—bone gap (ABG) may differ based on hearing loss etiology. For example, a small TM perforation may result in a small ABG, while ossicular discontinuity with an intact TM may result in a maximal conductive hearing loss.

In most cases, speech discrimination will not be affected by pure conductive pathology, and when speech is presented at an appropriate loudness for the patient's hearing loss, discrimination should be excellent. Fig. 6.4 outlines an example audiogram showing an air/bone gap from a 37-year-old patient with left-sided ossicular chain discontinuity following temporal bone fracture. Table 6.1 shows typical hearing loss severity and frequency dependence by the type of conductive lesion.

Tympanometry—Tympanometry may be performed to measure middle ear immittance, providing a quantitative measure of middle ear compliance that is more reliable than pneumatic otoscopy. The tympanometric waveform is typically obtained at 226 Hz and provides information about how sound energy enters the middle ear as a function of ear canal pressure. Head trauma may lead to conductive pathology that can be detected and differentiated via tympanometry. A normal, type A tympanogram indicates an intact TM and ossicular chain with middle ear pressure that is similar to ambient pressure (Fig. 6.5A). An ossicular discontinuity will result in a hypercompliant TM with a "sharp peak" as is seen in Fig. 6.5B. Middle ear fluid, such as hemotympanum, will result in a flat waveform with a normal ear canal volume, whereas a flat waveform with elevated ear canal volume is indicative of a TM perforation (Fig. 6.5C and D).

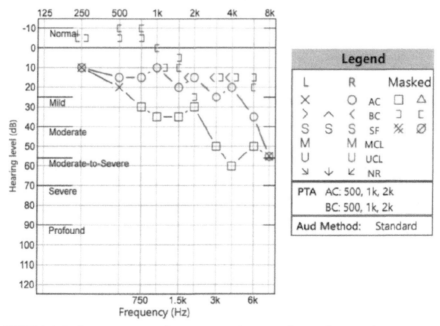

FIGURE 6.4 Audiogram demonstrating posttraumatic conductive hearing loss.

A 37-year-old man sustained bilateral temporal bone fractures after a motor vehicle accident. This resulted in a left-sided mild-to-moderate conductive hearing loss ranging from 15 to 45 dB due to a partial ossicular chain discontinuity. On the right, a small air bone gap was resolved with observation.

Table 6.1 Traumatic lesions of the conductive hearing pathway and expected air—bone gap.

Classification	Expected loss
Perforation of TM	10—40 dB, worse at low frequency and proportional to size of perforation[10,11]
Perforation of TM with ossicular interruption	>35 dB, greater losses imply discontinuity
Intact TM with partial (fibrous) ossicular interruption	30—40 dB, worse at high frequencies, primarily above 1 kHz (Farahmand et al. 2016)
Hemotympanum	10—30 dB
Ossicular interruption with intact TM	55—60 dB

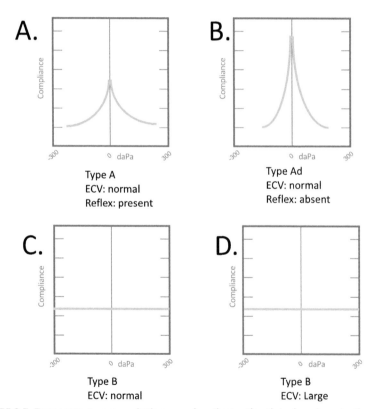

FIGURE 6.5 Tympanometry can assist in narrowing diagnostic etiologies of conductive hearing loss after head trauma.

Examples of common pathology and corresponding tympanometric findings shown. (A) Normal middle ear with present acoustic reflexes. (B) Hypercompliant middle ear: for example, ossicular discontinuity, with absent acoustic reflexes. (C) Flat tympanogram with normal ear canal volume: for example, middle ear effusion or hemotympanum. (D) Flat tympanogram with enlarged ear canal volume: for example, TM perforation (*ECV*, ear canal volume).

Otoacoustic emissions testing and auditory brainstem —Otoacoustic emissions (OAE) testing and auditory brainstem response (ABR) are objective audiometric tests that can be performed on patients who cannot undergo conventional audiometry, as neither test requires recording a patient's subjective response to sound.[12] Otoacoustic emissions are low-amplitude sound waves produced by the cochlea, transmitted across the middle ear to the external ear where they can be recorded.[13] A healthy cochlea produces OAEs, and both conductive and sensorineural hearing loss can affect OAEs.[12] Auditory brainstem response testing consists of an electrical response to an auditory stimuli to assess the auditory pathway from the ear through the brainstem to the auditory cortex.[14] ABR testing can distinguish between conductive and sensorineural hearing loss if bone conduction stimulation is used[15]; however, measurement of conductive losses with ABR is limited in frequency resolution, and severity and must be coupled with behavioral audiometry whenever possible.[12]

Imaging

Temporal bone imaging is frequently necessary in the evaluation of conductive hearing loss associated with head injury. Imaging allows for the evaluation of trauma to the temporal bone and soft tissues of the entire auditory pathway. Imaging can be performed with magnetic resonance imaging (MRI) or computed tomography (CT). Advantages to MRI include the avoidance of radiation exposure and sensitivity to soft tissue as well as central auditory abnormalities, while CT allows for precise spatial resolution of bony anatomy of the external, middle, and inner ear.

High-resolution computed tomography without contrast, including fine cuts in both the coronal and axial planes (0.6 mm), should be obtained in patients who are found to have obvious head, outer/middle ear trauma, peripheral nerve dysfunction, hemotympanum, periorbital or retroauricular hematoma, otorrhea or rhinorrhea containing CSF, or new-onset posttraumatic vestibular symptoms.[16] Fractures of the temporal bone are associated with a high incidence of conductive hearing loss in the acute phase due to blood within the external auditory canal or middle ear (hemotympanum). Persistent conductive hearing loss after temporal bone fracture should be evaluated radiographically to look for ear canal collapse or ossicular chain disruption. The radiologist and practitioner must work closely together to assess for subtle findings associated with posttraumatic conductive hearing loss.[17] If patients are found to have conductive hearing loss that does not improve after resolution of hemotympanum, repeat imaging may be indicated. See Fig. 6.6 for examples of ear trauma viewed on high-resolution CT.

Management

Management of conductive hearing loss associated with head injury depends on the source of conductive pathology. If the source of conductive hearing loss is transient, for example, from hemotympanum or an ear canal laceration, simple observation, or

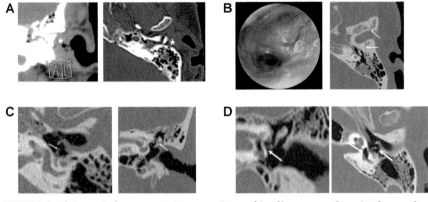

FIGURE 6.6 High-resolution computed tomography can identify sources of conductive or mixed hearing loss.

(A) Left ear canal collapse due to tympanic bone fracture in a 45-year-old man in coronal (*left*) and axial (*right*) view. The collapsed ear canal is noted with a star. (B) Endoscopic view showing blood behind the tympanic membrane indicative of hemotympanum in a 53-yearold man. Axial image from HR-CT showing responsible transverse left temporal bone fracture. (C) *Left* displaced incus at both incudostapedial (*left*) and incudomalleolar joints (*right*) due to temporal bone fracture in a 48-year-old man. (D) Coronal (*left*) and axial (*right*) images of a subluxed stapes and air in the vestibule of a 91-year-old woman caused by insertion of a foreign body (*Q*-tip) into the ear.

treatment with ototopical drops, is sufficient. However, persistent conductive hearing loss may require management with amplification or surgery. While conductive hearing loss is frequently seen following temporal bone fracture, a fracture is not necessary for many conductive lesions in head injury as will be discussed in the following. It is also important to note that immediately following injury, more than one lesion affecting the conductive pathway is frequently present in the same patient. Repeat examination and audiometry after a duration of 6—8 weeks is important to ensure resolution or to identify persistent lesions that need further evaluation and management.

External ear

Lesions of auricle

Sound localization begins when the sound reaches the visible portion of the auricle. Localization of sound is described in terms of 3-D position, which includes the horizontal angle, vertical angle, distance, and velocity of the sound. When trauma to the external ear occurs, auricular hematomas (Fig. 6.7) may form. Avulsed or contused auricles may result in abnormal sound localization, and large hematomas may even occlude the EAC, resulting in conductive hearing loss. After a diagnosis of hematoma is made, treatment may occur at the bedside or in the operating room depending on the severity and potential risks to the patient. Incision and drainage of the

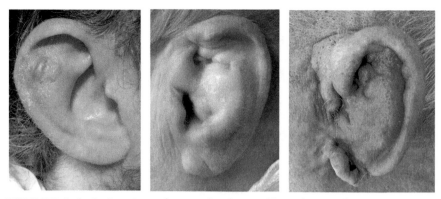

FIGURE 6.7 Auricular hematomas in several patients, with varying severity.

Mild hematomas (left) may only impact part of the auricle, while more severe cases can completely occlude the external ear canal and result in conductive hearing loss. (middle) If hematomas are not drained, they can lead to severe auricular deformity (cauliflower ear) with meatal collapse and associated conductive hearing loss (right).

hematoma is recommended to prevent cartilage remodeling and subsequent deformity of the auricle known colloquially as cauliflower ear.

Disorders of the external auditory canal

Disorders such as ear canal collapse, cerumen impaction, and ear canal hematoma may occur with head trauma, thereby causing disruption of sound passing through the external auditory canal. In severe cases of temporal bone fractures involving the tympanic bone, the anterior ear canal may be posteriorly displaced, thereby collapsing the canal (Fig. 6.6A). Stenting of the canal in the acute period is critical to ensure a displaced tympanic bone fracture does not result in long-term ear canal stenosis. In cases where the ear canal heals in an obliterated or collapsed form, surgical reopening via canaloplasty may be necessary to prevent keratosis obdurans and persistent conductive hearing loss.

Middle ear

Tympanic membrane perforation

Slap injury or blunt trauma to the head may cause a transient sharp elevation in ear canal pressure, leading to TM perforation (Fig. 6.8). Conductive hearing loss occurs with TM perforation, and the degree of conductive hearing loss depends upon the size but not the location of the perforation.[11] Small perforations cause the least amount of conductive hearing loss, while near-total perforations have a much higher chance of causing significant hearing loss.[10] Traumatic TM perforations heal spontaneously up to 94% of the time.[18] The vast majority of traumatic perforations, which will heal spontaneously, will do so by 3 months following the injury, after which point the likelihood of healing significantly declines.[19] Thus, if a perforation

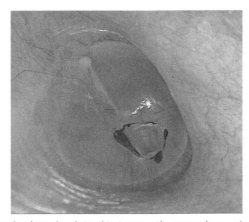

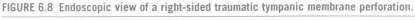

FIGURE 6.8 Endoscopic view of a right-sided traumatic tympanic membrane perforation.
Note the dried blood at the perforation site and the thickened edge of the perforation.

is present 3 months after a traumatic injury, it is reasonable to proceed with myringoplasty or tympanoplasty. If the patient does not report a history of chronic eustachian tube dysfunction or otorrhea, a simple fascia or perichondrium underlay technique will have a high chance of successfully closing the perforation. If no ossicular abnormalities are present, repair of a traumatic TM perforation will correct low- and mid-frequency conductive hearing losses effectively.[20]

Hemotympanum

If a basal skull fracture involving the temporal bone is present, hemotympanum may occur (Fig. 6.2A). Blood will increase the middle ear impedance and result in a conductive hearing loss from 10 to 30 dB. Conductive hearing losses larger than 30 dB with hemotympanum should raise the suspicion of a second source of conductive pathology, such as ossicular dislocation. Hemotympanum should be observed as most will clear through the Eustachian tube over several weeks. Patient should be seen 6−8 weeks after the injury for repeat examination and audiometry once the effusion has cleared. Intervention for isolated hemotympanum is typically not necessary.

Ossicular dislocation/fixation

Blunt trauma to the head may lead to ossicular dislocation within the middle ear (Fig. 6.9). A conductive hearing loss may range from mild to a maximal conductive hearing loss of up to 60 dB depending upon the degree of dislocation and the status of the TM (Table 6.1). In longitudinal temporal bone fractures, the incudomalleolar joint is prone to separate. This may result in a transient conductive hearing loss that improves with time as joint fibrosis occurs and sound transmission is reestablished. When ossicular dislocation is identified, it is prudent to wait 6−8 weeks to reevaluate the hearing to determine if the hearing loss will resolve. If an air−bone gap of at least 25 dB is present, the patient may be a candidate for amplification or

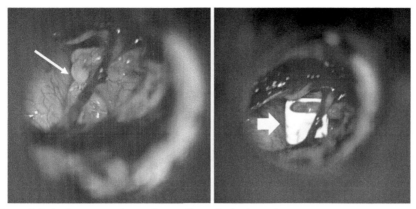

FIGURE 6.9 Ossiculoplasty for ossicular discontinuity following head trauma after a 32-year-old man fell from a ladder.

Note the air space between the lenticular process of the incus and the stapes capitulum (*white arrow*). An applebaum prosthesis is used to reconnect the incudostapedial joint (*white arrow head*).

exploratory tympanotomy with ossiculoplasty. Endoscopic ossiculoplasty for traumatic ossicular dislocation can be an ideal method to visualize the full range of ossicular dislocation and effectively reconstruct the middle ear sound conductive mechanism.

Traumatic cholesteatoma

Traumatic fractures of the ear canal and traumatic TM perforation may permit keratinizing epithelium to enter the mastoid air cells or the middle ear cleft. A traumatic cholesteatoma may consequently arise and lead to a conductive hearing loss through ear canal obstruction or ossicular erosion. For example, blast injury resulting in TM perforation has been noted to result in middle ear cholesteatoma from avulsed edges of the ruptured TM.[21] Evaluation of blast-induced TM perforations should include assessment for infolded perforation edges, which may require exteriorization. Typically, the time course for development of traumatic cholesteatoma is quite long, indicating a need to closely follow patients with significant temporal bone trauma for late sequela of their injury (Fig. 6.10). The management of traumatic cholesteatoma is a function of the temporal bone location affected and extent of disease. Canaloplasty, tympanoplasty, or tympanomastoidectomy may be necessary to remove the pathologic keratin and reestablish a barrier between the middle ear/mastoid and the keratin-lined external auditory canal.

Inner ear

Superior semicircular canal dehiscence

Superior semicircular canal dehiscence is an inner ear condition where the otic capsule over the superior canal neuroepithelium is dehiscent. Theories about its etiology range from a congenital lack of bone to progressive erosion of bone due to

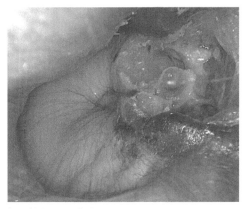

FIGURE 6.10 Traumatic middle ear cholesteatoma.

A traumatic perforation of tympanic membrane resulted in epithelial migration onto the medial surface of the tympanic membrane and obliteration of the middle ear cleft with cholesteatoma.

increased intracranial pressure. Superior canal dehiscence syndrome (SSCDS) has been well described to occur following head injury as symptoms may become "unmasked," a phenomenon noted to occur even following mild head trauma.[22] Blast-related head trauma caused by the Boston marathon bombings was noted to result in unmasking of SSCD in several patients.[21] Conductive hearing loss occurs in superior canal dehiscence because an altered inner ear impedance permits sound energy to travel through the vestibular system as compared with solely along the cochlear duct. Other third window symptoms, such as Tullio's phenomenon, autophony, pulsatile tinnitus, and hyperacusis, may also occur following head trauma in patients with preexisting superior canal dehiscence. Management options include observation, amplification, and surgery via canal resurfacing or plugging. Surgical management of superior canal dehiscence typically improves the attributed air–bone gap (Fig. 6.11).

Perilymphatic fistula

Head trauma, and more specifically, penetrating ear trauma, may result in trauma to the inner ear resulting in a perilymphatic fistula. Patients typically manifest a mixed hearing loss with acute vertigo. Imaging may identify pneumolabyrinth from a subluxed stapes or ruptured oval or round window. While most patients will respond to steroids and bedrest, some patients will experience continued symptoms and require surgical exploration. A subluxed stapes or ruptured oval or round window that does not spontaneously heal will benefit from soft tissue reinforcement (Figs. 6.6D and 6.12). Hearing does not typically return to baseline, but the conductive component to the hearing loss and the vestibular symptoms typically improve.

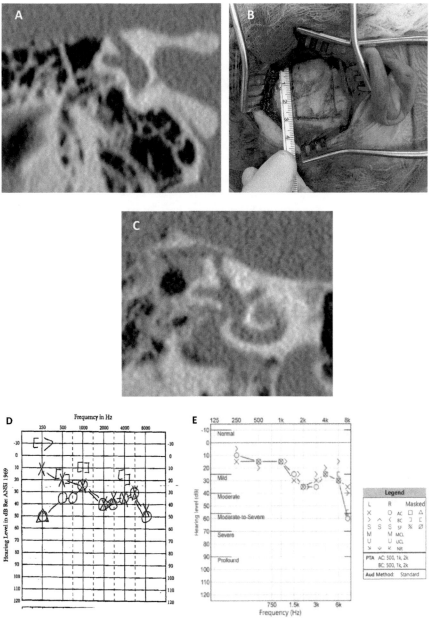

FIGURE 6.11 **Superior canal dehiscence.**

(A) Coronal CT view shows superior semicircular canal dehiscence in the right ear of a 56-year-old woman who developed a conductive hearing loss after mild head trauma. (B) A 3 × 2 cm bone flap created during superior canal dehiscence repair via a middle cranial fossa approach. Bone wax was used to plug the defect, and a split calvarial bone graft was used to reconstruct the middle fossa floor over the defect. (C) Postoperative coronal CT showing calvarial bone graft covering superior semicircular canal. (D) Preoperative audiogram for the patient demonstrates right-sided low-frequency conductive hearing loss. (E) Postoperative audiogram shows complete resolution of conductive hearing loss.

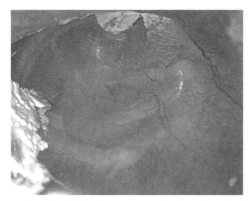

FIGURE 6.12 **Postoperative photo following tympanoplasty and repair of perilymphatic fistula.**

Patient was a 94-year-old woman who sustained a penetrating ear injury resulting in a subluxed stapes and pneumolabyrinth (see Fig. 6.6D).

Amplification of conductive hearing loss

Conductive hearing loss that persists for 3 months after head injury will likely not resolve with additional watchful waiting. Affected patients may benefit from amplification using an air or bone conducted hearing aid.

Traditional amplification

Traditional hearing aids including in-the-canal, in-the-ear, and behind-the-ear models may be considered for conductive hearing loss after head trauma. In cases of mixed hearing loss where the bone conduction thresholds are not in the normal range, a hearing aid should be considered in lieu of surgical correction of the air—bone gap. If, in such a scenario, a patient would still require a hearing aid after a conductive component of a mixed hearing loss was corrected, upfront amplication and avoidance of surgery is recommended. Consultation with an audiologist will provide the patient with a full range of hearing aid options.

Bone anchored hearing aids

Bone conduction hearing devices transfer sound by bone vibration directly to the cochlea, bypassing the outer and middle ear. With traumatic injury to the head, these may be especially useful when a hearing aid cannot be worn due to ongoing otorrhea, or a collapsed or obliterated external auditory canal. There are a variety of devices available, which can be broadly differentiated into percutaneous devices, where an abutment extends through the scalp tissue to directly connect to the external processor, and transcutaneous devices, where the processor sits external to the skin to stimulate the calvarium or osseointegrated implant through the skin. Decisions about which device is most appropriate are made by the patient, provider, and audiology team and must account for patient factors, such as the ability to maintain hygiene of a percutaneous device and the potential need for future MRI scans. Modern bone conduction hearing aids have low rates of complications and high rates of satisfaction.[23]

Conclusion

Conductive hearing loss can frequently occur as a result of traumatic head injury. A history and careful otomicroscopic exam along with audiometric testing can help evaluate hearing loss pathology. Imaging, including high-resolution CT, can help differentiate the source (or sources) of conductive pathology at the ear canal, middle, and inner ear level. Management of conductive hearing loss after trauma depends on the source and severity of conductive pathology. If the source of conductive hearing loss is transient, simple observation with repeat audiometry may be sufficient to confirm the return of normal hearing. Persistent mild conductive hearing loss may benefit from amplification. Moderate and severe conductive hearing losses may be successfully managed with middle ear surgery. In the absence of coincident Eustachian tube dysfunction, hearing improvement after middle ear surgery for traumatic conductive hearing loss can be excellent and durable.

References

1. Traumatic Brain Injury|Traumatic brain injury|CDC injury centereditor. *Cent Dis Control Prev*; 2021. https://www.cdc.gov/traumatic-braininjury/index.html. Accessed November 4, 2021.
2. Munjal SK, Panda NK, Pathak A. Audiological deficits after closed head injury. *J Trauma*. January 2010;68(1):13−18.
3. Kaul P, Manhas M, Bhagat A, et al. Otological assessment in head injury patients: a prospective study and review of literature. *Indian J Otolaryngol Head Neck Surg*. 2021; 74(1):658−667.
4. Burchhardt DM, David RJ, Eckert R, Robinette NL, Carron MA, Zuliani GF. Trauma patterns, symptoms, and complications associated with external auditory canal fractures: Burchhardt et al. *Laryngoscope*. 2015;125:1579−1582.
5. Chen JX, Lindeborg M, Herman SD, et al. Systematic review of hearing loss after traumatic brain injury without associated temporal bone fracture. *Am J Otolaryngol*. 2018 May−Jun;39(3):338−344.
6. Podoshin L, Fradis M. Hearing loss after head injury. *Arch Otolaryngol*. 1975;101(1): 15−18.
7. Kostiuk M, Burns B. Trauma assessment, 2022 May 4. In: *StatPearls [Internet]*. Treasure Island (FL): StatPearls Publishing; January 2022.
8. Van Hoecke H, Calus L, Dhooge I. Middle ear damages. *B-ENT*. 2016;Suppl 26(1): 173−183.
9. Sunder R, Tyler K. Basal skull fracture and the halo sign. *CMAJ (Can Med Assoc J)*. March 2013;185(5):416.

10. Mehta RP, Rosowski JJ, Voss SE, O'Neil E, Merchant SN. Determinants of hearing loss in perforations of the tympanic membrane. *Otol Neurotol*. February 2006;27(2): 136−143.

11. Voss SE, Rosowski JJ, Merchant SN, Peake WT. Middle-ear function with tympanic-membrane perforations. II. A simple model. *J Acoust Soc Am*. September 2001;110(3 Pt 1):1445−1452.

12. Young A, Cornejo J, Spinner A. Auditory brainstem response [Updated 2022 Feb 16]. In: *StatPearls [Internet]*. Treasure Island (FL): StatPearls Publishing; January 2022.

13. Richardson MP, Williamson TJ, Lenton SW, Tarlow MJ, Rudd PT. Otoacoustic emissions as a screening test for hearing impairment in children. *Arch Dis Child*. April 1995;72(4):294−297.

14. Kanji A, Khoza-Shangase K, Moroe N. Newborn hearing screening protocols and their outcomes: a systematic review. *Int J Pediatr Otorhinolaryngol*. December 2018;115: 104−109.

15. Bargen GA. Chirp-evoked auditory brainstem response in children: a review. *Am J Audiol*. December 2015;24(4):573−583.

16. Aguilar 3rd EA, Yeakley JW, Ghorayeb BY, et al. High resolution CT scan of temporal bone fractures: association of facial nerve paralysis with temporal bone fractures. *Head Neck Surg*. 1987;9:162.

17. Subramanian M, Chawla A, Chokkappan K, Lim T, Shenoy JN, Chin Guan Peh W. High-resolution computed tomography imaging in conductive hearing loss: what to look for? *Curr Probl Diagn Radiol*. 2018 Mar−Apr;47(2):119−124.

18. Lindeman P, Edström S, Granström G, et al. Acute traumatic tympanic membrane perforations: cover or observe? *Arch Otolaryngol Head Neck Surg*. 1987;113(12): 1285−1287.

19. Kronenberg J, Ben-Shoshan J, Wolf M. Perforated tympanic membrane after blast injury. *Am J Otol*. January 1993;14(1):92−94.

20. Polanik MD, Remenschneider AK. Medialized total ossicular replacement prosthesis. *OTO Open*. April 16, 2020;4(2), 2473974X20916432.

21. Remenschneider AK, Lookabaugh S, Aliphas A, et al. Otologic outcomes after blast injury: the Boston Marathon experience. *Otol Neurotol*. December 2014;35(10): 1825−1834.

22. McCrary HC, Babajanian E, Patel N, et al. Superior semicircular canal dehiscence syndrome following head trauma: a multi-institutional review. *Laryngoscope*. November 2021;131(11):E2810−E2818.

23. Kiringoda R, Lustig LR. A meta-analysis of the complications associated with osseointegrated hearing aids. *Otol Neurotol*. July 2013;34(5):790−794.

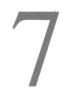

Medical and surgical management of temporal bone fractures

Matthew J. Wu, MD [1,2], **Elliott D. Kozin, MD** [1,3]

[1]*Department of Otolaryngology, Massachusetts Eye and Ear, Boston, MA, United States;*
[2]*Department of Otolaryngology-Head and Neck Surgery, Washington University School of Medicine in St Louis, St Louis, MO, United States;* [3]*Department of Otolaryngology, Harvard Medical School, Boston, MA, United States*

Introduction

Temporal bone fractures (TBFs) present complex diagnostic and management challenges. Due to the large amount of force required to fracture the temporal bone, several other injuries may also be present. The severity and number injuries may result in incomplete or evaluation of the temporal bone, which may delay diagnosis and proper follow-up care. The management of TBF overall focuses on restoring functional deficits and reducing regional and intracranial complications due to injury to structures within the TB. This chapter will provide an overview of the diagnosis and medical and surgical management of TBF.

Diagnosis

History

In the conscious patient, hearing loss is often the most immediately reported symptom following head and temporal bone injury.[1] Tinnitus may also be present and does not alter prognosis. Vestibular symptoms such as imbalance and dizziness often are exacerbated following ambulation. Symptoms of facial weakness, paralysis, and asymmetry suggest facial nerve injury, which warrant early surgical intervention.[2] Determining the temporality and onset of facial symptoms is critical as this will help guide treatment planning.[2,3]

In the unconscious patient, eliciting a detailed history is not possible and therefore relies on obtaining information from individuals who may have arrived with the patient and may help characterize the mechanism of injury. The nature and etiology of TBF may help dictate the urgency of interventions; TBF from penetrating trauma due to gunshot wounds may cause neurologic and vascular injury requiring more immediate attention than TBF from blunt trauma, such as motor vehicle accidents.

Otologic and Lateral Skull Base Trauma. https://doi.org/10.1016/B978-0-323-87482-3.00009-0

Physical examination and evaluation

Initial survey

Patients with suspected temporal bone trauma will be evaluated by the trauma team and assessed for life-threatening issues often before a complete temporal bone examination takes place. This consists of a full-body trauma assessment, including securing an airway, controlling hemorrhage and maintaining circulation, and examining neurologic status. The cervical spine should also be evaluated and stabilized.

Isolated TBFs are rare, which necessitates evaluation of the entire facial skeleton. Facial nerve function should be evaluated as soon as possible, particularly before muscle relaxants are administered, as this will affect examination accuracy and lose valuable prognostic information. An otologic exam should then be performed systematically, which focuses on the external and middle ear.

Otologic exam

The auricles and soft tissue are first inspected for exposed cartilage, hematomas, and lacerations. Hematomas should be incised and drained, and pressure bolsters are sutured to prevent "cauliflower ear" or auricular chondropathy.[4] Lacerations are cleaned and closed. Retroauricular hematoma, also known as the "Battle sign," may be present over the mastoid prominences, which is an arch-shaped bruising behind the auricle. This may point to a basilar skull fracture.

Next, the ear canal is inspected. Irrigation should not be used to remove cerumen or blood to avoid inadvertently introducing pathogens.[5] The presence of brain herniation, fracture of the roof of the external auditory canal, middle ear effusions (e.g., hemotympanum), scutum fracture, and color of otorrhea should be noted.[6] Otorrhea may be bloody or clear, which suggests a cerebrospinal fluid (CSF) leak.[6]

The tympanic membrane should also be assessed for perforations. Typically, traumatic tympanic membrane perforations heal spontaneously, and no immediate intervention is needed. Pneumatic otoscopy should be used judiciously and not be used in the early period following injury as this may introduce air or bacteria into the intracranial space or inner ear via a CSF fistula or otic capsule disrupting fracture.

An operating microscope may be used following stabilization to further evaluate the ear canal, tympanic membrane, or middle ear and may be required to remove a foreign body, if present. Packing of the ear canal is not generally initially needed unless significant hemorrhage is present. If profuse hemorrhage is present, management via balloon occlusion or carotid ligation may be used.

Hearing assessment

An early bedside evaluation with a 512-Hertz tuning fork allows for documenting baseline hearing function and potential hearing loss. The Weber test is performed by placing the base of a struck tuning fork on the forehead, nose, or teeth. The patient is then asked if the sound is louder on either side. Typically, a patient with unilateral sensorineural hearing loss (SNHL) will lateralize sound toward the unaffected side, whereas a patient with unilateral conductive hearing loss (CHL) will lateralize sound toward the affected side. There is no sound lateralization in a normal test.

The Rinne test is a follow-up test performed for each side by placing the base of a struck tuning fork on the mastoid and then held near the meatus. The patient is then asked if the tuning fork is louder near the meatus (evaluating air conduction) or when applied to the mastoid (evaluating bone conduction). A patient with a moderate CHL will report louder bone conduction than air conduction on the affected side. A patient with normal hearing will report louder air conduction than bone conduction (i.e., considered to be a positive Rinne) but does not exclude sensorineural hearing loss in the tested ear.

Combined results from the Weber and Rinne tests will help characterize the underlying nature of hearing loss. A patient may have CHL if the Weber test lateralizes to the affected ear and a negative Rinne is present. Patients with SNHL may have variable tuning fork findings. A Weber test that is louder on the affected side suggests SNHL and the Rinne test will generally be positive, unless if there is significant hearing loss. Audiograms are generally not obtained until the patient's condition is stabilized, unless if urgent complications such as CSF leak or facial paralysis are noted, which guides treatment approach in cases with residual hearing.

Vestibular assessment

Patients may report dizziness or imbalance following temporal bone trauma due to inner ear injury or neurologic injury. In addition to a detailed neurological evaluation, bedside vestibular testing should be performed. Patients who present in the setting of trauma should have cervical spine injuries ruled out before undergoing vestibular testing.

During the physical exam, the presence and type of nystagmus should be noted. Central causes of vertigo can present with purely vertical, horizontal, torsional, or direction-changing nystagmus.[7] Peripheral causes of vertigo may present with horizontal and/or torsional nystagmus.[7] Unlike central vertigo, nystagmus associated with peripheral vertigo is inhibited by eye fixation and is fatigable.[7] Peripheral vertigo is also generally more severe. The Dix-Hallpike maneuver can be used to assess for benign paroxysmal positional vertigo (BPPV), a common etiology of vertigo following traumatic brain injury, which will reveal transient torsional nystagmus.[7,8]

In most cases, posttraumatic vertigo will resolve spontaneously.[9] If vertigo persists, additional testing can be performed in the outpatient setting. The fistula test checks for abnormal communication between the middle and inner ear. Using a pneumatic otoscope, positive and negative pressure is applied in the ear canal. Presence of vertigo and nystagmus suggests evidence of a perilymphatic fistula.[10] Importantly, this test should never be performed if there is evidence of middle ear infection or CSF fistula, or in the acute setting to prevent introduction of air or infection in the inner ear.

Facial nerve

The complex anatomy of the facial nerve increases risk of injury following TBF. Notable anatomical features include tethering of the nerve at various points, such as the perigeniculate region and extremely narrow portions of the canal at the meatal foramen, which may lead to damage of the facial nerve via shearing, compression, and disruption.[11] Trauma leading to otic capsule or transverse TBF also increases risk of facial nerve injury due to the perpendicular direction of the fracture relative to the facial nerve.[11]

Evaluating facial nerve function

Asymmetrical facial movement in the setting of temporal bone trauma is likely due to facial nerve injury. Generally, more diffuse hemifacial weakness will be a result of injury to the intratemporal segments of the facial nerve compared with extratemporal segments. Patient should be instructed to perform several movements with their face, and asymmetries between sides should be noted: elevate their eyebrows to wrinkle their forehead, close their eyes tightly, smile, and puff out their cheeks. In patients who are unable to voluntarily complete these movements (e.g., altered mental status), a painful stimulus (e.g., sternal rub) may be used to assess facial movements. Significant edema may give the appearance of decreased facial function. It is important to note that a high degree of expression on the unaffected side may cause movement on the affected side near the midline. Physically limiting movement by pressing on the unaffected side and reassessing for movement on the suspected affected side can help ascertain if injury has occurred.

Characterizing facial nerve paralysis is important to determine future prognosis and treatment decision-making. Several scales for recording facial nerve function are available.[12,13] Regardless of which scale is used, it is important to determine if there is weakness (paresis) or no movement (paralysis) of the facial nerve.[13] The House—Brackmann (HB) 6-point scale is the most commonly used scale (Table 7.1).[14,15] A limitation of the HB scale is describing the distribution of which facial nerve branch is affected. As such, recording individual function of the facial nerve's extratemporal branches (temporal—forehead, zygomatic—eye closure, buccal—midface, marginal mandibular—mouth, and cervical—neck) can help localize the injury and dysfunction. Any patient with partial residual motor function is likely to have a good long-term outcome with conservative management.

Cerebrospinal fluid leak

Head injury and TBF may result in CSF leaks due to tears in the dura of the meninges. The primary reason to diagnose and manage a CSF leak is to decrease the risk of meningitis. Several diagnostic tests may be used to determine if a suspected fluid is CSF, such as detecting the presence of beta-2 transferrin or beta-trace protein.[16–19] Intrathecal fluorescein staining can additionally be used to detect

Table 7.1 House—Brackmann facial nerve grading system.

	Grade	Defined by
1	Normal	Normal facial function in all areas.
2	Mild dysfunction	Slight weakness noticeable only on close inspection. At rest: normal symmetry of forehead, ability to close eye with minimal effort and slight asymmetry, ability to move corners of mouth with maximal effort and slight asymmetry. No synkinesis, contracture, or hemifacial spasm.
3	Moderate dysfunction	Obvious but not disfiguring difference between two sides, no functional impairment; noticeable but not severe synkinesis, contracture, and/or hemifacial spasm. At rest: normal symmetry and tone. Motion: Slight to no movement of forehead, ability to close eye with maximal effort and obvious asymmetry, ability to move corners of mouth with maximal effort and obvious asymmetry. Patients who have obvious but no disfiguring synkinesis, contracture, and/or hemifacial spasm are grade III regardless of degree of motor activity.
4	Moderately severe dysfunction	Obvious weakness and/or disfiguring asymmetry. At rest: normal symmetry and tone. Motion: No movement of forehead; inability to close eye completely with maximal effort. Patients with synkinesis, mass action, and/or hemifacial spasm severe enough to interfere with function are grade IV regardless of motor activity.
5	Severe dysfunction	Only barely perceptible motion. At rest: possible asymmetry with droop of corner of mouth and decreased or absence of nasal labial fold. Motion: No movement of forehead, incomplete closure of eye and only slight movement of lid with maximal effort, slight movement of corner of mouth. Synkinesis, contracture, and hemifacial spasm usually absent.
6	Total paralysis	Loss of tone; asymmetry; no motion; no synkinesis, contracture, or hemifacial spasm.

a CSF leak by examining for the presence of discoloration or under Wood's lamp.[20] CT cisternography with contrast can be used to localize a CSF leak.[21]

Radiologic assessment

In the evaluation of a patient with suspected severe head trauma and temporal bone injuries, a CT is generally obtained by the trauma team to check for intracranial injury and hemorrhage. However, additional imaging of the temporal bone and skull base is needed if there is concern for CSF fistula, vascular injury, external auditory canal disruption, facial paralysis, ossicle displacement, or epithelial entrapment. Obtaining high-resolution computed tomography (HRCT) imaging with thin slice thickness in various reformats (axial, coronal) is recommended and is required for surgical planning and management of otologic complications. Isolated hearing loss does not require HRCT as immediate management does not affect prognosis for hearing function recovery. There is little role for conventional radiographs (e.g., X-ray) to assess for detailed structures of the temporal bone and skull base.

Review of the CT for course and fracture patterns of the temporal bone may help predict sequelae. The majority (70%–80%) of TBFs are longitudinal from impact near the parietal or temporal area of the skull.[22] Complications include facial paralysis, ossicular disruption, and hemotympanum and will often spare the otic capsule. Less commonly, transverse TBF will occur due to blows to the frontal or occipital bone.[22] These patients may have facial paralysis, SNHL due to disruption of the vestibulocochlear nerve and/or otic capsule, and vertigo.

Management

Head injury has the potential to lead to significant patient morbidity due to damage to structures closely associated within the temporal bone. This section will provide an overview of management strategies for sequelae of TBF. Additional details on management approaches are provided in later chapters.

Hearing loss

Initial audiometric evaluation often reveals CHL due to hemotympanum. Recording a baseline of hearing function is important to distinguish between hearing loss etiologies. Repeat audiometric testing is also performed 1–2 months after the initial injury to allow for hemotympanum to resolve and more accurate testing to occur following stabilization.

Patients who demonstrate early CHL do not require urgent surgical repair because hearing loss due to common etiologies such as hemotympanum may self-resolve. Early surgical intervention such as an ossiculoplasty can be considered if other surgical procedures will be performed (e.g., CSF leak repair). If however, CHL persists 3 months, elective surgical exploration can be performed. Persistent CHL should prompt suspicion for ossicular fracture (stapes superstructure or malleus fracture)[23] or dislocation (incudostapedial joint or incudomallear joint).[23–25] Children are also at increased risk of stapes fractures compared with adults due to greater deformability of the pediatric skull.[26]

Patients with lasting SNHL may be managed nonsurgically and surgically. Mild-to-moderate SNHL patients can benefit from standard amplification. For patients with unilateral profound SNHL, an option is to receive a bone-anchored hearing aid (BAHA), which can improve directional discrimination.[27] If patients are not satisfied with the appearance or performance of their BAHA, they can also choose to remove the external receiver. Another hearing rehabilitation option is to receive a cochlear implantation (CI). Candidates can have single-sided or bilateral several to profound SNHL. Anatomical prognostic factors of CI performance in this population includes intact cranial nerve VIII, minimal cochlear ossification, and bony discontinuity.[28-30].

Disequilibrium and vertigo

Following TBF, vertigo and dizziness are common and do not require urgent surgical intervention and can be treated at a later time with favorable outcomes. Posttraumatic vertigo often self-resolves, but several etiologies are considered if it persists.

BPPV is frequently experienced and is hypothesized to occur due to traumatic displacement of otoconia into the posterior semicircular canal.[7,8] Patients may have delayed presentation where symptoms appear days to weeks following injury. Undergoing treatment for BPPV is similar to management in nontraumatic settings and repositioning maneuvers such as the Epley maneuver will be curative in most cases.[31]

Perilymphatic fistula is another diagnosis and is managed surgically. Common locations of fistulae include the oval and round windows, which may be due to subluxation of the stapes footplate.[32,33] Surgical obliteration or patching of the oval and round window niches is performed to prevent further leakage of perilymphatic fluid.

Patients may also develop posttraumatic endolymphatic hydrops and have a late presentation. Treatment is primarily medical and supportive and similar to Meniere's disease, which includes oral corticosteroids, sodium restriction, and diuretics.

Unilateral vestibular loss due to injury-induced demyelination of the vestibulocochlear nerve, microischemic changes, or direct trauma to the labyrinth may occur in the setting of TBF.[34] Transverse TBFs compared with longitudinal TBFs have a greater chance of damaging the inner ear and vestibulocochlear nerve.[9] Treatment may initially include meclizine, ondansetron, or diazepam to improve nausea and vertigo. Persistent symptoms should include more extensive evaluation with videonystamography or electronystagmography.

Facial nerve injury

The duration and severity of facial nerve function deficit are two factors that will help guide management. Generally, partial facial paralysis compared with complete paralysis at presentation portends a favorable prognosis. Even if patients have initial partial facial paralysis that progresses to complete paralysis, these cases will generally self-recover. In cases where a patient is evaluated at a later point or the facial nerve injury timeline is unclear, electrophysiologic testing can be helpful to characterize the extent of injury.

Electrophysiologic testing

Two commonly used electrophysiologic tests to assess facial nerve integrity are electroneurography (ENoG) and electromyography (EMG) to help determine the prognosis of a facial nerve injury.[35] Both tests are indirect measures that quantify facial nerve function by recording action potentials and can be performed serially to assess improving or worsening nerve health. The timing of when to perform each test should also be considered. An ENoG should be performed after at least 3 days but within 2–3 weeks of injury to allow for Wallerian degeneration, whereas EMG can be performed at any time after the injury.[35]

ENoG is a noninvasive test that uses skin electrodes to measure evoked compound action potentials. Both sides of the face are assessed and compared to determine the percentage of degeneration of the affected side. Positive tests are generally considered to be greater than or equal to 90% degeneration of the affected side relative to the unaffected side.[15,36,37] Patients who have a normal ENoG study with facial paresis will generally have favorable return of facial nerve function.

EMG is a volitional test that uses needle electrodes positioned in the target muscle to assess action potentials while contracting. Findings include action potentials that portend a good prognosis, fibrillation potentials that suggest denervation, and polyphasic potentials that suggest reinnervation.[37] Eliciting an action potential generally rules out a complete nerve transection.

Treatment of early facial paralysis

There are several cases when early surgical intervention should be considered. Patients with immediate-onset paralysis and worsening ENoG functioning to less than 10% of the unaffected side[2,11] or immediate-onset paralysis and no recovery of facial nerve function within 1 week are surgical candidates. Visible severe nerve laceration on HRCT in the setting of paralysis is also an indicator for early surgery. If the timing of facial nerve paralysis onset is unclear, these cases can generally be managed as immediate onset.[38,39] If clinical exam findings of facial nerve paralysis are incomplete or electrophysiologic testing does not indicate severe nerve damage, high-dose corticosteroids given over 1–3 weeks followed by a taper can be used.[39,40]

Treatment of late and persistent paralysis

Patients who display continued facial paralysis several months after the initial injury are unlikely to regain complete spontaneous function in the future. An important complication of prolonged facial paralysis is exposure keratitis in the nonclosing eye, which can be managed with lubricating eye drops or gold weight lid implants. Grading with the HB scale can help guide further management. Patients with HB grades I to II are generally satisfied with their cosmetic appearance and functional outcome, lending to no further management. HB grades III to IV do not require direct surgical repair of the facial nerve. Management focuses on augmentation procedures such as botulinum injection for synkinesis or brow lifts. Patients with HB grades V to VI can undergo reinnervation and reanimation procedure 1 year after the injury to allow for maximal spontaneous recovery of the facial nerve. Another option is decompression of the facial nerve and is performed several months after the initial injury, which has shown to recover patients to HB grade I or II.[41]

Cerebrospinal fluid leak

Management of traumatic CSF leaks following a head injury starts with conservative treatment. The goal of initial management is focused on reducing intracranial pressure and leakage. Patients should be limited to bed rest, elevate their head, and avoid coughing, nose blowing or straining of stool.[42] In most cases, CSF leaks will resolve within a week without intervention and do not generally require antibiotics.[43] If a CSF leak persists for greater than 1 week, however, the risk of meningitis increases and further management is needed.[43] Following a continuing CSF leak after a week, consultation with neurosurgery for surgical repair of a CSF leak and infectious disease for antibiotic management is recommended. Preoperative imaging with an HRCT will determine the size of the defect and presence of intracranial contents, which will guide surgical decision-making.

Vascular injury

Vascular injury to the carotid artery is a potential complication of head injury and may result as from fracture of the carotid canal. Patients should undergo a carotid angiography if a cervical bruit is present on exam, fracture through the carotid canal, or the neurologic exam is inconsistent with the temporal bone CT findings.[44] Patients may demonstrate Horner's syndrome (single eye with droopy lid and small pupil) or symptoms suggesting lateralization: weakness, numbness. Traumatic head injuries may also form a carotid cavernous fistula, which is an abnormal connection between the carotid artery and/or its branches and the cavernous sinus. Patients will may present with chemosis, ocular bruit, and exophthalmos. Treatment may include endovascular approaches utilizing balloon occlusion and embolization.

Cholesteatoma

Cholesteatoma is a rare complication of TBF that may develop several years later. The pathophysiology of cholesteatoma development is due to entrapment of epithelium and may occur with both penetrating and blunt temporal bone trauma.[45] The entrapped epithelium located in the soft tissue may subsequently lead to cholesteatoma development.[45] Determining level of risk of cholesteatoma development is a diagnostic challenge unless overt evidence of epithelial entrapment is present. Patients with increased risk are those significant injury of the external auditory canal or penetrating mechanisms.

Management for cholesteatoma prevention is dependent on the degree of epithelium entrapment. In cases with gross entrapment, patients should undergo early canalplasty and mastoidectomy. Patients with less severe injuries may undergo observation with clinical follow-ups and serial CT to monitor for delayed cholesteatoma development. External auditory canal stenosis commonly occurs for head injury, and the EAC lumen should be maintained using ear wicks saturated with antibiotic drops. Later, a canalplasty and tympanoplasty can be performed to prevent future cholesteatoma formation.

References

1. Lyos AT, Marsh MA, Jenkins HA, Coker NJ. Progressive hearing loss after transverse temporal bone fracture. *Arch Otolaryngol Head Neck Surg*. 1995;121(7):795−799.
2. Nosan DK, Benecke Jr JE, Murr AH. Current perspective on temporal bone trauma. *Otolaryngol Head Neck Surg*. 1997;117(1):67−71.
3. Yanagihara N, Murakami S, Nishihara S. Temporal bone fractures inducing facial nerve paralysis: a new classification and its clinical significance. *Ear Nose Throat J*. 1997; 76(2):79−80, 83−76.
4. Jones SE, Mahendran S. Interventions for acute auricular haematoma. *Cochrane Database Syst Rev*. 2004;2:CD004166.
5. Rubin J, Yu VL, Kamerer DB, Wagener M. Aural irrigation with water: a potential pathogenic mechanism for inducing malignant external otitis? *Ann Otol Rhinol Laryngol*. 1990;99(2 Pt 1):117−119.
6. Hicks GW, Wright Jr JW, Wright 3rd JW. Cerebrospinal fluid otorrhea. *Laryngoscope*. 1980;90(11 Pt 2 Suppl. 25):1−25.
7. Labuguen RH. Initial evaluation of vertigo. *Am Fam Phys*. 2006;73(2):244−251.
8. Hanley K, O'Dowd T. Symptoms of vertigo in general practice: a prospective study of diagnosis. *Br J Gen Pract*. 2002;52(483):809−812.
9. Fife TD, Giza C. Posttraumatic vertigo and dizziness. *Semin Neurol*. 2013;33(3): 238−243.
10. Choi JE, Moon IJ, Kim H, Lee K, Cho YS, Chung WH. Diagnostic criteria of barotraumatic perilymph fistula based on clinical manifestations. *Acta Otolaryngol*. 2017;137(1): 16−22.
11. Coker NJ, Kendall KA, Jenkins HA, Alford BR. Traumatic intratemporal facial nerve injury: management rationale for preservation of function. *Otolaryngol Head Neck Surg*. 1987;97(3):262−269.
12. Terzis JK, Noah ME. Analysis of 100 cases of free-muscle transplantation for facial paralysis. *Plast Reconstr Surg*. 1997;99(7):1905−1921.
13. Burres S, Fisch U. The comparison of facial grading systems. *Arch Otolaryngol Head Neck Surg*. 1986;112(7):755−758.
14. Yen TL, Driscoll CL, Lalwani AK. Significance of House-Brackmann facial nerve grading global score in the setting of differential facial nerve function. *Otol Neurotol*. 2003;24(1):118−122.
15. House JW. Facial nerve grading systems. *Laryngoscope*. 1983;93(8):1056−1069.
16. Tubbs RS, Shoja MM, Loukas M, Oakes WJ, Cohen-Gadol A. William Henry Battle and Battle's sign: mastoid ecchymosis as an indicator of basilar skull fracture. *J Neurosurg*. 2010;112(1):186−188.
17. Pretto Flores L, De Almeida CS, Casulari LA. Positive predictive values of selected clinical signs associated with skull base fractures. *J Neurosurg Sci*. 2000;44(2):77−82. discussion 82−73.
18. Meurman OH, Irjala K, Suonpaa J, Laurent B. A new method for the identification of cerebrospinal fluid leakage. *Acta Otolaryngol*. 1979;87(3−4):366−369.
19. Meco C, Oberascher G, Arrer E, Moser G, Albegger K. Beta-trace protein test: new guidelines for the reliable diagnosis of cerebrospinal fluid fistula. *Otolaryngol Head Neck Surg*. 2003;129(5):508−517.

20. Raza SM, Banu MA, Donaldson A, Patel KS, Anand VK, Schwartz TH. Sensitivity and specificity of intrathecal fluorescein and white light excitation for detecting intraoperative cerebrospinal fluid leak in endoscopic skull base surgery: a prospective study. *J Neurosurg*. 2016;124(3):621−626.

21. Stone JA, Castillo M, Neelon B, Mukherji SK. Evaluation of CSF leaks: high-resolution CT compared with contrast-enhanced CT and radionuclide cisternography. *AJNR Am J Neuroradiol*. 1999;20(4):706−712.

22. Goodwin Jr WJ. Temporal bone fractures. *Otolaryngol Clin*. 1983;16(3):651−659.

23. Cannon CR, Jahrsdoerfer RA. Temporal bone fractures. Review of 90 cases. *Arch Otolaryngol*. 1983;109(5):285−288.

24. Ghorayeb BY, Yeakley JW, Hall 3rd JW, Jones BE. Unusual complications of temporal bone fractures. *Arch Otolaryngol Head Neck Surg*. 1987;113(7):749−753.

25. Wysocki J. Cadaveric dissections based on observations of injuries to the temporal bone structures following head trauma. *Skull Base*. 2005;15(2):99−106. discussion 106−107.

26. Singh S, Salib RJ, Oates J. Traumatic fracture of the stapes suprastructure following minor head injury. *J Laryngol Otol*. 2002;116(6):457−459.

27. Baguley DM, Bird J, Humphriss RL, Prevost AT. The evidence base for the application of contralateral bone anchored hearing aids in acquired unilateral sensorineural hearing loss in adults. *Clin Otolaryngol*. 2006;31(1):6−14.

28. Camilleri AE, Toner JG, Howarth KL, Hampton S, Ramsden RT. Cochlear implantation following temporal bone fracture. *J Laryngol Otol*. 1999;113(5):454−457.

29. Simons JP, Whitaker ME, Hirsch BE. Cochlear implantation in a patient with bilateral temporal bone fractures. *Otolaryngol Head Neck Surg*. 2005;132(5):809−811.

30. Kozin ED, Lubner RJ, Knoll RM, Remenschneider A, Nadol Jr JB. Are cochlear implants a viable option following temporal bone fracture? *Laryngoscope*. 2020;130(7): 1613−1615.

31. Gordon CR, Levite R, Joffe V, Gadoth N. Is posttraumatic benign paroxysmal positional vertigo different from the idiopathic form? *Arch Neurol*. 2004;61(10):1590−1593.

32. Kita AE, Kim I, Ishiyama G, Ishiyama A. Perilymphatic fistula after penetrating ear trauma. *Clin Pract Cases Emerg Med*. 2019;3(2):115−118.

33. Ederies A, Yuen HW, Chen JM, Aviv RI, Symons SP. Traumatic stapes fracture with rotation and subluxation into the vestibule and pneumolabyrinth. *Laryngoscope*. 2009; 119(6):1195−1197.

34. Chiaramonte R, Bonfiglio M, D'Amore A, Viglianesi A, Cavallaro T, Chiaramonte I. Traumatic labyrinthine concussion in a patient with sensorineural hearing loss. *NeuroRadiol J*. 2013;26(1):52−55.

35. Lee DH. Clinical efficacy of electroneurography in acute facial paralysis. *J Audiol Otol*. 2016;20(1):8−12.

36. May M, Blumenthal F, Klein SR. Acute Bell's palsy: prognostic value of evoked electromyography, maximal stimulation, and other electrical tests. *Am J Otol*. 1983;5(1):1−7.

37. Sittel C, Stennert E. Prognostic value of electromyography in acute peripheral facial nerve palsy. *Otol Neurotol*. 2001;22(1):100−104.

38. Brodie HA, Thompson TC. Management of complications from 820 temporal bone fractures. *Am J Otol*. 1997;18(2):188−197.

39. Darrouzet V, Duclos JY, Liguoro D, Truilhe Y, De Bonfils C, Bebear JP. Management of facial paralysis resulting from temporal bone fractures: our experience in 115 cases. *Otolaryngol Head Neck Surg*. 2001;125(1):77−84.

40. Dahiya R, Keller JD, Litofsky NS, Bankey PE, Bonassar LJ, Megerian CA. Temporal bone fractures: otic capsule sparing versus otic capsule violating clinical and radiographic considerations. *J Trauma*. 1999;47(6):1079−1083.

41. Quaranta A, Campobasso G, Piazza F, Quaranta N, Salonna I. Facial nerve paralysis in temporal bone fractures: outcomes after late decompression surgery. *Acta Otolaryngol*. 2001;121(5):652−655.

42. Oh JW, Kim SH, Whang K. Traumatic cerebrospinal fluid leak: diagnosis and management. *Korean J Nutr*. 2017;13(2):63−67.

43. Santos SF, Rodrigues F, Dias A, Costa JA, Correia A, Oliveira G. [Post-traumatic meningitis in children: eleven years' analysis]. *Acta Med Port*. 2011;24(3):391−398.

44. Dempewolf R, Gubbels S, Hansen MR. Acute radiographic workup of blunt temporal bone trauma: maxillofacial versus temporal bone CT. *Laryngoscope*. 2009;119(3):442−448.

45. Lin HC, Shih CP, Chen HC, et al. Risk of acquired cholesteatoma and external auditory canal stenosis in traumatic brain injury: a nationwide population-based cohort study. *Int J Environ Res Publ Health*. 2020;17(18).

Labyrinthine concussion: diagnosis and management

Renata M. Knoll, MD [1,2], **Elliott D. Kozin, MD** [1,2]

[1]*Department of Otolaryngology, Massachusetts Eye and Ear, Boston, MA, United States;*
[2]*Department of Otolaryngology, Harvard Medical School, Boston, MA, United States*

Since the 20th century, the term "labyrinthine concussion"[1−3] or "inner ear concussion"[4−6] has been used to describe sensorineural hearing loss following head trauma in the absence of temporal bone fracture and is generally defined as head trauma resulting in sensorineural hearing loss without evidence of fracture involving the labyrinth. Although poorly reported in the medical literature, it does not seem to be a rare complication of head trauma, occurring in as many as 58% of patients.[7] This chapter will provide an overview of the diagnosis and management of labyrinthine concussion.

Diagnosis

The diagnosis of labyrinthine concussion is typically a diagnosis of exclusion with often no physical exam or imaging findings to suggest an etiology of sensorineural hearing loss.

History and symptoms

The initial investigation should begin with a comprehensive history, including not only auditory symptomatology but also a proper description of the mechanism of injury. It is important to determine the nature of the head trauma, whether it was caused by direct impact, sudden or rapid acceleration and deceleration, penetrating injury or blast injury, and whether there have been prior episodes of head trauma. Additionally, prior otologic symptoms, general medical and surgical history, and any other relevant information that may help to elucidate the diagnosis of the auditory dysfunction should be inquired.

In terms of symptomatology, complaints of patients with labyrinthine concussion are nonspecific and may include new onset of unilateral or bilateral hearing loss, aural fullness, tinnitus, and hyperacusis following head trauma. These symptoms might also occur in conjunction with vestibular dysfunction. Additionally, hearing loss related to labyrinthine concussion may not be permanent as some level of recovery has been already reported in prior clinical and experimental studies.[8−10].

Otologic and Lateral Skull Base Trauma. https://doi.org/10.1016/B978-0-323-87402-3.00008-3

Physical examination and evaluation

The physical examination generally includes otoscopy, which may be useful to assess other potential causes of hearing loss such as cerumen impaction, middle ear effusion, or tympanic membrane perforation. Additionally, a fistula test may be performed in the setting of vestibular symptomatology, as traumatic perilymphatic fistula should be considered in the differential diagnosis. Tunning forks can be also used for the assessment of hearing loss, in which a Weber test in a patient with unilateral sensorineural hearing loss will lateralize sound toward the unaffected side, and Rinne test should be positive unless significant hearing loss to the tested ear exists.

Objective audiometric testing may demonstrate variable severity of sensorineural hearing loss depending on the extent of neurosensory injury. Clinical and experimental studies have suggested that hearing loss due to labyrinthine concussion is typically more severe in high frequencies, in particular the range from 3 to 8 KHz, resembling an acoustic trauma.[8,9,11] This finding is thought to be a result from perilymph and endolymph vibrating waves generated by the concussive trauma associated to an inherent fragility in the upper region of the basal turn, or to physical properties of the impulse.[12]

Radiologic assessment

In the evaluation of a patient with sensorineural hearing loss following head trauma, a high-resolution computed tomography (HRCT) is the initial imaging modality recommended to check for fractures through the temporal bone involving the otic capsule, or pneumolabyrinth that may suggest a perilymphatic fistula. In the setting of a negative HRCT study, diagnosis of labyrinthine concussion is more likely. A complementary magnetic resonance imaging (MRI) may be also obtained to look for intralabyrinthine hemorrhage and cranial nerves integrity. If intralabyrinthine bleeding occurs as a result of concussion, high signal intensity in the inner ear may be seen on T1-weighted and fluid-attenuated inversion-recovery (FLAIR) imaging.[13,14]

Management

There is no specific treatment for labyrinthine concussion. One option is to manage it expectantly as spontaneous recovery has been reported for some individuals.[8,15] However, in the presence of associated vestibular symptomatology (e.g., vertigo), there seems to be a greater possibility of permanent hearing loss.[8] Another possibility is to treat labyrinthine concussion as in idiopathic sudden sensorineural hearing loss, though use of corticosteroid remains controversial in this setting. To date, the application of steroids for labyrinthine concussion has been largely based on case reports,[16] and it is not known whether improvements in hearing thresholds may be a response to empirical corticotherapy or just spontaneous recovery.

Regarding long-term management of permanent hearing loss resulted from laby-rinthine concussion, there are multiple options to compensate for hearing loss and improve daily function and well-being, such as assistive listening devices, hearing aids, and auditory training. Cochlear implantation has been also effective for pa-tients with profound sensorineural hearing loss, especially for those with short dura-tion of severe or profound hearing impairment.[17−19].

References

1. Hofmann L. Fracturen der schlafenbein pyramide. *Zbl Ohrenh.* 1925;7:539.
2. Koch J. Studien über Veränderungen des Gehörorgans, insbesondere Störungen der Inne-nohrfunktion nach Schädelunfällen mit und ohne Verletzung des Schläfenbeins. *Arch f Ohrenh.* 1933;137(2):105−160.
3. Klingenberg A. Die Isolierte Schneckenfractur bei Schadelbasisbruchen. *Z Hals Nas Orenheilk.* 1929;22:452.
4. Stenger P. Beitrag zur Kenntnis der nach Kopfverletzungen auftretenden Veränderungen im inneren. *Ohr Arch Ohrenheilk.* 1909;79:43−69.
5. Brunner H. Disturbances of the function of the ear after concussion of the brain. *Laryngoscope.* 1940;50:921.
6. Voss O. *Die Chirurgie der Schädelbasisfrakturen.* Leipzig: Ambrosius Barth; 1936.
7. Chen JX, Lindeborg M, Herman SD, et al. Systematic review of hearing loss after trau-matic brain injury without associated temporal bone fracture. *Am J Otolaryngol.* 2018; 39(3):338−344.
8. Choi MS, Shin SO, Yeon JY, Choi YS, Kim J, Park SK. Clinical characteristics of laby-rinthine concussion. *Korean J Audiol.* 2013;17(1):13−17.
9. Schuknecht HF, Davison RC. Deafness and vertigo from head injury. *AMA Arch Otolaryngol.* 1956;63(5):513−528.
10. Gros JC. The ear in skull trauma. *South Med J.* 1967;60(7):705−711.
11. Ulug T, Ulubil SA. Contralateral labyrinthine concussion in temporal bone fractures. *J Otolaryngol.* 2006;35(6):380−383.
12. Bartholomew RA, Lubner RJ, Knoll RM, et al. Labyrinthine concussion: historic otopa-thologic antecedents of a challenging diagnosis. *Laryngoscope Investig Otolaryngol.* 2020;5(2):267−277.
13. Maillot O, Attye A, Boyer E, et al. Post traumatic deafness: a pictorial review of CT and MRI findings. *Insights Imaging.* 2016;7(3):341−350.
14. Chiaramonte R, Bonfiglio M, D'Amore A, Viglianesi A, Cavallaro T, Chiaramonte I. Traumatic labyrinthine concussion in a patient with sensorineural hearing loss. *NeuroRa-diol J.* 2013;26(1):52−55.
15. Schuknecht HF. A clinical study of auditory damage following blows to the head. *Ann Otol Rhinol Laryngol.* 1950;59(2):331−358.
16. Villarreal IM, Mendez D, Silva JM, Del Alamo PO. Contralateral cochlear labyrinthine concussion without temporal bone fracture: unusual posttraumatic consequence. *Case Rep Otolaryngol.* 2016;2016:2123182.
17. Lubner RJ, Knoll RM, Trakimas DR, et al. Long-term cochlear implantation outcomes in patients following head injury. *Laryngoscope Investig Otolaryngol.* 2020;5(3):485−496.

18. Medina M, Di Lella F, Di Trapani G, et al. Cochlear implantation versus auditory brainstem implantation in bilateral total deafness after head trauma: personal experience and review of the literature. *Otol Neurotol*. 2014;35(2):260−270.
19. Khwaja S, Mawman D, Nichani J, Bruce I, Green K, Lloyd S. Cochlear implantation in patients profoundly deafened after head injury. *Otol Neurotol*. 2012;33(8):1328−1332.

The neurosurgical management of lateral skull base trauma

Aaron Plitt, MD[1], Scott Connors, MD[1], Tomas Garzon-Muvdi, MD, MSc[2], Kalil Abdullah, MD, MSc[3,4]

[1]*Department of Neurological Surgery, University of Texas Southwestern Medical Center, Dallas, TX, United States;* [2]*Department of Neurological Surgery, Emory University, Atlanta, GA, United States;* [3]*Department of Neurosurgery, University of Pittsburgh School of Medicine, Pittsburgh, PA, United States;* [4]*Hillman Comprehensive Cancer Center, University of Pittsburgh Medical Center, Pittsburgh, PA, United States*

Introduction

The lateral skull base is comprised predominantly of the dense, pyramid-shaped petrous temporal bone. Fractures of the petrous temporal bone comprise approximately 20% of all skull fractures.[1] Given the density of the petrous temporal bone, fractures are caused by high-impact trauma and are nearly uniformly associated with traumatic brain injury (TBI). In addition, 8%−29% of temporal bone fractures are bilateral, resulting in significant morbidity.[2,3]

These fractures are typically caused by direct impact and compression mechanisms and, historically, have been classified as either transverse or longitudinal depending on the orientation of the fracture along the long axis of the temporal bone. More recent classification, however, has focused on the relationship of the fracture to the otic capsule as this represents a more clinically relevant distinction.[4] In this scheme, fractures are either otic capsule sparing (OCS) or otic capsule disrupting (OCD). OCS fractures are more common, comprising approximately 95% of fractures, and typically result from direct impact on the temporoparietal convexity. Resultant fractures are through the posterior wall of the external auditory canal (EAC), mastoid air cells, middle ear, mastoid tegmen, and tegmen tympani. As a result, OCS injuries are associated with conductive or mixed hearing loss. In contrast, OCD fractures are typically from impact to the occiput with a fracture line from the foramen magnum through the petrous pyramid. These fractures can involve the jugular foramen, internal auditory canal, and foramen lacerum. OCD fractures lead to an obligate, often profound, and sensorineural hearing loss (SNHL)[5] (Fig. 9.1).

Fractures of the lateral skull base are a source of significant morbidity. They can lead to cerebrospinal fluid (CSF) leak, facial nerve injury, meningitis, hearing loss

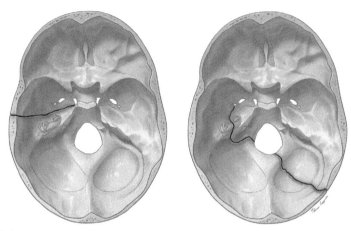

FIGURE 9.1

(*Left*) Otic capsule sparing fractures result from impact on the temporoparietal convexity, leading to a fracture line through the petrous temporal bone, but without violation of the otic capsule. (*Right*) Otic capsule disrupting fractures are typically from impact to the occiput with a fracture line from the foramen magnum through the petrous temporal bone and the otic capsule.

(both conductive and sensorineural), and cerebrovascular injury. As such, early recognition is important to allow for appropriate management.

Clinical evaluation and diagnosis

Temporal bone fractures are typically the result of high-impact trauma. Often these fractures occur in patients who also have TBI and polytrauma. Therefore, it is common for temporal bone fractures to be initially diagnosed on a CT of the head. A temporal bone fracture should also be suspected in an awake posttrauma patient with facial weakness, dizziness, or hearing loss, or in an obtunded posttrauma patient with ecchymosis over the mastoid prominence (Battle's sign) or otorrhea.

The physical exam is critical for acute diagnosis and management of these fractures. Otoscopy should be performed on any patient with a suspected fracture. Evaluation should begin with inspection of the external ear. Superficial lacerations will often heal without intervention. Circumferential lacerations of the EAC, however, may lead to stenosis in the future and should be repaired. The canal should also be inspected for brain parenchyma (rare) and CSF leak (more common). The integrity of the tympanic membrane (TM) should be assessed. The most common findings are hemotympanum if the TM is intact, and bloody otorrhea if the TM is perforated. Similarly, in the case of a CSF leak, otorrhea will be present if the TM is perforated, but if the membrane is intact, the fluid drains through the eustachian tube producing rhinorrhea.

Pneumatic otoscopy should be deferred in the acute setting to avoid introduction of air and bacteria into the subarachnoid space.

Evaluation and documentation of facial movement is also imperative in the acute setting as it has significant prognostic value[6–8]. By necessity, facial movement evaluation is often delayed, however, as patients may be intubated and unable to participate in an examination or other injuries may take priority. Those patients who cannot be examined immediately should be considered to have indeterminate onset of facial weakness. The House–Brackmann scale is a simple and consistent grading scale that can be utilized for long-term follow-up.[9] Patients with immediate, acute-onset complete facial paralysis have a much worse prognosis for recovery than those with delayed-onset weakness. Recovery of incomplete facial paralysis is seen in nearly 100% of cases.[6,8,10,11]

Hearing should also be tested at bedside with a 512-Hz tuning fork. The Rinne and Weber tests can help differentiate conductive hearing loss from SNHL. Audiometry is typically delayed for several weeks after initial trauma to allow for resolution of middle ear fluid unless the patient requires an urgent surgical intervention.

Disruption of the otic capsule can present with vertigo and nystagmus. For that reason, an examination of extraocular movements should be performed to assess for nystagmus in addition to cranial nerve III, IV, and VI palsies. An abducens palsy is common in TBI and can be associated with temporal bone fractures, especially fractures extending into the clivus.

High-resolution temporal bone CT is not routinely necessary unless patients develop persistent CSF leaks, hearing loss, or facial weakness. It should also be obtained prior to any planned surgical intervention. CT angiography should also be considered in the setting of temporal bone fractures as the petrous segment of the internal carotid is at risk for injury as are the transition points between the relatively mobile cervical and petrous segments and the petrous to lacerum segments.

Management and outcomes

Management of lateral temporal bone fractures hinges on the indications for surgical intervention. In general, early surgery should be considered for open, depressed squamous temporal fractures or any mass occupying lesions with a poor neurologic exam, such as a large temporal lobe contusion or an epidural hematoma. The goal of acute surgical intervention is preservation of neurologic function and decompression of the brainstem. In contrast, delayed surgical intervention is reserved for persistent CSF leaks and facial nerve decompression.

Cerebrospinal fluid leak

CSF leak occurs in approximately 17% of temporal bone fractures.[2,10,12–14] It significantly increases the patient's risk of meningitis and ensuing morbidity. Evidence of a CSF fistula may be present initially on examination, but also commonly develops several days following an injury as posttraumatic soft tissue edema resolves. It may present as either clear otorrhea or rhinorrhea depending on the integrity of the TM. In OCS fractures, the CSF fistula typically occurs through a fracture in the tegmen tympani or mastoideum, whereas in OCD fractures, the leak typically results from injury to the posterior fossa dura creating a direct fistula from the posterior fossa subarachnoid space into the middle ear via the otic capsule.[5] The leak can be confirmed as CSF by evaluating the fluid for the presence of Beta2-transferrin, which is only present in CSF, perilymph, and aqueous humor.[15]

Initially, the treatment for a CSF fistula should be conservative, using measures to decrease intracranial pressure and diminish any pressure gradient as a fibrous layer forms to seal the dural defects. Such measures include elevation of the head of bed, stool softeners, avoidance of sneezing, and nose blowing as well as avoiding situations requiring the equivalent of a Valsalva maneuver. Temporary CSF diversion with repeated lumbar punctures or a lumbar drain can also be employed. With conservative management, 57%–85% of CSF fistulae will resolve within 1 week of initial injury.[2,11,12,16,17]

After 1 week, the risk of meningitis increases significantly, ranging from 88% to 100% among those with persistent CSF leaks.[2,5,18] Among these patients, *Pneumococcus*, *Streptococcus*, and *Haemophilus influenzae* are the most common pathogens.[18] With such a high incidence of meningitis, persistent CSF leak is an indication for operative repair. To facilitate surgery, further investigation should be directed toward identifying the site of the leak. A high-resolution CT of the temporal bone is able to locate the site of CSF egress in 70% of cases.[14] If the CT is inconclusive, then an intrathecal fluorescein evaluation can be performed to localize the site of the leak. Surgical repair should ensue after the site of the leak has been identified.

The surgical approach for repair of a CSF fistula is determined by the site of the leak and the hearing status of the patient. In OCD fractures with profound SNHL, a complete mastoidectomy with removal of ossicular chain, obliteration of the eustachian tube, and oversewing of the EAC is recommended to treat the leak. The approach for CSF leak repair in OCS fractures with salvageable hearing, on the other hand, is dictated by the location of the leak. The most common site of leak is the tegmen tympani. For these locations, a middle fossa craniotomy and a temporalis fascia flap overlay are the approaches of choice. For other sites of leak, a transmastoid, labyrinth-sparing approach allows for repair of the fistula while preserving hearing.[19,20]

Due to the risk of meningitis resulting from CSF fistula, consideration has been given to the use of prophylactic antibiotic therapy. Historically, practice has varied widely regarding the use, duration, and agents used for prophylactic therapy. However, a metaanalysis performed in 2011 by Ratilal et al.[21] found no reduction in the frequency of meningitis, all-cause mortality, meningitis-related mortality, or need for surgical correction between antibiotic use and nonuse in those with a CSF leak. Therefore, in the absence of concern for meningitis, antibiotic prophylaxis is not generally recommended for those with a CSF leak.

Facial nerve injury

Facial nerve injury occurs in 6%—7% of temporal bone fractures. Of those with facial nerve injury, 27% will initially present with facial weakness, while the other 73% will develop delayed-onset facial weakness within 1—16 days after the injury. Most patients will develop partial facial weakness, with only 25% presenting with acute-onset complete paralysis (i.e., House—Brackman 6 facial weakness).[2] Regardless of severity and timing of weakness onset, the initial treatment should be with 7—14 days of systemic glucocorticoid treatment.

Delayed facial weakness and incomplete weakness are associated with better long-term outcomes than acute-onset, complete facial paralysis. Ninety-four percent of delayed facial weakness patients completely recover, and up to 100% of patients with incomplete facial weakness will completely recover.[6,10,11] Therefore, surgical decompression of the facial nerve is reserved for acute-onset, complete facial weakness with poor prognosis for recovery. Prognosis is determined electrophysiologically, using electroneurography (ENoG) and voluntary electromyography (EMG). ENoG measures the compound muscle action potential generated by an electrical stimulus at the stylomastoid foramen. These muscle action potentials are the result of synchronous discharge of multiple viable nerve fibers, and decreased amplitudes suggest Wallerian degeneration. Voluntary EMG measures the motor response via needle electrodes when a patient attempts to make facial muscle contractions. EMG is typically used in patients for whom ENoG has demonstrated >90% degeneration to evaluate for active motor units that may be too asynchronous in their activity to produce a compound action motor potential. The presence of asynchronous active motor units suggests recovering nerve fibers and portends a better prognosis.[22] Electrophysiologic testing should be delayed for at least 3 days to allow Wallerian degeneration to occur because patients with complete nerve disruption will retain distal stimulability for 3—5 days after initial injury.[11] Moreover, testing is not typically performed after 14 days as those with >90% degeneration after 2 weeks do not show favorable response to surgical intervention, while those who have not met the 90% degeneration threshold have a high chance of recovery.[22]

The most common site of injury is the perigeniculate facial nerve in the fallopian canal. For OCS fractures, surgical approach is typically transmastoid, supralabyrinthine to expose the distal labyrinthine segment down to the mastoid segment of the facial nerve and to decompress it in the fallopian canal. Alternatively, a middle fossa craniotomy can be performed with direct decompression of the perigeniculate facial nerve by identifying the greater superficial petrosal nerve and following it proximally to the geniculate ganglion. For OCD fractures, as a consequence of the SNHL, a translabyrinthine approach can be used to decompress the facial nerve. In all cases, the goal is to remove any bony fragments compressing the perineurium or to repair a transected nerve.[10,11] In cases of facial nerve transection, primary anastomosis between facial nerve ends has the most favorable results in motor outcomes. However, when the facial nerve is too damaged to repair primarily, then a "cable graft" can be performed. In this procedure, a section of donor nerve is harvested and used as an interposition graft to restore the continuity of the facial nerve. Common donor nerves include the greater auricular nerve, sural nerve, and the medial and lateral antebrachial cutaneous nerves.[23] Alternatively, a hypoglossal-facial anastomosis can be performed.[7,24,25] In cases where the facial nerve does not recover, then facial reanimation can be performed in a delayed fashion.

The most important aspect of preventative care for a patient with facial weakness is eye protection. As the facial nerve recovers, the patient is at high risk for exposure keratitis and corneal abrasions, which can comprise vision. Artificial tears, ointment, and moisture chambers should be utilized. Lateral tarsorrhaphy can be utilized to augment eye closure in incomplete injuries. In complete paralysis, a gold weight should be considered in the upper eyelid.

Hearing loss

Hearing loss is common with temporal bone fractures. Depending on the fracture, it can be conductive, SNHL, or mixed. While OCS fractures can present with conductive or mixed hearing loss, OCD fractures are uniformly SNHL, which is the type that has the worst prognosis for recovery. As previously mentioned, an audiogram should be delayed for 4–6 weeks postinjury to allow for resolution of middle ear fluid.

Conductive hearing loss is typically secondary to middle ear effusion or hemotympanum but in up to 20% of patients can be due to ossicular chain disruption.[26] For those with persistent conductive hearing loss lasting for longer than 6 months, an exploratory tympanotomy with possible ossiculoplasty can be considered. These patients may also benefit from hearing aids or amplifiers. Repair should not be attempted earlier because scar formation around the ossicular chain and resorption of middle ear fluid often resolves the hearing loss.

SNHL has a worse prognosis for recovery than conductive hearing loss. It can also occur in patients with TBI without temporal bone fractures. Surgical intervention is typically not indicated, but those with bilateral profound SNHL can be treated with cochlear implants.[27]

Vertigo

Vertigo and dizziness are common with temporal bone fractures and TBI, in general. The most common type of vertigo is benign paroxysmal positional vertigo.[28] The patient should initially be treated with vestibular rehabilitation. For most patients, the vertigo, and resultant nystagmus, will resolve within 4–6 weeks of initial injury. For patients with OCD fractures, vestibular rehabilitation may be required for a longer period of time.

Vascular injury

High-impact trauma to the head and neck region is associated with traumatic dissections to cerebral vasculature. These traumatic dissections are a nidus for clot formation and as a result place the patient at risk for stroke. Arterial transition points are particularly vulnerable to injury, including the entry of the cervical internal carotid artery into the petrous temporal bone. For this reason, any patient with lateral skull base trauma should also be considered for a CT angiogram of the head and neck to assess for arterial injury. Internal carotid artery dissection with at least 25% stenosis, pseudoaneurysm formation, or occlusion is typically treated with antiplatelets or anticoagulation.[29]

Additional considerations

Patients who sustain an injury to the EAC or have undergone ear surgery are at increased risk for external canal stenosis and cholesteatoma formation, both of which can lead to impaired hearing. Cholesteatoma formation can occur following trauma by one of four possible mechanisms: skin epithelial entrapment in a fracture line, ingrowth of epithelium in an unhealed fracture line or disrupted TM, traumatic implantation of epithelium in middle ear, or trapping of skin epithelium medial to an EAC stenosis.[30] Therefore, patients require continued, long-term monitoring after temporal bone fractures for cholesteatoma formation and EAC stenosis. If the patient develops EAC stenosis, then it is recommended to stent the stenosis or perform a canaloplasty to prevent cholesteatoma formation and augment hearing.

Conclusions

Petrous temporal bone fractures are caused by high-impact trauma and can result in significant morbidity. The most common complications are facial nerve injury, CSF leak, and hearing loss. The timing of onset of facial weakness and degree of injury is the most critical initial evaluation to determine next step in management. Overall, most complications can be managed conservatively with favorable outcomes. Following temporal bone fracture, patients require long-term monitoring for delayed cholesteatoma formation.

References

1. Lemole M, Behbahani M. Retrospective study of skull base fracture: a study of incidents, complications, management, and outcome overview from trauma-one-level institute over 5 years. *J Neurol Surg Part B Skull Base.* 2013;74(S 01):A239.
2. Brodie HA, Thompson TC. Management of complications from 820 temporal bone fractures. *Am J Otol.* 1997;18(2):188–197.
3. Griffin JE, Altenau MM, Schaefer SD. Bilateral longitudinal temporal bone fractures: a retrospective review of seventeen cases. *Laryngoscope.* 1979;89(9 Pt 1):1432–1435.
4. Ishman SL, Friedland DR. Temporal bone fractures: traditional classification and clinical relevance. *Laryngoscope.* 2004;114(10):1734–1741.
5. Diaz RC, Cervenka B, Brodie HA. Treatment of temporal bone fractures. *J Neurol Surg Part B Skull Base.* 2016;77(5):419–429.

6. Chang CY, Cass SP. Management of facial nerve injury due to temporal bone trauma. *Am J Otol.* 1999;20(1):96−114.
7. May M. Facial reanimation after skull base trauma. *Am J Otol.* 1985;Suppl:62−67.
8. Ulug T, Arif Ulubil S. Management of facial paralysis in temporal bone fractures: a prospective study analyzing 11 operated fractures. *Am J Otolaryngol.* 2005;26(4):230−238.
9. House JW, Brackmann DE. Facial nerve grading system. *Otolaryngol Head Neck Surg.* 1985;93(2):146−147.
10. Feldman JS, Farnoosh S, Kellman RM, Tatum 3rd SA. Skull base trauma: clinical considerations in evaluation and diagnosis and review of management techniques and surgical approaches. *Semin Plast Surg.* 2017;31(4):177−188.
11. Patel A, Groppo E. Management of temporal bone trauma. *Craniomaxillofacial Trauma Reconstr.* 2010;3(2):105−113.
12. Bell RB, Dierks EJ, Homer L, Potter BE. Management of cerebrospinal fluid leak associated with craniomaxillofacial trauma. *J Oral Maxillofac Surg.* 2004;62(6):676−684.
13. Friedman JA, Ebersold MJ, Quast LM. Post-traumatic cerebrospinal fluid leakage. *World J Surg.* 2001;25(8):1062−1066.
14. Stone JA, Castillo M, Neelon B, Mukherji SK. Evaluation of CSF leaks: high-resolution CT compared with contrast-enhanced CT and radionuclide cisternography. *AJNR Am J Neuroradiol.* 1999;20(4):706−712.
15. Meurman OH, Irjala K, Suonpää J, Laurent B. A new method for the identification of cerebrospinal fluid leakage. *Acta Otolaryngol.* 1979;87(3−4):366−369.
16. Lewin W. Cerebrospinal fluid rhinorrhea in nonmissile head injuries. *Clin Neurosurg.* 1964;12:237−252.
17. Prosser JD, Vender JR, Solares CA. Traumatic cerebrospinal fluid leaks. *Otolaryngol Clin.* 2011;44(4):857−873 (vii).
18. MacGee EE, Cauthen JC, Brackett CE. Meningitis following acute traumatic cerebrospinal fluid fistula. *J Neurosurg.* 1970;33(3):312−316.
19. Kruse JJ, Awasthi D. Skull-base trauma: neurosurgical perspective. *J Craniomaxillofac Trauma.* 1998;4(2):8−14. discussion 17.
20. Kveton JF. Obliteration of mastoid and middle ear for severe trauma to the temporal bone. *Laryngoscope.* 1987;97(12):1385−1387.
21. Ratilal BO, Costa J, Sampaio C, Pappamikail L. Antibiotic prophylaxis for preventing meningitis in patients with basilar skull fractures. *Cochrane Database Syst Rev.* 2011; 8:Cd004884.
22. Sun DQ, Andresen NS, Gantz BJ. Surgical management of acute facial palsy. *Otolaryngol Clin.* 2018;51(6):1077−1092.
23. Humphrey CD, Kriet JD. Nerve repair and cable grafting for facial paralysis. *Facial Plast Surg.* 2008;24(2):170−176.
24. do Nascimento Remigio AF, Salles AG, de Faria JCM, Ferreira MC. Comparison of the efficacy of onabotulinumtoxinA and abobotulinumtoxinA at the 1: 3 conversion ratio for the treatment of asymmetry after long-term facial paralysis. *Plast Reconstr Surg.* 2015; 135(1):239−249.
25. Samii M, Tatagiba M. Skull base trauma: diagnosis and management. *Neurol Res.* 2002; 24(2):147−156.
26. Yoganandan N, Pintar FA, Sances Jr A, et al. Biomechanics of skull fracture. *J Neurotrauma.* 1995;12(4):659−668.
27. Mack KF, Kempf HG, Lenarz T. [Patients with trauma-induced deafness—rehabilitation using a cochlear implant]. *Wien Med Wochenschr.* 1997;147(10):249−251.

28. Schuknecht HF. Mechanism of inner ear injury from blows to the head. *Ann Otol Rhinol Laryngol*. 1969;78(2):253–262.
29. Carney N, Totten AM, O'Reilly C, et al. Guidelines for the management of severe traumatic brain injury, fourth edition. *Neurosurgery*. 2017;80(1):6–15.
30. Goldfarb A, Eliashar R, Gross M, Elidan J. Middle cranial fossa cholesteatoma following blast trauma. *Ann Otol Rhinol Laryngol*. 2001;110(11):1084–1086.

Vascular injury following lateral skull base trauma: diagnosis and management

10

Syeda Maheen Batool[1,a], **Robert M. Gramer**[1,a], **Justin E. Vranic**[1,2], **Christopher J. Stapleton**[1]

[1]*Department of Neurosurgery, Massachusetts General Hospital, Boston, MA, United States;*
[2]*Department of Radiology, Massachusetts General Hospital, Boston, MA, United States*

Introduction

Head trauma has been cited as the most frequent clinical presentation in the emergency department. According to a 2013 survey by American College of Surgeons, nearly 800 trauma admissions were reported across different healthcare facilities in the United States. Additionally, skull base injuries were seen in one-third of the patients.[1] The reported incidence is even greater in the developing countries or regions of limited healthcare access. Traumatic brain injury (TBI) therefore represents a global health problem contributing to high rates of in-hospital morbidity and mortality.

Etiology

The etiology can be broadly classified into penetrating and nonpenetrating trauma. Nonpenetrating injuries have been identified as the leading causes of skull base fractures with a prevalence of 7%—16%.[2] This usually includes high-velocity trauma including motorized vehicle collisions (MVCs), blunt cerebrovascular injury (BCVI) via falls, and assaults. Penetrating trauma (mostly gunshot wounds) accounts for less than 10% of the cases.[2,3] Identification of skull base fractures often prompts assessment of coexisting orbital and facial fractures in addition to intracranial lesions. The extent of potential vascular complications and resulting management depends on the location and pattern of the fracture, which is in turn determined by the mechanism of injury and type of impact.

---

[a] These authors are co-first authors.

Skull base anatomy

The skull base is made up of seven bones, the paired frontal and temporal bones, and the unpaired ethmoid, sphenoid, and occipital bones. It is divided into anterior, central, and posterior regions, which form the floor of the anterior, middle, and posterior cranial fossae.

The anterior skull base (ASB), formed by the frontal and ethmoid bones, separates the anterior and inferior frontal lobes and olfactory structures within the anterior cranial fossa from the orbits and the sinonasal cavity. Anterior fossa is bound by important structures: The lateral and anterior borders are formed by the frontal bone and frontal sinus, and floor is formed by the cribriform plates and roof of the ethmoid sinuses. Lesser wing of the sphenoid bone, including the clinoid process, forms the posterior border between the anterior and central skull base. Anterior and posterior ethmoid artery foramina are located in ASB.

The central skull base (CSB), formed by the sphenoid and anterior temporal bones, is closely related to the pituitary gland, cavernous sinuses, and the temporal lobes superiorly, and the sphenoid sinus anteriorly and inferiorly. The anterior border of the CSB is formed by the posterior margin of the lesser wing of the sphenoid bone, clinoid process, and tuberculum sella. The floor is formed by the greater wing and central body of the sphenoid bone, the sphenoid sinus, and the sella. The posterior border between the central and posterior skull base is formed by the superior margin of the petrous ridge of the temporal bone, the basi sphenoid portion of the clivus, and the dorsum sella. Important vascular structure in this par includes the internal carotid artery.

The posterior skull base (PSB) is formed by the posterior temporal bone and the occipital bone. The anterior border is formed by the petrous ridge of the temporal bone superiorly, and the clivus (basi occiput portion) inferiorly. Foramen magnum located in the PSB transmits the vertebral artery.

According to Van Huijzen's classification, extension lines from the suborbital fissure and the petrooccipital fissure intersect at the apex of the nasopharynx inside, pointing outward to the zygomatic bone and posterior margin of the mastoid process, respectively. The triangular area between the two lines is described as a lateral skull base and includes parapharyngeal space, infratemporal fossa, and pterygopalatine fossa. The lateral skull base houses important neurovascular structures including internal carotid artery, the lateral sinus, and sigmoid that will give the vein jugular, and petrosal sinus.[4]

A 5-year retrospective study of 1606 patients with skull base trauma reported the highest frequency of temporal bone (40%) involvement followed by orbital roof (24.1%), sphenoid (22.6%), occipital (15.4%), ethmoid (10.8%), and clival bone (1.03%).[5]

Blunt cerebrovascular injury classification

The diagnosis of vascular injury in association with skull base trauma is closely tied to the screening criteria used for patient evaluation. This then facilitates and determines the choice of diagnostic modalities and subsequent management.[6] Biffl et al. proposed a grading scale, Denver criteria, to assess blunt cerebrovascular injuries (BCVIs) and subsequent neurological outcomes: grade I (mild intimal injury or irregular intima), grade II (dissection with raised intimal flap/intramural hematoma/intraluminal thrombosis with luminal narrowing >25%), grade III (pseudoaneurysm), grade IV (vessel occlusion/thrombosis), and grade V (vessel transection).[7] This is commonly used for classification of blunt injury in carotid and vertebral arteries. A total of 76 patients presenting with blunt carotid arterial injury were included in the analysis. Grade I injuries were associated with the best prognosis, with two-thirds of cases resolving spontaneously. On the other hand, vascular transection (grade V) was shown to be refractory to any intervention. Based on their findings, Biff et al. recommended endovascular repair for grade II, III, IV, and V lesions in addition to systemic anticoagulation. Isolated heparin therapy was associated with progressing dissections (grade II) and less than 10% of pseudoaneurysms (grade III) healing.[7] Another clinically relevant tool is Memphis criteria.

Both Memphis (Table 10.1) and Denver criteria (Table 10.2) have been modified to further improve the utility of these tools in diagnostic settings.[8] Overall, introduction of the screening criteria in combination with advanced imaging has significantly improved the sensitivity of BCVI identification.

Trauma to the vertebral artery

Neurological compromise following vertebral artery injury can be significant secondary to ensuing ischemic and embolic sequelae. Vertebral artery injury usually presents as dissection with or without pseudoaneurysm formation, luminal stenosis, or an arteriovenous fistula formation. Blunt vertebral artery injuries are associated with 14%−24% morbidity and 8%−18% mortality[9−11].

Grade 1 (vessel lumen stenosis <25%) and grade 2 (luminal stenosis between 25% and 50%) injuries are the most common form of blunt vertebral artery (VA) injury. These low-grade injuries in hemodynamically stable patients can be managed

Table 10.1 Memphis screening criteria for blunt cerebrovascular injury (BCVI).

Modified memphis criteria
◆ Basilar skull fracture with involvement of the carotid canal
◆ Basilar skull fracture with involvement of petrous bone
◆ Cervical spine fracture
◆ Neurological exam not explained by brain imaging
◆ Horner's syndrome
◆ LeFort II or III fracture pattern
◆ Neck soft tissue injury (seatbelt sign or hanging or hematoma)

Table 10.2 Denver screening criteria for blunt cerebrovascular injury (BCVI).

Modified denver criteria

Signs and symptoms

◆ Potential arterial hemorrhage from the neck, nose, or mouth
◆ Cervical bruit in patients <50 y of age
◆ Expanding neck hematoma
◆ Focal neurologic deficit (transient ischemic attack, hemiparesis, vertebrobasilar symptoms, Horner's syndrome)
◆ Neurologic deficit not explained by imaging findings
◆ Stroke CT or MRI**High-energy trauma and additional risk factors:**
◆ Le Fort II or III displaced midface fracture
◆ Mandibular fracture
◆ Complex skull fracture
◆ Base of skull fracture (sphenoid, petrous temporal, clivus, and occipital condyle fractures)
◆ Scalp degloving
◆ Cervical spine fracture, subluxation, or ligamentous injury
◆ Severe traumatic brain injury with Glasgow Coma Scale <6
◆ Near hanging with hypoxic–ischemic brain injury
◆ Clothesline-type injury or seat belt abrasion with significant swelling, pain, or altered mental status
◆ Traumatic brain injury with thoracic injuries including upper rib fractures, thoracic vascular injuries, and cardiac rupture

by pharmacological treatment, including acetylsalicylic acid or other antiplatelet or anticoagulant. One study, analyzing a similar group of patients, reported radiological improvement (stable/improved/resolved) in 97.4% of low-grade blunt VA injuries after conservative management.[12] Endovascular therapy with stent placement is preferred in selected situations: (1) hemodynamically unstable dissection, (2) recurrent thromboembolic events, and (3) contraindication to anticoagulant therapy.[13] However, there is no general consensus on the practices related to screening, management, and follow-up of VA injuries. Important variables to consider include the duration of the anticoagulation and risk of posterior circulation strokes. In a retrospective study, Scott et al. reported posterior circulation strokes in only 1.7% of the cases. Interestingly, these infarcts were demonstrated by neuroimaging in the acute period of hospitalization (within 4 days of injury) and showed no correlation to the pharmacological treatment.[12] Another study also reported similar findings in Biffl grade V VA injuries with stroke rates unrelated to the presence of emboli or antiplatelet drugs.[14]

High-grade traumatic vertebral artery injury (TVAI) is most difficult to treat and can lead to a potentially fatal posterior circulation stroke. The variable clinical presentation and lack of widely accepted diagnosis and management guidelines make it a clinical challenge. Patients may have a delayed onset of neurological symptoms including headache, hemiplegia, gait ataxia, and/or position-associated dizziness.[15] However, due to compensatory mechanisms, the majority of the cases of TVAI are asymptomatic, therefore making early screening important. Cerebral catheter angiography (CTA) is considered to be the gold standard for TVAI diagnosis. A high sensitivity of 99% and the ability to initiate timely treatment make it the most widely used screening modality.[16] While medical therapy with anticoagulation is aimed at reducing disease progression and thrombotic sequelae, studies have reported complications of stroke (1.8%–3.8%, first or recurrent) and intracranial hemorrhage (0.5%).[17] However, antiplatelet therapy does help prevent in-stent stenosis. Surgical treatments include ligation and vascular reconstruction.[18] Revascularization is performed in cases of no bleeding and small aneurysm. Life-threatening neurological deterioration with uncontrollable hemorrhage warrants an open surgery. Direct open surgery otherwise is not routinely performed due to vertebral artery anatomy and its location within the transverse foramen, limiting exposure and access.[19] There is extensive literature advocating the safety of adopting an endovascular approach. The minimally invasive and effective treatment modality has shown to be associated with good clinical and angiographic outcomes with no stent-related complications and new-onset neurological symptoms during follow-ups.[20,21] Common interventions include stent placement, stent-assisted coiling, and vessel occlusion. A study discussed important variables to consider to devise endovascular treatment strategies. Based on their findings, two approaches were proposed depending on the diameter of the parent artery (D) and caliber of the neck of the aneurysm (d): (1) $D > d$, exclusive stenting and (2) $D < d$, combined endovascular tools (stent angioplasty, coils, balloon, liquid glue) to maintain steady blood flow dynamics.[15] This is because an aneurysmal wall is subject to greater stress from blood flow when the parent artery is thinner, thereby increasing the risk of aneurysm rupture, which requires filling in the sac. Randomized clinical trials and long-term follow-up studies are needed to establish conclusive findings about endovascular management of high-grade TVAI.

Direct vertebral arteriovenous fistula may result from penetrating trauma (stab wounds, projectile injury, iatrogenic). The fistulous connection of the injured vertebral artery is usually occluded using detachable endovascular coils, placed proximal and distal to the site of fistula formation. Often, proximal occlusion combined with a retrograde microcatheter from the contralateral vertebral artery is sufficient. Assessment of fistula recurrence is made using long-term follow-up with delayed angiography to ensure no collateral pathways develop.[13]

Carotid-cavernous fistulas

Sphenoid body fractures (seen in 50% of sphenoid fractures), including sellar and clival involvement, are associated with increased risk of carotid injury. Carotid-cavernous (CC) fistula represents a pathologically created direct communication between carotid artery and venous channels in the cavernous sinus, thereby creating a high-flow fistula (Fig. 10.1). An anatomical–radiographic (Barrow et al.) classification can be used for patient evaluation: (1) type A, high-flow shunts between the

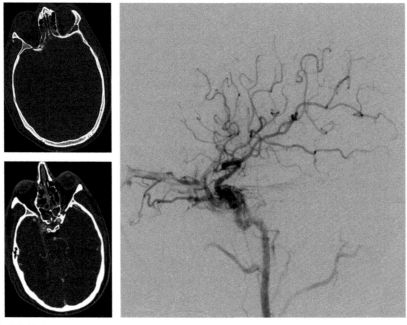

FIGURE 10.1

Traumatic right carotid-cavernous fistula (CCF) following motor vehicle accident (MVA).

internal carotid artery (ICA) and the cavernous sinus, (2) type B, between meningeal branches of the iICA and the cavernous sinus, (3) type C, between meningeal branches of the external carotid artery (ECA) and the cavernous sinus, and (4) type D, between meningeal branches of both ICA and ECA and the cavernous sinus.[22] Further subclassification of traumatic CC fistulas (Barrow type A) can be performed via angiographic evaluation of the opacification of anterior cerebral artery (ACA) and middle cerebral artery (MCA): small-size (opacification of both ACA and MCA), medium-size (opacification of either ACA or MCA), and large-size fistula (opacification of neither ACA nor MCA).[23]

Depending on the type of injury, the onset of symptoms may be within hours (direct shunt) or weeks to months (indirect shunt) after injury. CC fistulas usually present with Dandy's triad of exophthalmos, bruit, and conjunctival chemosis. Other clinical manifestations include ophthalmoplegia (cranial nerves III, IV, VI), epistaxis, diplopia, and progressive visual loss.[24,25] Pathologic mechanisms contributing to visual decline include reversal of venous drainage, arterial flow into the superior ophthalmic vein, increased intraocular venous pressure, and eventually ischemic optic neuropathy. The incidence in untreated CC fistulas can be as high as 89%, thereby warranting an early intervention.[26] Prior studies have reported high morbidity (32%–67%) and mortality (17%–38%).[27]

The gold standard for diagnosis of CC fistulas is four-vessel digital subtraction cerebral angiography. With evolution in the treatment strategies, endovascular embolization is the intervention of choice. Prior to endovascular treatment, management of Barrow type A CC fistulas comprised muscle occlusion and/or carotid artery ligation. In addition to procedural risks, these methods were associated with a high recurrence rate due to collaterals.[28,29] There are multiple approaches to endovascular treatment. One group described the transarterial route through the carotid artery. Approaches that could aid better localization of rent in the carotid artery include use of higher magnification rates and use of a microwire for exploration of the carotid artery wall. Following access to fistula, access is maintained using a microcatheter advanced into the cavernous sinus. This is followed by the placement of long coils into the cavernous sinus. One method to prevent coil placement in carotid artery lumen is use of a balloon in carotid-cavernous artery to help distinguish cavernous sinus from ICA. Both coils and detachable balloons can be used for embolization of the fistula. The selection of detachable balloon as an embolic material has shown to be cheaper. However, studies have demonstrated higher failure rates (5% −10%).[30] Additionally, unexpected balloon detachment can lead to embolism and stroke. Therefore, anticipation of embolic materials and understanding of fistula size is crucial to avoid unfavorable outcomes.[23] If direct transarterial approach is not feasible due to inability to advance the microcatheter through the rent in the carotid artery, embolization can be performed via venous access through the inferior petrosal sinus or superior ophthalmic vein. Small patient population−based studies using superior ophthalmic vein have reported no complications.[31] Superior ophthalmic vein can be accessed through direct puncture or ophthalmologic cutdown.[32,33] As a last resort, the carotid artery may be sacrificed to occlude the CC fistula.

Traumatic intracranial aneurysms

Traumatic aneurysms of the intracranial arteries are rare, accounting for less than 1% of all cerebral aneurysms. However, in injuries secondary to penetrating trauma, the incidence can be as high as 20%−50%.[34,35] Common etiologies include motor vehicle accidents and falls. These include both true aneurysms with all three arterial wall layers or pseudoaneurysms with no wall layers. The risk of rupture of untreated intracranial aneurysms is highest in the first 3 weeks postinjury, with a mortality of 50%. The risk of mortality is even greater with conservative versus surgical treatment.

The pathologic outpouching of vessel walls commonly involves intracavernous ICA, infraclinoid carotid artery, and vertebrobasilar artery. Infraclinoid segment represents the transitional zone between the relatively fixed cavernous and mobile supraclinoid segments of ICA.[36] In distal circulation, anterior cerebral artery (ACA, pericallosal, and callosomarginal segments) and, less frequently, middle cerebral artery (MCA) are involved.[37] Fleischer et al. reported 41 cases of traumatic aneurysms, with distal branches of MCA involved in 50% cases.[38] Traumatic intracranial aneurysms (TICAs) can be classified based on location relative to circle of Willis: proximal to circle of Willis (supraclinoid carotid, infraclinoid carotid, and vertebrobasilar arteries), distal to circle of Willis (subcortical and cortical arteries).[36] Mao et al. further classify TICAs into perifalx and distal cortical aneurysmal. Perifalx aneurysms are located on distal ACA, posterior cerebral artery, and superior cerebellar artery. Distal cortical aneurysms involve cortical branches of MCA or ACA.[39]

Common clinical features include cranial nerve palsies, epistaxis, subarachnoid hemorrhage, and mass effect. Average duration to the onset of hemorrhage from injury is 3 weeks. Clinical presentation can vary depending on the location of the aneurysm.[35,40] Infraclinoid ICA aneurysms usually present acutely with epistaxis, progressive cranial nerve palsies, and diabetes insipidus.[35,37] Supraclinoid ICA, distal ACA, and distal cortical aneurysm have a delayed onset of severe symptoms. The patient may report sudden onset of headache and/or altered sensorium secondary to subarachnoid hemorrhage.[41,42] It is important to look for signs of intracerebral bleed in these cases. Buckingham et al. reported findings from 11 patients presenting with distal cortical aneurysms. Subarachnoid hemorrhage was seen in 63% of the cases, with only 20% of the aneurysms being diagnosed before rupture.[37]

Intracranial aneurysms are a rare complication of skull base trauma. At present, CT scans are more commonly employed as primary investigation tools in closed head injury. This versus cerebral angiography may lead to more intracranial aneurysms being overlooked or misdiagnosed. There is no general consensus on the timing of performing cerebral angiography. While multiple studies have recommended different time frames, clinical presentation and risk of impending hemorrhage are important factors to consider. CT angiography (CTA) has emerged as a noninvasive screening tool for TICAs. However, given the limited sensitivity, some studies suggest use of digital subtraction angiography (DSA) following negative findings on CTA as a necessary confirmation tool.[43,44]

The high risk of aneurysm rupture warrants treatment. Overall, surgical management of TICAs is challenging due to its pathological complexity and close anatomical relations to the skull base. As the mainstay treatment of intracranial aneurysms, clipping is also an important surgical intervention for TICAs. However, for TICAs, it may not always be feasible due to absence of neck, poorly defined wall, and arachnoidal adhesions. These anatomic features present a higher risk of intraoperative rupture of TICAs during clipping.[45] Therefore, it is important to plan ahead of the procedure. Alternative interventions include trapping, excision, and wrapping of the aneurysm. To be noted, studies have shown high prevalence of recurrence and rupture with wrapping.[46] For PICA aneurysms, one option is PICA-PICA bypass and sacrifice of the vertebral artery given adequate flow in the contralateral circulation.[47] Both surgical clipping and endovascular occlusion can be challenging for management of infraclinoid ICA aneurysm. It is helpful to determine the feasibility of proximal ICA ligation or external carotid–internal carotid (EC-IC) bypass before securing ICA. This can be done preoperatively using a balloon test occlusion.[36] Endovascular occlusion can also be performed if anatomy favors coiling. However, TICAs tend to be small with no true arterial wall, leading to risk of rupture. A study assessed the outcomes of endovascular approach in 13 patients presenting with TICAs

(MCA = 7, ACA = 2, ICA = 4). Glasgow Outcome Scale (GOS) was determined: five patients with a score of 5, seven patients scored 7, and one patient had 3.[48]

Trauma to the middle meningeal artery

Temporal bone fractures are commonly associated with complication of middle meningeal artery (MMA) lesions. Common clinical presentations of MMA lesion include the formation of an epidural or subdural hematoma. It is important to note that while MMA rupture classical presents as epidural hemorrhage, this pathology can be multifactorial and occur secondary to lesions involving middle meningeal vein, diploic veins, and venous sinuses.[49] Fishpool et al. reported important anatomical observations of MMA vasculature at the level of greater wing of sphenoid bone and foramen spinosum. Investigation of 29 cadaveric specimens revealed that dural venous sinuses accompany MMA throughout its course forming a plexiform arrangement around the artery caudal to the foramen spinosum.[50] The authors therefore postulated that epidural hemorrhage was less likely due to an exclusive MMA lesion.[50] Clinical presentation can be divided into three phases: consciousness, lucid interval, and rapid neurological deterioration.

Pseudoaneurysms as previously described commonly involve carotid arteries. However, skull base trauma can also lead to rare MMA pseudoaneurysms. Around 70%–90% of cases occur secondary to fractures of temporal bone.[51] The pathogenesis involves a tear in the MMA, which is in turn sealed by a clot. This is followed by recanalization and formation of a false lumen. The resulting pseudoaneurysm enlarges over time and can lead to epidural hematoma if ruptured[52–55]. Very rarely, traumatic pseudoaneurysm of MMA (TPMMA) can also present as intraparenchymal hemorrhage (IPH). While the exact pathogenesis remains unclear, a study hypothesized that progressive thinning of dura secondary to TPMMA enlargement may contribute to delayed IPH.[56] Less than 10 cases have been reported in literature.[53,56] There are two case reports presenting findings of acute IPH secondary to ruptured TPMMA. In both cases, there was a dural defect secondary to dual contact with ruptured TPMMA.[57,58] Sudden and abrupt neurological deterioration in a patient with temporal bone fracture should raise a strong suspicion for TPMMA. This manifestation usually occurs following a latent period of 10–21 days from the initial injury. Studies have also reported clinical presentation of intractable epistaxis secondary to arterial wall weakening and adjacent bony erosion.[59,60]

Middle meningeal arteriovenous fistulas (MMAVFs) are rare and likely underreported lesions occurring between middle meningeal artery and neighboring veins (diploic vein, meningeal vein, cortical vein) or dural venous sinuses (petrosal sinus)[61–66]. Freckmann et al. investigated 446 angiograms of patients presenting with trauma. In this population, the incidence of MMAVFs was 1.8%.[63] These lesions pose a high risk of intracranial hemorrhage and may explain manifestations of nonaneurysmal SAH. Sakata et al. reported findings of diffuse, basal SAH preceded by a progressively enlarging MMAVF with dilated intracranial venous drainage. This was postulated to occur secondary to formation and rupture of a venous aneurysm.[67]

Initial screening modality is computed tomography (CT). It is important to mention that since routine arteriography has now largely been replaced by CT in the initial management, a large proportion of lesions go misdiagnosed. Therefore, there has been an increase in the number of cases presenting with delayed intracranial hemorrhage following skull base trauma. Main treatment modalities for TPMMA include surgical excision, endovascular treatment with detachable coils, and N-butyl-cyanoacrylate. Selective embolization of the parent artery has several advantages: better localization and visualization of the feeding vessels, greater access to distal vessels, rapid turnover, and preservation of ECA branches.[68,69]

For management of MMAVFs there is no comprehensive comparison of prognosis following conservative versus surgical intervention. The natural history of the lesion is therefore unclear. However, some studies have reported successful outcomes following endovascular obliteration. Liquid embolic agents (onyx) and more dilute preparations (e.g., n-BCA) have been proposed depending on several anatomic considerations: location and size of fistula, degree of vessel tortuosity, and feasibility of navigation.[70]

Venous epidural hematomas

As previously described, most epidural hematomas result from the MMA lesion (Fig. 10.2). Less frequently, epidural hematoma (EDH) can also originate from rupture of arachnoid granulations, diploic emissary veins, and dural sinuses. They have been described as bifrontal (detach first third of sagittal sinus), biparietal or vertex, and bioccipital (detach posterior third of sagittal longitudinal sinus) EDH[71-73]. Presence of adequate collateral venous drainage is associated with lower mortality in anterior superior sagittal sinus (SSS, 17%) versus central and posterior lesions (50%).[74,75] Goal of intervention is to decompress neural structures and arrest bleeding. The closer the EDH is located to the midline, the slower the bleeding. On exposure, the external surface of dura presents with diffuse bleeding, making it difficult to locate the bleeding source. Surgical management of venous sinus–related EDH is traditionally a craniotomy and evacuation of the clot. This has been well described for transverse sinus.[76,77] However, this poses a greater risk of damage to sinus and limited visibility to identify the bleeding spot. Hence, multiple studies have reported using a strip of bone overlying the sinus. In this technique, strip craniotomy, clot is then progressively resected from the periphery.[77,78]

Cerebral venous sinus thrombosis

Cerebral venous sinus thrombosis (CVST) most commonly manifests secondary to skull base fracture occurring close to dural sinus or jugular bulb[79-82]. Fractures of the petrous temporal bone are usually associated with injury to transverse sinus,

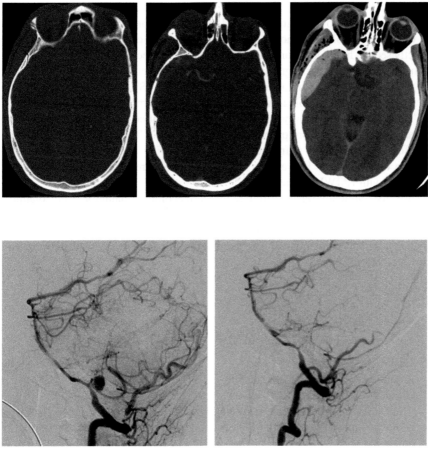

FIGURE 10.2

Epidural hematoma secondary to middle meningeal artery (MMA) lesion following a fall.

sigmoid sinus, and jugular bulb. Occipital bone fractures usually can extend to superior sagittal sinus.[79] The pathogenesis remains poorly understood. It is hypothesized that endothelial injury caused by direct compression of the sinus triggers activation of the coagulation cascade.[37,83] Other proposed mechanisms include extension of thrombus from injured emissary vein, compression of sinus from intracranial edema, and intramural hemorrhages.[79]

Clinical presentation is variable and nonspecific, closely related to the location of thrombus and extent of elevation of intracranial pressure (ICP). CVST has often been associated with delayed intracerebral hemorrhage (ICH).[79,81] Hence, timely diagnosis is of paramount importance and requires a high index of clinical suspicion since imaging modalities may report normal findings due to subacute clinical course.[84] Around 40% patients present with a stroke-like syndrome within 48 h of symptom onset, greater than 50% present within 1 month, and less than 10% present with chronic symptoms of greater than 1-month duration.[85]

CT is the radiological modality of choice. In some cases, the thrombus can be directly seen as hyperdense on plain CT. However, indirect signs are more frequently seen and include delta sign, cord/dense sign, and empty delta sign (contrast CT).[80,84,86,87] If the CT findings are suggestive of CVST, CT venography (CT-V) can be performed to reliably identify the occlusion in cerebral veins and sinuses.[88,89]

Treatment predominantly consists of systemic anticoagulation to prevent secondary complications from propagation of thrombus.[90] There is evidence in literature for the use of both unfractionated heparin (UFH) and low-molecular-weight heparin (LMWH).[91,92] However, a single-center RCT reported significantly lower mortality with LMWH versus UFH.[93]

It is also clinically relevant to initiate pharmacologic (mannitol, acetazolamide, hypertonic saline) treatment for lowering of ICP.[94] Lastly, if there is worsening neurological deterioration or poor response to treatment, surgical decompression or endovascular treatments such as chemical thrombolysis or mechanical thrombectomy can also be considered.[95]

General management

Clinical presentation

- History and exam
- Assessment of hemodynamic stability
- Glasgow Coma Scale (GCS) score
- Clinical findings (periorbital ecchymosis, Battle sign [postauricular ecchymosis], hemotympanum, epistaxis, CSF otorrhea or rhinorrhea, and cranial nerve deficits)

Imaging modalities

CT remains the first-line imaging modality in acute trauma. Thin-slice (0.6–1.0 mm) axial images extend from the skull vertex through the facial bones. Coronal and sagittal reformatted images can be utilized for assessing injuries to the anterior and central skull base (ASB and CSB)[96–98].

Additional imaging using CT angiography (CTA) can be performed for assessment of vascular injuries, fractures through the carotid canal (CSB), or clivus. It can also be helpful in diagnosis and/or management of dissection, traumatic pseudoaneurysm, or presence of carotid-cavernous fistula.[96,97,99] This modality is commonly used in blunt trauma based on Denver and Memphis criteria.[96]

CT venogram is performed in skull base fractures (e.g., posterior fossa) extending into the major venous sinuses (transverse sinus, sigmoid sinus, jugular foramen).[96] It is usually used for confirmation of venous sinus thrombosis following presence of equivocal findings on initial CT.

Magnetic resonance imaging (MRI) is not routinely used for initial diagnosis. However, it provides important prognostic information on the extent of primary lesions and secondary complications.[96]

Bibliography

1. Baugnon KL, Hudgins PA. Skull base fractures and their complications. *Neuroimaging Clin N Am*. 2014;24:439−465. vii−viii.
2. Yilmazlar S, Arslan E, Kocaeli H, et al. Cerebrospinal fluid leakage complicating skull base fractures: analysis of 81 cases. *Neurosurg Rev*. 2006;29:64−71.
3. Samii M, Tatagiba M. Skull base trauma: diagnosis and management. *Neurol Res*. 2002; 24:147−156.
4. van Huijzen C. Anatomy of the skull base and the infratemporal fossa. *Adv Oto-Rhino-Laryngol*. 1984;34:242−253.
5. Lemole M, Behbahani M. Retrospective study of skull base fracture: a study of incidents, complications, management, and outcome overview from trauma-one-level institute over 5 years. *J Neurol Surg B Skull Base*. 2013;74.
6. Burlew CC, Biffl WL, Moore E, Barnett CC, Johnson JL, Bensard DD. Blunt cerebrovascular injuries: redefining screening criteria in the era of noninvasive diagnosis. *J Trauma Acute Care Surg*. 2012;72, 330−5; discussion 336−7, quiz 539.
7. Biffl WL, Moore EE, Offner PJ, Brega KE, Franciose RJ, Burch JM. Blunt carotid arterial injuries: implications of a new grading scale. *J Trauma*. 1999;47:845−853.
8. Ciapetti M, Circelli A, Zagli G, et al. Diagnosis of carotid arterial injury in major trauma using a modification of Memphis criteria. *Scand J Trauma Resuscitation Emerg Med*. 2010;18:61.
9. Miller PR, Fabian TC, Bee TK, et al. Blunt cerebrovascular injuries: diagnosis and treatment. *J Trauma*. 2001;51:279−285. discussion 285−6.
10. Timpone V, Schneider BE, Sherman PM. Screening CT angiography for detection of blunt carotid and vertebral artery injury in the setting of combat-related trauma. *Mil Med*. 2013;178:416−420.
11. Biffl WL, Moore EE, Elliot JP, et al. The devastating potential of blunt vertebral arterial injuries. *Ann Surg*. 2000;231:672−681.
12. Scott WW, Sharp S, Figueroa SA, Madden CJ, Rickert KL. Clinical and radiological outcomes following traumatic Grade 1 and 2 vertebral artery injuries: a 10-year retrospective analysis from a Level 1 trauma center. *J Neurosurg*. 2014;121:450−456.
13. Dahlin BC, Waldau B. Surgical and nonsurgical treatment of vascular skull base trauma. *J Neurol Surg B Skull Base*. 2016;77:396−403.
14. Morton RP, Hank BW, Levitt MR, et al. Blunt traumatic occlusion of the internal carotid and vertebral arteries. *J Neurosurg*. 2014;120:1446−1450.
15. Mei Q, Sui M, Xiao W, et al. Individualized endovascular treatment of high-grade traumatic vertebral artery injury. *Acta Neurochir*. 2014;156:1781−1788.
16. Eastman AL, Chason DP, Perez CL, McAnulty AL, Minei JP. Computed tomographic angiography for the diagnosis of blunt cervical vascular injury: is it ready for primetime? *J Trauma*. 2006;60:925−929. discussion 929.
17. Edwards NM, Fabian TC, Claridge JA, Timmons SD, Fischer PE, Croce MA. Antithrombotic therapy and endovascular stents are effective treatment for blunt carotid injuries:

results from longterm followup. *J Am Coll Surg*. 2007;204:1007−1013. discussion 1014−5.

18. Yamada K, Hayakawa T, Ushio Y, et al. Therapeutic occlusion of the vertebral artery for unclippable vertebral aneurysm: relationship between site of occlusion and clinical outcome. *Neurosurgery*. 1984;15:834−838.

19. Eskander MS, Drew JM, Aubin ME, et al. Vertebral artery anatomy: a review of two hundred fifty magnetic resonance imaging scans. *Spine*. 2010;35:2035−2040.

20. Lee Y-J, Ahn JY, Han IB, Chung YS, Hong CK, Joo JY. Therapeutic endovascular treatments for traumatic vertebral artery injuries. *J Trauma*. 2007;62:886−891.

21. Wang H, Orbach DB. Traumatic dissecting aneurysm at the vertebrobasilar junction in a 3-month-old infant: evaluation and treatment strategies. Case report. *J Neurosurg Pediatr*. 2008;1:415−419.

22. Barrow DL, Spector RH, Braun IF, Landman JA, Tindall SC, Tindall GT. Classification and treatment of spontaneous carotid-cavernous sinus fistulas. *J Neurosurg*. 1985;62:248−256.

23. Chi CT, Nguyen D, Duc VT, Chau HH, Son VT. Direct traumatic carotid cavernous fistula: angiographic classification and treatment strategies. Study of 172 cases. *Intervent Neuroradiol*. 2014;20:461−475.

24. Li J, Lan Z-G, Xie X-D, You C, He M. Traumatic carotid-cavernous fistulas treated with covered stents: experience of 12 cases. *World Neurosurgery*. 2010:73 514−519.

25. Vadivelu S, Bell RS, Crandall B, DeGraba T, Armonda RA. Delayed detection of carotid-cavernous fistulas associated with wartime blast-induced craniofacial trauma. *Neurosurg Focus*. 2010;28:E6.

26. King Jr GL. Pulsating exophthalmos. *Am J Ophthalmol*. 1931;14:786−791.

27. Fabian TC, Patton JH, Croce MA, Minard G, Kudsk KA, Pritchard FE. Blunt carotid injury. Importance of early diagnosis and anticoagulant therapy. *Ann Surg*. 1996;223, 513−22; discussion 522−5.

28. Brooks B. The treatment of traumatic arteriovenous fistula. *South Med J*. 1930;23:100−106.

29. Parkinson D. Carotid cavernous fistula: direct repair with preservation of the carotid artery. Technical note. *J Neurosurg*. 1973;38:99−106.

30. Naesens R, Mestdagh C, Breemersch M, Defreyne L. Direct carotid-cavernous fistula: a case report and review of the literature. *Bull Soc Belge Ophtalmol*. 2006:43−54.

31. Monsein LH, Debrun GM, Miller NR, Nauta HJ, Chazaly JR. Treatment of dural carotid-cavernous fistulas via the superior ophthalmic vein. *AJNR Am J Neuroradiol*. 1991;12:435−439.

32. Dashti SR, Fiorella D, Spetzler RF, Albuquerque FC, McDougall CG. Transorbital endovascular embolization of dural carotid-cavernous fistula: access to cavernous sinus through direct puncture: case examples and technical report. *Oper Neurosurg*. 2011:68 ons75−ons83.

33. Wolfe SQ, Cumberbatch NMA, Aziz-Sultan MA, Tummala R, Morcos JJ. Operative approach via the superior ophthalmic vein for the endovascular treatment of carotid cavernous fistulas that fail traditional endovascular access. *Neurosurgery*. 2010;66:293−299. discussion 299.

34. Rosenfeld JV, Bell RS, Armonda R. Current concepts in penetrating and blast injury to the central nervous system. *World J Surg*. 2015;39:1352−1362.

35. Larson PS, Reisner A, Morassutti DJ, Abdulhadi B, Harpring JE. Traumatic intracranial aneurysms. *Neurosurg Focus*. 2000;8:e4.

36. Bhaisora KS, Behari S, Godbole C, Phadke RV. Traumatic aneurysms of the intracranial and cervical vessels: a review. *Neurol India*. 2016;64(Suppl):S14−S23.

37. Buckingham MJ, Crone KR, Ball WS, Tomsick TA, Berger TS, Tew Jr JM. Traumatic intracranial aneurysms in childhood: two cases and a review of the literature. *Neurosurgery*. 1988;22:398−408.

38. Fleischer AS, Patton JM, Tindall GT. Cerebral aneurysms of traumatic origin. *Surg Neurol*. 1975;4:233−239.

39. Mao Z, et al. Traumatic intracranial aneurysms due to blunt brain injury-a single center experience. *Acta Neurochir*. 2012;154:2187−2193. discussion 2193.

40. Holmes B, Harbaugh RE. Traumatic intracranial aneurysms: a contemporary review. *J Trauma*. 1993;35:855−860.

41. Parkinson D. Traumatic aneurysms. *Surg Neurol*. 1985;23:453−454.

42. Bavinzski G, Killer M, Knosp E, Ferraz-Leite H, Gruber A, Richling B. False aneurysms of the intracavernous carotid artery—report of 7 cases. *Acta Neurochir*. 1997;139: 37−43.

43. Dubey A, Sung W-S, Chen Y-Y, et al. Traumatic intracranial aneurysm: a brief review. *J Clin Neurosci*. 2008;15:609−612.

44. Cohen JE, Gomori JM, Segal R, et al. [p 476] results of endovascular treatment of traumatic intracranial aneurysms. *Neurosurgery*. 2008;63:N4.

45. Levy ML, Rezai A, Masri LS, et al. The significance of subarachnoid hemorrhage after penetrating craniocerebral injury: correlations with angiography and outcome in a civilian population. *Neurosurgery*. 1993;32:532−540.

46. He Y, Wang L, Ou Y, et al. Surgical treatment of traumatic distal anterior cerebral artery aneurysm: a report of nine cases from a single centre. *Acta Neurochir*. 2020;162: 523−529.

47. Korja M, Sen C, Langer D. Operative nuances of side-to-side in situ posterior inferior cerebellar artery-posterior inferior cerebellar artery bypass procedure. *Neurosurgery*. 2010;67:471−477.

48. Cohen JE, et al. Results of endovascular treatment of traumatic intracranial aneurysms. *Neurosurgery*. 2008;63:476−485. discussion 485−6.

49. Aguiar G, Silva J, Souza R, Acioly MA. Skull base fracture involving the foramen spinosum - an indirect sign of middle meningeal artery lesion: case report and literature review. *Turk Neurosurg*. 2015;25:317−319.

50. Fishpool SJC, Suren N, Roncaroli F, Ellis H. Middle meningeal artery hemorrhage: an incorrect name. *Clin Anat*. 2007;20:371−375.

51. Kawaguchi T, Kawano T, Kaneko Y, Ooasa T, Ooigawa H, Ogasawara S. Traumatic lesions of the bilateral middle meningeal arteries—case report. *Neurol Med Chir*. 2002;42: 221−223.

52. Gu J, Lu J, Wang X, Liu Z, Gao G, Zhang S. Traumatic middle meningeal artery pseudoaneurysms presenting with intractable epistaxis: a rare case report and review of literature. *Clin Med Insights Case Rep*. 2015;04:28−31.

53. Wu X, Jin Y, Zhang X. Intraparenchymal hematoma caused by rupture of the traumatic pseudoaneurysm of middle meningeal artery. *J Craniofac Surg*. 2014;25:e111−e113.

54. de Andrade AF, Figueiredo EG, Caldas JG, et al. Intracranial vascular lesions associated with small epidural hematomas. *Neurosurgery*. 2008;62:416−420. discussion 420−1.

55. Roski RA, Owen M, White RJ, Takaoka Y, Bellon EM. Middle meningeal artery trauma. *Surg Neurol*. 1982;17:200−203.

56. Montanari E, Polonara G, Montalti R, et al. Delayed intracerebral hemorrhage after pseudoaneurysm of middle meningeal artery rupture: case report, literature review, and forensic issues. *World Neurosurg.* 2018;117:394−410.

57. Kumar RJ, Sundaram PK, Gunjkar JD. Traumatic giant pseudoaneurysm of the middle meningeal artery causing intracerebral hematoma. *Neurol India.* 2011;59:921−922.

58. Moon JU, Youn SH, Suh J-H, Kim MS. Acute intraparenchymal hemorrhage caused by rupture of a traumatic pseudoaneurysm of the middle meningeal artery: a case report. *Interdiscip Neurosurg.* 2020;22:100801.

59. Chen D, Concus AP, Halbach VV, Cheung SW. Epistaxis originating from traumatic pseudoaneurysm of the internal carotid artery: diagnosis and endovascular therapy. *Laryngoscope.* 1998;108:326−331.

60. Zhang CW, Xie XD, You C, et al. Endovascular treatment of traumatic pseudoaneurysm presenting as intractable epistaxis. *Korean J Radiol.* 2010;11:603−611.

61. Chandrashekar HS, Nagarajan K, Srikanth SG, Jayakumar PN, Vasudev MK, Pandey P. Middle meningeal arteriovenous fistula and its spontaneous closure. A case report and review of the literature. *Intervent Neuroradiol.* 2007;13:173−178.

62. Fincher EF. Arteriovenous fistula between the middle meningeal artery and the greater petrosal sinus; case report. *Ann Surg.* 1951;133:886−888.

63. Freckmann N, Sartor K, Herrmann HD. Traumatic arteriovenous fistulae of the middle meningeal artery and neighbouring veins or dural sinuses. *Acta Neurochir.* 1981;55:273−281.

64. Ishii R, Ueki K, Ito J. Traumatic fistula between a lacerated middle meningeal artery and a diploic vein; case report. *J Neurosurg.* 1976;44:241−244.

65. Liu AH, Lv X, Li Y, Lv M, Wu Z. Traumatic middle meningeal artery and fistula formation with the cavernous sinus: case report. *Surg Neurol.* 2008;70:660−663.

66. Markham JW. Arteriovenous fistula of the middle meningeal artery and the greater petrosal sinus. *J Neurosurg.* 1961;18:847−848.

67. Sakata H, Nishimura S, Mino M, et al. Serial angiography of dynamic changes of traumatic middle meningeal arteriovenous fistula: case report. *Neurol Med Chir.* 2009;49:462−464.

68. Mehta S, Alawi A, Edgell RE-. 073 endovascular treatment of a traumatic middle meningeal artery pseudoaneurysm with onyx LES: a case report and review of literature. *J Neurointerventional Surg.* 2014;6. A73−A73.

69. Singam P, Thanabalan J, Mohammed Z. Superselective embolisation for control of intractable epistaxis from maxillary artery injury. *Biomed Imaging Interv J.* 2011;7:e3.

70. Almefty RO, Kalani MYS, Ducruet AF, Crowley RW, McDougall CG, Albuquerque FC. Middle meningeal arteriovenous fistulas: a rare and potentially high-risk dural arteriovenous fistula. *Surg Neurol Int.* 2016;7:S219−S222.

71. Guha A, Perrin RG, Grossman H, Smyth HS. Vertex epidural hematomas. *Neurosurgery.* 1989;25:824−828.

72. Jones TL, Crocker M, Martin AJ. A surgical strategy for vertex epidural haematoma. *Acta Neurochir.* 2011;153:1819−1820.

73. Ceylan S, Kuzeyli K, Baykal S, Akturk F. Bilateral posterior fossa epidural hematoma—report of two cases. *Neurol Med Chir.* 1992;32.

74. Kim Y-S, Jung S-H, Lim D-H, Kim T-S, Kim J-H, Lee J-K. Traumatic dural venous sinus injury. *Korean J Nutr.* 2015;11:118−123.

75. Meirowsky AM. Wounds of dural sinuses. *J Neurosurg.* 1953;10:496−514.

76. Fernandes-Cabral DT, Kooshkabadi A, Panesar SS, et al. Surgical management of vertex epidural hematoma: technical case report and literature review. *World Neurosurg*. 2017; 103:475−483.

77. Parker SL, Cabana AA, Conner CR, et al. Management of venous sinus-related epidural hematomas. *World Neurosurg*. 2020;138:e241−e250.

78. Bimpis A, Marcus HJ, Wilson MH. Traumatic bifrontal extradural haematoma resulting from superior sagittal sinus injury: case report. *JRSM Open*. 2015;6, 2054270415579137.

79. Delgado Almandoz JE, Kelly HR, Schaefer PW, Lev MH, Gonzalez RG, Romero JM. Prevalence of traumatic dural venous sinus thrombosis in high-risk acute blunt head trauma patients evaluated with multidetector CT venography. *Radiology*. 2010;255: 570−577.

80. Lakhkar B, Lakhkar B, Singh BR, Agrawal A. Traumatic dural sinus thrombosis causing persistent headache in a child. *J Emergencies, Trauma, Shock*. 2010;3:73−75.

81. Hsu P-J, Lee C-W, Tang S-C, Jeng J-S. Pearls & Oysters: delayed traumatic intracerebral hemorrhage caused by cerebral venous sinus thrombosis. *Neurology*. 2014;83: e135−e137.

82. Awad A-W, Bhardwaj R. Acute posttraumatic pediatric cerebral venous thrombosis: case report and review of literature. *Surg Neurol Int*. 2014;5:53.

83. Dalgiç A, Secer M, Ergungor F, Okay O, Akdag R, Ciliz D. Dural sinus thrombosis following head injury: report of two cases and review of the literature. *Turk Neurosurg*. 2008;18:70−77.

84. Weimar C, Masuhr F, Hajjar K. Diagnosis and treatment of cerebral venous thrombosis. *Expert Rev Cardiovasc Ther*. 2012;10:1545−1553.

85. Ferro JM, Canhao P, Stam J, Bousser M-G, Barinagarrementeria F, ISCVT Investigators. Prognosis of cerebral vein and dural sinus thrombosis: results of the international study on cerebral vein and dural sinus thrombosis (ISCVT). *Stroke*. 2004;35:664−670.

86. Selim M, Caplan LR. Radiological diagnosis of cerebral venous thrombosis. *Front Neurol Neurosci*. 2008;23:96−111.

87. Coutinho JM, van den Berg R, Zuurbier SM, et al. Small juxtacortical hemorrhages in cerebral venous thrombosis. *Ann Neurol*. 2014;75:908−916.

88. Khandelwal N, Agarwal A, Kochhar R, et al. Comparison of CT venography with MR venography in cerebral sinovenous thrombosis. *AJR Am J Roentgenol*. 2006;187: 1637−1643.

89. Casey SO, Alberico RA, Patel M, et al. Cerebral CT venography. *Radiology*. 1996;198: 163−170.

90. Coutinho J, de Bruijn SF, Deveber G, Stam J. Anticoagulation for cerebral venous sinus thrombosis. *Cochrane Database Syst Rev*. 2011:CD002005.

91. Einhäupl KM, Villringer A, Meister W, et al. Heparin treatment in sinus venous thrombosis. *Lancet*. 1991;338:597−600.

92. de Bruijn SF, Stam J. Randomized, placebo-controlled trial of anticoagulant treatment with low-molecular-weight heparin for cerebral sinus thrombosis. *Stroke*. 1999;30: 484−488.

93. Misra UK, Kalita J, Chandra S, Kumar B, Bansal V. Low molecular weight heparin versus unfractionated heparin in cerebral venous sinus thrombosis: a randomized controlled trial. *Eur J Neurol*. 2012;19:1030−1036.

94. Saposnik G, Barinagarrementeria F, Brown Jr RD, et al. Diagnosis and management of cerebral venous thrombosis: a statement for healthcare professionals from the American Heart Association/American Stroke Association. *Stroke*. 2011;42:1158−1192.

95. Canhão P, Falcão F, Ferro JM. Thrombolytics for cerebral sinus thrombosis: a systematic review. *Cerebrovasc Dis*. 2003;15:159−166.

96. Adams A. Imaging of skull base trauma: fracture patterns and soft tissue injuries. *Neuroimaging Clin N Am*. 2021;31:599−620.

97. Skull base and facial trauma overview. In: *Imaging in Otolaryngology*. Elsevier; 2018: 384−387.

98. Skull base trauma. In: *Imaging in Otolaryngology*. Elsevier; 2018:390.

99. Greinwaldjr J. Temporal bone and skull base trauma. In: Neurotology *1070−1088*. Elsevier; 2005.

Facial nerve injury following temporal bone fracture: diagnosis and management

11

Yohan Song, MD[1], Amy F. Juliano, MD[2], Felipe Santos, MD[1]

[1]*Department of Otolaryngology-Head and Neck Surgery, Massachusetts Eye and Ear, Harvard Medical School, Boston, MA, United States;* [2]*Department of Radiology, Massachusetts Eye and Ear, Harvard Medical School, Boston, MA, United States*

Background

Temporal bone trauma accounts for 5% of all facial palsy cases[1,2] and 3% of all bilateral facial palsy.[3] Only 7% of temporal bone fractures result in facial palsy and 25% of those result in complete facial paralysis.[4] Historically, temporal bone fractures have been classified as either longitudinal or transverse, a classification scheme that refers to the direction of the fracture with respect to the long axis of the petrous temporal bone.[5] Another classification scheme differentiates a fracture based on whether it involves or spares the otic capsule.[6] Approximately 30% −50% of patients with a transverse fracture pattern have facial nerve injury resulting in paralysis.[7,8] The transverse fracture pattern is associated with more severe facial nerve injury and portends a poorer prognosis when compared with the longitudinal fracture pattern.[9] Facial nerve injury occurs in only 10%−20% of patients with longitudinal fractures in comparison.[7,9,10] Otic capsule violating fractures are quite rare (less than 6%) compared with otic capsule sparing fractures (>94%), and facial nerve injury is twice as common in otic capsule violating fractures than in its counterpart.[6,11]

Evaluation

It is estimated that close to 1900 lbs of force is necessary to fracture a temporal bone.[12] As such, patients presenting with facial palsy following a temporal bone fracture often present with other injuries. A CT temporal bone protocol with 0.625-mm-thick slices is best suited to evaluate the fracture pattern. Multiplanar formats can be created to enable fracture pattern interpretation that may be difficult to see on routine axial and coronal planes.[13]

In an awake and cooperative patient, a careful history and physical exam should be performed. Patients lucid enough to provide an accurate history should be asked about the mechanism of injury, any lapses in memory or loss of consciousness, vision changes, presence of hearing loss or vertigo, or clear rhinorrhea or otorrhea. A full head and neck examination should be performed. One of many findings may be visible on otoscopic exam including a fracture extending into the EAC with disruption of the canal skin, rupture of the tympanic membrane, ossicular dislocation, clear otorrhea, and hemotympanum. A tuning fork exam may demonstrate sensorineural hearing loss, particularly for fractures violating the otic capsule. Conductive hearing loss may be present for patients with ossicular disruption or middle ear fluid or blood. A full cranial nerve examination should be performed. Documenting the initial facial nerve function is important in predicting nerve recovery, determining need for further electrodiagnostic studies, and deciding on the candidacy for surgical decompression.

In light of the degree of force necessary to cause a temporal bone fracture, many patients present with other concomitant injuries that necessitate intubation and sedation. In an intubated and sedated patient, a physical examination may be very limited. A sternal rub may stimulate the patient enough so that a grimace can be elicited. However, until the sedation can be held and the patient's medical condition is stabilized, it may not be possible to obtain an accurate facial nerve examination in the acute setting.

Timing and extent of facial paralysis

Traumatic facial nerve injury can be classified into immediate-onset complete paralysis or delayed-onset or incomplete paralysis.[4,14] Patients with immediate-onset complete facial nerve paralysis have a poor prognosis of achieving full recovery. A systematic review of 35 studies showed that only 36% of patients with immediate-onset paralysis recovered fully without intervention, while 80% of patients with delayed-onset paralysis recovered fully.[15] Similarly, only 57% patients with complete facial nerve paralysis achieved full facial nerve recovery without intervention compared with 82% of patients with partial facial nerve paralysis. Some studies cite recovery rates of delayed-onset incomplete paralysis as >90%.[16,17]

Patients with incomplete paralysis have excellent long-term outcomes, and patients with <90% degeneration on electroneurography (ENOG) testing expected to regain close to or normal facial function.[4,18] As such, while patients with immediate-onset complete paralysis should undergo electrodiagnostic studies to determine if they are operative candidates, patients with delayed-onset or incomplete paralysis may be observed since there is a high likelihood of full facial nerve recovery.

It is often not possible to determine the nature and onset of the paralysis due to a patient's intubation status or other coexisting injuries. In patients whose history and exam are unreliable, electrodiagnostic studies are important to determine whether surgical decompression would be beneficial.

Fallopian canal fracture pattern

The course of the facial nerve can be anatomically divided into five segments: (1) intracranial, (2) internal auditory canal, (3) labyrinthine, (4) tympanic, and (5) mastoid. The facial nerve traverses through the bony fallopian canal, which can be variably dehiscent. Various fallopian canal fracture patterns have been described (Fig. 11.1). The perigeniculate region between the labyrinthine and tympanic segment is the most common site of facial nerve injury in temporal bone fractures.[19−23] It is affected in approximately 80%−90% of cases. The next most common site is the mastoid segment making up 10%−20% of cases.[11,21] Tympanic segment fractures are the least common, with a prevalence of around 5%.[11,21] The perigeniculate region is thought to the be the most prone area to facial nerve injury not only because the nerve is tethered by the greater superficial petrosal nerve as the labyrinthine segment turns into the tympanic segment, but also because the meatal foramen and labyrinthine segment are the narrowest portions of the fallopian canal that can predispose the nerve to ischemic injury from perineural edema.[24] Facial nerve injury from temporal fractures can also result from extratemporal and internal auditory canal fractures.

Electrodiagnostic tests

Electrodiagnostic testing is indicated for patients with immediate-onset or unknown onset of facial paralysis as it can help determine the prognosis of nerve recovery and identify patients who may be candidates for surgical decompression. The utility of electrodiagnostic testing has been studied most extensively in acute facial paralysis resulting from Bell's palsy[25−27]. Many facial nerve injuries resulting from temporal bone trauma can have a similar pathophysiology and pathway of nerve degeneration as Bell's palsy and can be managed similarly.[28] These types of injuries are typically more subtle on imaging and likely result from perineural edema leading to a similar nerve degeneration cascade as that seen in Bell's palsy. Electrodiagnostic testing could be helpful in these cases. In more severe injuries with obvious nerve displacement or transection on imaging, electrodiagnostic testing may be of limited utility since the extent of the injury may already indicate the need for surgical exploration and possible nerve repair. Electrodiagnostic testing is not indicated in patients with incomplete or delayed paralysis since those patients carry a favorable prognosis. ENOG and electromyography (EMG) are the two most useful electrophysiologic tests available.

Wallerian degeneration, wherein the axon distal to the site of injury degenerates, begins 72 h after injury and continues for about 2 weeks.[11] ENOG estimates the proportion of nerve fibers that have degenerated and is useful between day 4−14 after

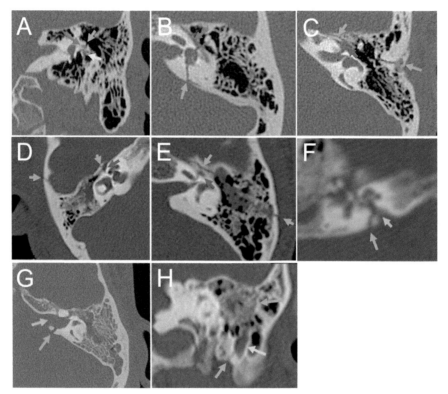

FIGURE 11.1

(A) coronal CT image of the left temporal bone showing a fracture through the second genu of the fallopian canal. Tympanic segment of the facial nerve is labeled with *orange arrow*, and vertical segment of the facial nerve is labeled with a *yellow arrow*. *Blue arrow* labels the fracture line. (B) Axial scan of a left temporal bone fracture (*blue arrow*) through the vestibule and tympanic segment of the facial nerve (*orange arrow*). (C) Axial scan of a left temporal bone with a longitudinal fracture (*blue arrow*) from the mastoid cavity extending anteriorly lateral to the geniculate ganglion (*red arrow*). (D) Axial scan of a right temporal bone with a longitudinal fracture (*blue arrow*) involving the geniculate ganglion (*red arrow*). (E) Axial scan of a left temporal bone with a longitudinal fracture (*blue arrow*) involving the peri-geniculate region. Geniculate ganglion marked by red arrow. (F) Axial scan of a right temporal bone with a transverse fracture (*blue arrow*) involving the internal auditory canal (*green*). (G) Axial scan of a left temporal bone with a fracture (*blue arrow*) through the internal auditory canal (*green*). (H) Coronal scan of a left temporal bone with a fracture (*blue arrow*) through the mastoid segment of the facial nerve (*yellow arrow*).

the onset of injury.[29] Electrodiagnostic testing is not performed before day 4 since it takes 72 h for Wallerian degeneration to begin. Moreover, testing is typically not performed after 14 days since if the ENOG continues to be favorable up to 14 days, the chance of recovery to HB 1 or 2 has been shown to be nearly 100%,[18] and patients are not considered to be candidates for surgery. However, a recent study by Remenschneider et al. argues for longer serial electrodiagnostic testing of up to 2 months for facial palsy resulting from temporal bone trauma since some patients with initially favorable testing can develop degeneration beyond 2 weeks.[30]

ENOG is performed by applying a supramaximal electrical current at the stylomastoid foramen and measuring the response as a compound muscle action potential (CMAP), while EMG measures voluntary motor activity by placing electrodes in the orbicularis oculi and oris muscles. The CMAP in ENOG estimates the number of remaining nerve fibers after Wallerian degeneration that remain viable.[31] The CMAP on the affected side is compared with that of the unaffected side, and a percentage is calculated.[32] If 90% or greater degeneration is reached within 14 days of the injury, an EMG is performed to determine the presence of "deblocking."[33] Deblocking refers to the process by which asynchronous discharge of actively regenerating nerve fibers and motor units can cause phase cancellation of the overall electrical output and thereby reduce the CMAP amplitude. The presence of deblocking suggests a favorable prognosis for nerve recovery. Patients with deblocking on EMG should be observed despite the degree of degeneration seen on ENOG.

Management

The management of facial palsy depends on the timing and degree of paralysis (Fig. 11.2). Patients with delayed-onset or incomplete facial paralysis should be treated nonsurgically with high-dose corticosteroids.[6,11,34] Patients can be started on 1 mg/kg per day of prednisone or an equivalent dose of steroid with a 1–3 week taper.[6] As mentioned before, these patients have an excellent prognosis in achieving full recovery.

Patients with immediate-onset complete paralysis or those with an uncertain onset can undergo further electrodiagnostic testing to determine the prognosis of facial nerve recovery and surgical candidacy. It is important to note that much of the data establishing the utility of electrodiagnostic testing in stratifying surgical versus nonsurgical patients in the setting of acute facial palsy have been derived from Bell's palsy studies.[25−27,32,33] Depending on the type of injury, traumatic facial nerve palsy can have similarities and differences in pathophysiology as that in Bell's palsy. Traumatic facial nerve palsies that are a result of a stretch or shear injury from nondisplaced uncomplicated fallopian canal fracture may have a nerve injury undergoing a degenerative cascade similarly seen in Bell's palsy as the nerve swells in an enclosed bony canal. These types of facial palsies can be worked up and managed similarly as Bell's palsy with electrodiagnostic testing between days 4−14, and considering surgical decompression if ENOG shows >90% degeneration and there

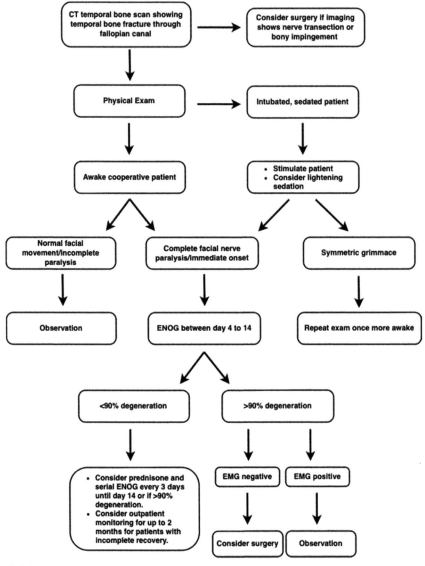

FIGURE 11.2

Flowchart demonstrating management options following fallopian-canal involving temporal bone fractures.

is absence of deblocking on EMG.[28] Surgical decompression in these cases would be focused on the site of injury based on the fracture pattern (Figs. 11.3 and 11.4). In contrast, in traumatic facial nerve palsies with imaging showing complete nerve transection or evidence of a penetrating injury from displaced bony fragments,

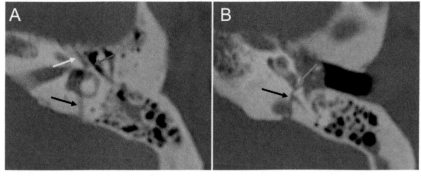

FIGURE 11.3

(A) CT temporal bone fracture demonstrating fracture line (*black arrow*) through lateral semicircular canal and through the horizontal (tympanic) segment of the facial nerve (*red arrow*). Horizontal segment of the facial nerve is labeled with *yellow arrow*. (B) Fracture line (*black arrow*) involving the round window niche (*orange arrow*).

surgical intervention would be favored for exploration and potential nerve repair. The algorithm for managing Bell's palsy may not be applicable in these cases.

In patients with immediate-onset complete paralysis, a surgical decompression and nerve repair may offer a chance for improved facial nerve outcomes of HB III or better. Cannon et al.[35] reported a retrospective review of 18 patients who underwent MF surgical decompression for labyrinthine, perigeniculate, and tympanic segment injuries and a mastoidectomy for descending segment injuries. Indications for surgery in this study included immediate-onset complete facial paralysis (HB VI), >90% degeneration on ENOG testing, and no voluntary EMG responses, presenting within 14 days of injury. For irreversible injuries or nerve transection, a nerve graft was placed. All 18 patients achieved a facial nerve recovery of HB 3 or better. In patients with intact facial nerves, 73% of patients achieved normal or near normal facial nerve function within 1 year. All patients who required nerve grafting improved to an HB III.

Controversy exists regarding the ideal timing for surgical decompression. In general, decompression and nerve repair in patients meeting surgical criteria should be done within 14 days of the injury.[35] Several studies have shown that early decompression <14 days was associated with improved facial nerve recovery[36–38]. Hato et al. demonstrated that there was a 93% rate of recovery to HB I and HB II if patients were decompressed within 2 weeks, compared with only a 63% rate of achieving the same recovery for patients decompressed after 2 weeks.[38] However, others have reported a 78% rate of recovery to HB I and HB II in patients decompressed 1–3 months after injury.[39] Another study did not find a significant difference in facial nerve recovery between early (within 1 month) decompression compared with decompression in 2–3 months.[40] These studies suggest that while patients with traumatic facial palsy may benefit from early decompression (within 14 days), those who present later may also benefit from surgical decompression.

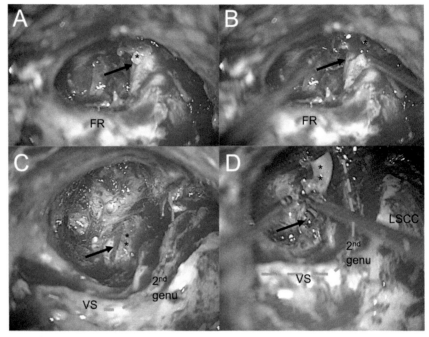

FIGURE 11.4

Intraoperative photographs of a canal wall down cavity from patient with CT scan shown in Fig. 11.3. (A) *Black arrow* points to the fracture line through the tympanic segment of the fallopian canal. *Asterisk marks* flail bone segment. FR = facial ridge. (B) *Black arrow* points to the fracture line through the horizontal segment of the fallopian canal. *Asterisk marks* flail bone segment. Facial nerve is unroofed. FR = facial ridge. (C) *Black arrow* points to fracture line through the round window niche. *Double asterisk* labels a flail otic capsule bone. *Dotted green lines* show the course of the facial nerve. VS = vertical segment (of the fallopian canal). (D) *Black arrow* points to fracture line through round window niche. *Double asterisk* labels the flail bone segment, now displaced anteriorly exposing the basilar membrane. *Dotted green lines* show the course of the facial nerve VS = vertical segment (of the fallopian canal). LSCC = lateral semi-circular canal.

Conclusion

The management of facial palsy from temporal bone trauma depends critically on the timing and extent of paralysis. Patients with incomplete and delayed paralysis can have excellent outcomes and can be managed nonsurgically, while those with complete and immediate-onset paralysis can be worked up similarly as seen in Bell's palsy with electrodiagnostic testing assuming no obvious structural injuries to the nerve such as complete transection or nerve impingement by a bony fragment. Evidence suggests that surgical decompression can offer a chance of recovery in select patients. Every intervention should be customized for each patient with detailed counseling on the risks and benefits.

References

1. Hohman MH, Hadlock TA. Etiology, diagnosis, and management of facial palsy: 2000 patients at a facial nerve center. *Laryngoscope*. 2014;124(7). https://doi.org/10.1002/lary.24542.
2. Steenerson RL. Bilateral facial paralysis. *Am J Otol*. 1986;7(2):99−103. https://doi.org/10.1111/j.1525-1497.2006.00466.x.
3. Glasscock ME, Wiet RJ, Jackson CG, Dickins JRE. Rehabilitation of the face following traumatic injury to the facial nerve. *Laryngoscope*. 1979;LXXXIX(9):1389−1404. https://doi.org/10.1288/00005537-197909000-00004.
4. Brodie HA, Thompson TC. Management of complications from 820 temporal bone fractures. *Am J Otol*. 1997;18(2):188−197.
5. Tos M. Course of and sequelae to 248 petrosal fractures. *Acta Otolaryngol*. 1973;75(2−6):353−354. https://doi.org/10.3109/00016487309139745.
6. Dahiya R, Keller JD, Litofsky NS, Bankey PE, Bonassar LJ, Megerian CA. Temporal bone fractures: otic capsule sparing versus otic capsule violating clinical and radiographic considerations. *J Trauma Inj Infect Crit Care*. 1999;47(6):1079−1083. https://doi.org/10.1097/00005373-199912000-00014.
7. Grove WE. Skull fractures involving the ear. A clinical study of 211 cases. *Laryngoscope*. 1939;49(8):678−707. https://doi.org/10.1288/00005537-193908000-00005.
8. MCHUGH HE. Facial paralysis in birth injury and skull fractures. *Arch Otolaryngol*. 1963;78:443−455. https://doi.org/10.1001/archotol.1963.00750020455006.
9. Harker LA, McCabe BF. Temporal bone fractures and facial nerve injury. *Otolaryngol Clin*. 1974;7(2):425−431. https://doi.org/10.1016/s0030-6665(20)32849-8.
10. Kettel K. Management of peripheral facial palsies due to trauma. *Proc Roy Soc Med*. 1959;52:1069−1074.
11. Darrouzet V, Duclos JY, Liguoro D, Truilhe Y, De Bonfils C, Bebear JP. Management of facial paralysis resulting from temporal bone fractures: our experience in 115 cases. *Otolaryngol Head Neck Surg*. 2001;125(1):77−84. https://doi.org/10.1067/mhn.2001.116182.
12. Johnson F, Semaan MT, Megerian CA. Temporal bone fracture: evaluation and management in the modern era. *Otolaryngol Clin*. 2008;41(3):597−618. https://doi.org/10.1016/j.otc.2008.01.006.
13. Juliano AF, Ginat DT, Moonis G. Imaging review of the temporal bone: Part II. Traumatic, postoperative, and noninflammatory nonneoplastic conditions. *Radiology*. 2015;276(3):655−672.
14. Diamond C, Frew I. *The Facial Nerve*. Oxford University Press; 1979.
15. Nash JJ, Friedland DR, Boorsma KJ, Rhee JS. Management and outcomes of facial paralysis from intratemporal blunt trauma: a systematic review. *Laryngoscope*. 2010;120(suppl. 4). https://doi.org/10.1002/lary.21681.
16. Maiman DJ, Cusick JF, Anderson AJ, Larson SJ. Nonoperative management of traumatic facial nerve palsy. *J Trauma Inj Infect Crit Care*. 1985;25(7):644−648. https://doi.org/10.1097/00005373-198507000-00012.
17. McKennan KX, Chole RA. Facial paralysis in temporal bone trauma. *Am J Otol*. 1992;13(2):167−172.

18. Sillman JS, Niparko JK, Lee SS, Kileny PR. Prognostic value of evoked and standard electromyography in acute facial paralysis. *Otolaryngol Neck Surg.* 1992;107(3): 377−381. https://doi.org/10.1177/019459989210700306.

19. Coker NJ. Management of traumatic injuries to the facial nerve. *Otolaryngol Clin.* 1991; 24(1):215−227. https://doi.org/10.1016/s0030-6665(20)31176-2.

20. Coker NJ, Kendall KA, Jenkins HA, Alford BR. Traumatic infratemporal facial nerve injury: management rationale for preservation of function. *Otolaryngol Neck Surg.* 1987;97(3):262−269. https://doi.org/10.1177/019459988709700303.

21. Lambert P, Brackmann D. Facial paralysis in longitudinal temporal bone fractures: a review of 26 cases. *Laryngoscope.* 1984;94(8):1022−1026.

22. Lindeman RC. Temporal bone trauma and facial paralysis. *Otolaryngol Clin.* 1979; 12(2):403−413. https://doi.org/10.1016/s0030-6665(20)32474-9.

23. Schubiger O, Valavanis A, Stuckmann G, Antonucci F. Temporal bone fractures and their complications—examination with high resolution CT. *Neuroradiology.* 1986;28(2): 93−99. https://doi.org/10.1007/BF00327878.

24. Ge X-X, Spector GJ. Labyrinthine segment and geniculate ganglion of facial nerve in fetal and adult human temporal bones. *Ann Otol Rhinol Laryngol.* 1981;90(4 II Suppl. 85):1−12. https://doi.org/10.1177/00034894810900s401.

25. Gantz BJ, Rubinstein JT, Gidley P, Woodworth GG. Surgical management of Bell's palsy. *Skull Base Surg.* 1999;9(4):308. https://doi.org/10.1097/00129492-200200001-00079.

26. Fisch U. Surgery for Bell's palsy. *Arch Otolaryngol.* 1981;107(1):1−11. https://doi.org/10.1001/archotol.1981.00790370003001.

27. Fisch U. Prognostic value of electrical tests in acute facial paralysis. *Am J Otol.* 1984; 5(6):494−498.

28. Sun DQ, Andresen NS, Gantz BJ. Surgical management of acute facial palsy. *Otolaryngol Clin.* 2018;51(6):1077−1092. https://doi.org/10.1016/j.otc.2018.07.005.

29. Gantz BJ. Traumatic facial paralysis. In: *Current Therapy in Otolaryngology Head and Neck Surgery.* BC Decker; 1987.

30. Remenschneider AK, Michalak S, Kozin ED, et al. Is serial electroneuronography indicated following temporal bone trauma? *Otol Neurotol.* 2017;38(4):572−576. https://doi.org/10.1097/MAO.0000000000001337.

31. Krarup C. Compound sensory action potential in normal and pathological human nerves. *Muscle Nerve.* 2004;29(4):465−483. https://doi.org/10.1002/mus.10524.

32. Gantz BJ, Holliday M, Gmuer AA, Fisch U. Electroneurographic evaluation of the facial nerve: method and technical problems. *Ann Otol Rhinol Laryngol.* 1984;93(4):394−398. https://doi.org/10.1177/000348948409300422.

33. Fisch U. Maximal nerve excitability testing vs electroneuronography. *Arch Otolaryngol.* 1980;106(6):352−357. https://doi.org/10.1001/archotol.1980.00790300040008.

34. Nosan DK, Benecke J, Murr AH. Current perspective on temporal bone trauma. *Otolaryngol Head Neck Surg.* 1997;117(1):67−71. https://doi.org/10.1016/S0194-5998(97)70209-2.

35. Cannon RB, Thomson RS, Shelton C, Gurgel RK. Long-term outcomes after middle fossa approach for traumatic facial nerve paralysis. *Otol Neurotol.* 2016;37(6): 799−804. https://doi.org/10.1097/MAO.0000000000001033.

36. Fisch U. Facial paralysis in fractures of the petrous bone. *Laryngoscope.* 1974;84(12): 2141−2154.

37. Fisch U. Management of intratemporal facial nerve injuries. *J Laryngol Otol.* 1980; 94(1):129−134. https://doi.org/10.1017/S0022215100088575.
38. Hato N, Nota J, Hakuba N, Gyo K, Yanagihara N. Facial nerve decompression surgery in patients with temporal bone trauma: analysis of 66 cases. *J Trauma Inj Infect Crit Care.* 2011;71(6):1789−1792. https://doi.org/10.1097/TA.0b013e318236b21f.
39. Quaranta A, Campobasso G, Piazza F, Quaranta N, Salonna I. Facial nerve paralysis in temporal bone fractures: outcomes after late decompression surgery. *Acta Otolaryngol.* 2001;121(5):652−655. https://doi.org/10.1080/000164801316878999.
40. Xu P, Jin A, Dai B, Li R, Li Y. Surgical timing for facial paralysis after temporal bone trauma. *Am J Otolaryngol—Head Neck Med Surg.* 2017;38(3):269−271. https://doi.org/10.1016/j.amjoto.2017.01.002.

Management of cerebrospinal fluid leak following lateral skull base trauma

Ricky Chae, BA [1,2]**, David H. Jung, MD, PhD** [3,4]**, Divya A. Chari, MD** [1,2,3,4]

[1]*T.H. Chan School of Medicine, University of Massachusetts Chan Medical School, Worcester, MA, United States;* [2]*Department of Otolaryngology-Head and Neck Surgery, University of Massachusetts Chan Medical School, Worcester, MA, United States;* [3]*Department of Otolaryngology-Head and Neck Surgery, Harvard Medical School, Boston, MA, United States;* [4]*Department of Otolaryngology-Head and Neck Surgery, Massachusetts Eye and Ear, Boston, MA, United States*

Introduction

Leakage of cerebrospinal fluid (CSF) can occur when a defect of the skull base and dura results in an abnormal communication between the subarachnoid space and nasal or middle ear cavities.[1,2] This pathologic entity was first reported by St Clair Thompson in 1899 and can occur in the nose (CSF rhinorrhea) or the ear (CSF otorrhea).[3] CSF leaks are further classified into traumatic and nontraumatic.[4] Traumatic cases account for 80% to 90% of CSF leaks and more commonly present with rhinorrhea (80%) than with otorrhea (20%) in adult patients.[1,3] Most traumatic CSF leaks are clinically evident within the first 2 days of injury and almost all within the first 3 months.[5,6]

CSF leaks that occur secondary to skull base fractures account for 2%−3% of all closed head injuries.[7−10] The most common fractures associated with posttraumatic CSF leakage involve the anterior skull base, including the frontal sinus and lateral lamella of the cribriform plate.[11,12] Approximately 12%−30% of patients with anterior skull base fractures develop a CSF leak,[13−15] which include those with a mild head injury as rated by the Glasgow Coma Scale.[8] Therefore, all closed head injuries should be evaluated for CSF leak. In addition, the incidence of anterior skull base CSF leaks is five to six times higher compared with that of the lateral skull base.[8,16] This is attributed to the firmer attachment of the dura to the anterior skull base, which may increase the likelihood of dural lacerations.[6]

In the setting of a lateral skull base trauma, CSF leakage typically courses through the middle cranial fossa (tegmen tympani and mastoideum) and into the epitympanic recess, antrum, and mastoid air cell tract.[17] Temporal bone fractures along the petrous bone and middle ear associated with dural defects may lead to CSF otorrhea if there is a perforation within the tympanic membrane, or CSF rhinorrhea via the Eustachian tube if the tympanic membrane is intact. In a retrospective study of 1773 patients with posttraumatic CSF leaks from the Taiwan Traumatic Brain Injury Registry System, the temporal bone was the most common fracture site (40.3%) for those with CSF otorrhea.[18] The mortality rate in patients with CSF otorrhea was 8.5%, and CSF rhinorrhea was 10.9% (33/302). These patients also had a higher rate of intracranial hemorrhage (64.7%) compared with those without CSF leakage (28.8%, $P < .001$). Furthermore, in a study of 13,861 pediatric patients admitted to the hospital with skull fractures, 1.46% of patients developed CSF leaks, of whom 58.4% presented with CSF otorrhea and 41.6% presented with rhinorrhea. Notably, patients with CSF leaks were more likely to have longer average hospitalizations (9.6 vs. 3.7 days, $P < .0001$) and higher rates of neurologic deficits (5.0% vs. 0.7%, $P < .0001$), meningitis (5.5 vs. 0.3%, $P < .0001$), and hospital readmission (24.7% vs. 8.5%, $P < .0001$) at 90 days.[19] Taken together, these studies elucidate the importance of diagnosing and managing skull base CSF leaks following traumatic injury.

Lateral skull base CSF leaks tend to have a higher likelihood of spontaneous resolution than anterior skull base CSF leaks.[15,20] In a review of 81 cases of posttraumatic CSF leaks, 17/28 (60.7%) of lateral skull base CSF leaks resolved spontaneously, compared with only 14/53 (26.4%) of anterior skull base leaks.[8] Similarly, in a retrospective study of 699 patients with 820 temporal bone fractures and 122 CSF leaks, 95/122 (77.9%) CSF leaks resolved spontaneously in less than 1 week, 21/122 (17.2%) in less than 2 weeks, and only 5/122 (4.1%) persisted.[21] Despite the higher rates of spontaneous resolution, lateral skull base CSF leak following traumatic injury must be appropriately evaluated and managed to reduce the risk of meningitis and other complications.

Spontaneous CSF leaks represent cases that present without distinct etiologies for the leak, such as trauma, surgery, and congenital anomalies. Recent studies have noted an increase in the incidence of spontaneous CSF leaks, exploring associations with rising obesity rates, obstructive sleep apnea, idiopathic intracranial hypertension, and superior semicircular canal dehiscence.[22–26] Unlike traumatic or intraoperative CSF leaks, spontaneous CSF leaks can have a more insidious presentation with nonspecific symptoms of otorrhea, hearing loss, and aural fullness.[27–30] The etiology underlying spontaneous lateral CSF leaks is not entirely well elucidated, but one theory posits that arachnoid granulations within the temporal bone respond to CSF pulsations, causing erosion of the skull base over time.[31]

History and physical exam

Unlike spontaneous CSF leaks in which the history can be vague, traumatic CSF leaks arise, by definition, from head trauma with associated skull base fractures. Nevertheless, while a CSF leak may be suspected, determining whether the otorrhea or rhinorrhea contains CSF can be challenging. When combined with blood, a CSF leak may stain as a "ring" or "halo" on an absorbent material. Caution must be taken when interpreting this finding, since a mixture of blood and other clear fluids can also present a similar stain.[32] Patients with traumatic injuries may also present with occult and delayed CSF leaks, with an average of 13 days posttrauma (range 1−30 days).[15] This delayed presentation could be due to herniation of dura into the bony defect, hematoma blocking CSF flow and leakage, slow resolution of edema, progressive increase in intracranial pressure, or wound contraction.[6,17] Patients with delayed presentation of CSF leak would also be at a risk of delayed meningitis. Signs of extensive skull base trauma including fractures of the otic capsule, facial nerve weakness, and ossicular chain discontinuity should increase suspicion for a traumatic CSF leak.

Physical exams should include a complete neurological and otologic exam, including an otoscopic exam to identify fluid. The tympanic membrane should be examined for a perforation or middle ear effusion. Nasal endoscopy can be used to identify whether there is transgression of clear rhinorrhea down the Eustachian tube into the nasopharynx.[30] Patients may describe a salty or sweet taste in their mouth, most commonly in a position of standing or learning forward. It is important to note that CSF rhinorrhea can present intermittently and even mimic other rhinologic pathologies including allergies, creating difficulties for diagnostic testing.[6] Furthermore, history and physical exam can be limited by the patient's physical and mental status secondary to the traumatic injury. Patients may have severe intracranial injuries or require intubation, which present challenges to the diagnostic evaluation of CSF leak.

An audiogram is an essential component of the workup to guide management for patients with a traumatic injury of the lateral skull base. In a retrospective review of pediatric patients with temporal bone fractures, 2.9% with otic capsule-sparing fractures developed sensorineural hearing loss, while 47.1% developed conductive hearing loss. Notably, conductive hearing loss often resolves over a period of 6 weeks to 3 months.[33−35] For example, a retrospective study of 173 patients with otic capsule-sparing temporal bone fractures demonstrated that the air−bone gap closed from 27.2 dB (average 22 days posttrauma) to 19.6 dB (average 80 days posttrauma) without surgical intervention.[33] Closure of the air−bone gap may be related to resolution of a middle ear effusion and/or a fibrous reattachment of the ossicles. All patients with otic capsule-violating fractures had sensorineural hearing loss, and 20% had CSF leaks.[36] In another study, Magliulo et al. reported that 42.5% of patients with otic capsule-violating injuries had CSF leaks.[37] The presence of a CSF effusion in the middle ear can cause a conductive hearing loss, which should resolve with management of the CSF leak.[38]

The diagnostic evaluation often involves confirmation of CSF leak by beta-2 transferrin analysis.[2] Beta-2 transferrin is a glycoprotein detected in CSF but not in nasal or middle ear drainage or tissue.[32] This allows beta-2 transferrin to be a marker for CSF rhinorrhea and otorrhea with a high sensitivity and specificity. In a prospective study on 205 patients with suspected CSF leak, 35 tested positive for beta-2 transferrin. Of those who tested positive, 34 were confirmed to be true positives through evaluating the patient's history, using radionuclide cisternography, and intraoperative visualization.[39] Additional advantages of beta-2 transferrin testing include its noninvasive approach and relatively low cost. However, disadvantages of this approach include the amount of fluid needed for the assay and the turnaround time, which can take up to 2 days.[40]

High-resolution computed tomography (HRCT) scan is a noninvasive modality for diagnosing CSF leak. This modality has been reported to be 87% accurate in demonstrating the presence of a CSF leak.[2] In a prospective study of 45 patients with suspected CSF rhinorrhea, HRCT accurately detected the presence or absence of CSF leak in 93% of patients.[41] This is attributed to the utility of HRCT in identifying bony defects and fractures that may indicate the site of CSF leakage. In particular, thin fractures within the temporal bone can be readily visualized with HRCT and increase confidence of a suspected diagnosis of CSF otorrhea or rhinorrhea. This includes determining whether the fracture spares (Fig. 12.1) or violates the otic capsule (Fig. 12.2), which will be important for clinical management. For traumatic injuries of the lateral skull base, physicians may be able to more easily identify the site of leakage using HRCT compared with a spontaneous CSF leak.

Magnetic resonance imaging (MRI) is another radiologic study that can be helpful in the diagnosis of CSF leak. This modality is noninvasive and involves detection of CSF on T2-weighted images with fat suppression. MRI has been associated with a sensitivity of 87%, though the combination of MRI and HRCT has been shown to

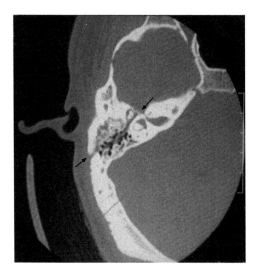

FIGURE 12.1

Axial-cut high-resolution computed tomography scan of an otic capsule–sparing temporal bone fracture. *Black arrow* indicates a longitudinal fracture line.

Adapted from Brodie HA. Management of temporal bone trauma. Cummings Otolaryngol Head Neck Surg. *2010; 2036–2047.*

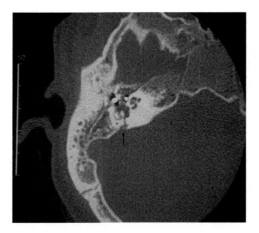

FIGURE 12.2

Axial-cut high-resolution computed tomography scan of an otic capsule—violating temporal bone fracture. *Black arrow* indicates a traverse fracture line.

Adapted from Brodie HA. Management of temporal bone trauma. Cummings Otolaryngol Head Neck Surg. 2010; 2036–2047.

have a sensitivity of 93% and specificity of 100%—all of which are slightly lower or comparable with those of HRCT.[42,43]

Other imaging modalities have been described, though these are not widely employed. Radionuclide cisternography involves intrathecal administration of a radiotracer isotope, indium-III diethylene-triaminepentaacetic acid, to assess CSF leaks. Notably, this technique requires patient follow-up over a period of 2–3 days following the injection.[44] In a retrospective review of 42 patients with CSF rhinorrhea and/or otorrhea, radionuclide cisternography had a sensitivity of 76% compared to 100% for high-resolution CT. Additionally, radionuclide cisternography did not detect CSF leaks in 29% of patients who had clinical evidence of CSF leaks. Other studies report a false positive rate of 33% and accuracy of 28% for patients with inactive leaks.[14,45] Considering the discomfort caused by intrathecal administration, need for follow-up, and relatively low sensitivity and accuracy, radionuclide cisternography should be reserved for patients with multiple skull base fractures, or clinical scenarios where the diagnosis may be otherwise uncertain. CT cisternography with contrast presents a similar case and involves an intrathecal administration of radiopaque contrast. As observed for radionuclide cisternography, the sensitivity of CT cisternography is low (48%)[44] compared with that of high-resolution CT (58.8%–100%).[42] The density of the dye may also lead to difficulties in locating the bony defect. Therefore, this imaging modality should primarily be used for active CSF leaks to increase its sensitivity. When there is concordance between clinical findings and high-resolution CT imaging, CT cisternography is typically unnecessary considering its poorer sensitivity and discomfort of intrathecal contrast for patients.

Intrathecal fluorescein can be used preoperatively or intraoperatively to identify and localize CSF leaks. This technique involves placing a lumbar subarachnoid catheter and administering an intrathecal injection of fluorescein. Although its use has not been approved by the U.S. Food and Drug Administration, several studies have shown that using a low dose of intrathecal fluorescein resulted in an acceptable safety profile and allowed for successful identification of CSF leaks, ranging from 59.7% to 80.5%.[46–48] For example, one study involving 419 patients undergoing endonasal endoscopic skull base surgery reported a sensitivity and specificity of 92.9% and 100%, respectively, for identification of intraoperative CSF leak using intrathecal fluorescein.[47] However, intraoperative fluorescein visualization should not be used alone to localize CSF leaks due to the presence of false negatives, which can be as high as 26.2%.[48] Additionally, safety concerns remain, with complications including seizure, hydrocephalus muscle paralysis, and radicular symptoms. To avoid these complications, intrathecal application of fluorescein should be limited to 2.5–50 mg (less than 5% concentration).[46]

Management

Management of lateral skull base CSF leaks following traumatic injury should be tailored according to the fracture characteristics, leakage site, and associated intracranial defects. An algorithm for management has been summarized in Fig. 12.3. Most lateral skull base CSF leaks spontaneously resolve.[8] To facilitate spontaneous resolution of the leak, intracranial pressure should be reduced by elevating the head of bed at least 30 degrees, encouraging total bed rest, ordering stool softeners, and informing the patient to avoid Valsalva maneuvers, sneezing, and nose blowing.[21] Conservative management can be employed for up to 10 days following the traumatic injury, with a goal of reducing active flow through the leak.[20] Physicians should be aware that strict bed rest increases the risk of deep vein thrombosis. These risks can be mitigated with the use of sequential compressive devices applied to the lower extremity.[49]

CSF may also be diverted with a lumbar drain or ventriculostomy to avoid infections and decompress the leak.[50,51] Acetazolamide is a carbonic anhydrase inhibitor that decreases CSF production and is used as a first-line treatment in idiopathic intracranial hypertension.[52,53] The use of acetazolamide in combination with CSF diversion has been reported to significantly reduce intracranial pressure within 4–6 h of drug administration.[53] Despite relatively widespread use of lumbar drains in the conservative management of CSF leaks, they are not without risk and may lead to increased hospital length of stay and costs, pneumocephalus, herniation, infection, and severe headaches if the drainage rate is too high.[20,32,54] In particular, studies have found a 5%–7% infection rate with lumboperitoneal or ventriculoperitoneal shunts.[55,56]

Conservative management may also include use of prophylactic antibiotics to reduce the risk of meningitis, though the timing and effectiveness of antibiotics

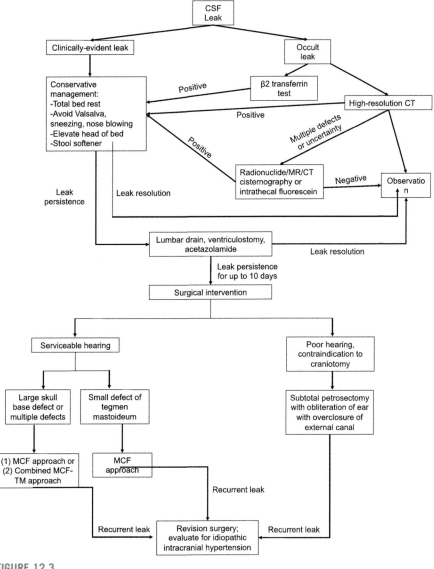

FIGURE 12.3

Algorithm for management of CSF leak.

remain controversial. Although most CSF leaks related to trauma will spontaneously resolve, 7%–30% of leaks may result in meningitis.[57] Some studies have found that using prophylactic antibiotics for CSF leaks in the skull base does not significantly decrease the risk of meningitis.[58–60] On the other hand, Friedman et al. found that only 10% of CSF leak patients treated with prophylactic antibiotics developed meningitis, compared with 21% of those who were not treated with antibiotics, though this was not statistically significant.[15] In a large metaanalysis, Brodie reported that the incidence of meningitis was 2.5% among 237 patients who received prophylactic antibiotics, compared with 10% among those who did not receive prophylaxis ($P = .006$).[61] The conflicting data between different studies may be attributed to including patients whose leaks spontaneously resolved within 24 h. One author has suggested using antibiotics for 72 h after the active leak has resolved, though more evidence is needed prior to widespread implementation of this practice pattern.[20]

If patients do not respond to conservative management within 7–10 days[60,61] or present with other complications related to the trauma, such as facial nerve paralysis and/or brain herniation, surgical intervention should be considered.[21] The most common intervention is a middle cranial fossa approach (48%–50%), followed by a combined transmastoid and middle cranial fossa approach (24%–29%), and transmastoid approach alone (20%–22%).[57,62] Selection of surgical approach is based on the size, location, number of skull base defects, and surgeon preference. In general, a middle fossa craniotomy is useful for large bony defects involving the tegmen tympani or petrous ridge.[63] A major advantage of this approach is the visualization of the entire middle cranial fossa floor when multiple defects are present (including asymptomatic defects) and the ability to place multiple layers of grafts.[22] However, elderly patients may be more susceptible to dural tears due to adherence of dura to the middle cranial fossa floor or thinning of dura over the defects.[64] Perioperative risks are low but include stroke, seizures, and intracranial and extracranial hematomas.[54]

The combined middle fossa craniotomy–transmastoid approach is typically used for large defects involving the tegmen tympani and mastoideum. This combined approach has been associated with the lowest leak recurrent rates[57] and is increasingly utilized in the recent literature.[65,66] This approach allows for a wide mastoidectomy to carefully inspect the middle cranial fossa floor and minimize the chance of overlooking other leak sites.[67]

The transmastoid approach can be effective for small tegmen mastoideum dehiscences. The primary advantage of this approach is that it avoids the risks of a craniotomy. One prospective study on temporal bone CSF leaks reported that 9 out of 15 patients were treated with the transmastoid approach and no leak was observed at follow-up.[64] Other studies report a 2%–14.5% recurrence rate of CSF leaks in transmastoid approaches.[66–68] In addition, the transmastoid approach has been associated with lower morbidity and shorter hospital length of stay compared with that of a middle cranial fossa approach (1.7 vs. 6.3 days),[69] though these findings may be confounded by the fact that craniotomy approaches could be favored in patients with greater preoperative trauma. Both middle cranial fossa and transmastoid approaches have been shown to result in acceptable hearing outcomes.[70,71] Nevertheless, the transmastoid approach presents with limitations for large tegmen tympani defects located anteriorly toward the petrous apex or at the level of the anterior epitympanum, which is less well visualized via this approach than an MCF approach, even if the ossicular chain is removed.[71]

Mastoid obliteration for management of a CSF leak is a definitive option. A major disadvantage of a mastoid obliteration, however, is that the patient is left with a maximal conductive hearing loss. In patients with ipsilateral severe or profound sensorineural hearing loss, a mastoid obliteration may therefore be the preferred surgical approach, but in patients with less severe hearing loss, other approaches may be preferable.[20,37,72,73] For patients with poor hearing (congenital or due to trauma), high risk of recurrent leaks (e.g., idiopathic intracranial hypertension, thinning of tegmen tympani and tegmen mastoideum, prior surgery, use of anticoagulants), medical comorbidities that contraindicate craniotomy, or bony defects with minimal chance of successful repair using the aforementioned surgical approaches, a subtotal petrosectomy with obliteration of ear with or without overclosure of external canal can be considered.[72,74]

Selection of reconstructive materials depends on the size and location of the defect and surgeon preference. Fascia, cartilage, pericranium, calvarial bone, synthetic materials such as hydroxyapatite bone cement and fibrin glue, rotational flaps, and free tissue transfer have all been used for repair of lateral skull base defects, both individually and in combination.[63,65,75−77] Notably, the choice of reconstructive material does not appear to significantly impact clinical outcomes for CSF leaks of the lateral skull base.[57,78] An exception is the use of artificial titanium mesh to reconstruct the middle fossa floor. In their retrospective review of 86 patients undergoing CSF leak repair, Carlson et al. report that the titanium mesh was associated with an increased risk of wound infection ($P = .039$), recurrent CSF leak ($P = .004$), and meningitis ($P = .014$).[79] If the CSF leak involves brain herniation, a three-layer closure technique can be employed: temporalis fascia as an extradural inlay graft, placement of intracranial bone graft, and temporalis fascia an extracranial onlay graft.[21] In a retrospective review of 92 patients undergoing repair of CSF leaks, the success rate was 100% for surgeries involving a multilayer closure technique, whereas the success rate was 76% for those involving a single-layer closure.[80]

Postoperative care for patients undergoing middle cranial fossa and combined approaches should involve admission to the intensive care unit with neurointensive monitoring.[57] Patients undergoing a transmastoid only approach can be admitted for brief observational admission. Pressure dressings may also be used for 48−72 h after surgery to reduce the risk of CSF leak or pseudomeningocele formation.[49,81] Patients should also be evaluated for idiopathic intracranial hypertension to reduce the risk of persistent or recurrent CSF leaks.

Considering that traumatic brain injury accounts for 10%−20% of symptomatic epilepsy,[82] seizure prophylaxis is paramount to decreasing the incidence of posttraumatic seizures. In the setting of a traumatic injury, the risk of seizure may be elevated when considering temporal lobe damage, cerebral ischemia, or intracerebral hemorrhage.[83] A randomized double-blind study has shown that phenytoin significantly reduces the risk of seizures in patients with serious head trauma if administered during the first week after injury.[84] However, the incidence of seizures occurring postoperatively after CSF leak repair is relatively low. In a case series of 65 patients undergoing the middle cranial fossa approach for spontaneous CSF leaks, only one patient developed a seizure postoperatively.[54] A similar outcome was observed in a retrospective study of 50 patients with CSF leaks.[76] For patients undergoing the middle cranial fossa approach, Stevens et al. have advocated for intraoperative seizure prophylaxis with 1000 mg of levetiracetam and additional indications for extended temporal lobe retraction.[57] Yet, Zampella et al. report that levetiracetam does not reach prophylactic levels at standard dosing regiments, compared with phenytoin which did reach levels required for seizure prophylaxis.[85] Further studies are needed on determining criteria for seizure prophylaxis following traumatic CSF leak in the lateral skull base.

Recurrent leaks

Recurrent CSF leaks are defined as leaks detected after postoperative day 3. These leaks can present as otorrhea in the external canal or emerge through the Eustachian tube as rhinorrhea or a postnasal drip.[57] They can be detected with a head hanging test or Valsalva maneuver and confirmed with beta-2 transferrin testing. Recurrent CSF leaks have been found to be more common in cases where the transmastoid approach was used alone.[57,65] The leaks were often found anterior to the initial repair site.[65,75] Recurrent leaks can be managed with a middle cranial fossa approach or a combined approach.[28] More aggressive approaches include a subtotal petrosectomy with obliteration with overclosure of the external auditory canal. CSF may also be diverted with lumbar drains and ventriculoperitoneal shunts, though this may increase risk of infection.

In addition, comorbid idiopathic intracranial hypertension should be considered in the differential diagnosis as it has been associated with increased risk of leak recurrence.[57,86] Due to a "pressure relief valve" effect, where the CSF leak may serve as a temporary release valve lowering the intracranial pressure, a diagnostic lumbar puncture can be performed 6−8 weeks after leak repair in patients with active leaks.[6,76] Furthermore, a pseudomeningocele may form as a collection of CSF deep to a closed wound. While it is not considered a leak, pseudomeningocele can increase the risk of transcutaneous leak formation, which can be managed conservatively with antibiotics and a lumbar drain.

Conclusion

CSF leak following lateral skull base trauma may present as rhinorrhea via the Eustachian tube or otorrhea if there is a perforation within the tympanic membrane. Considering the high morbidity and healthcare costs associated with CSF leaks, appropriate diagnosis and management is imperative to reduce the risk of meningitis and other complications. Patients can present with facial nerve weakness, ossicular chain discontinuity, and skull base fractures involving the otic capsule, which should be evaluated using an audiogram and high-resolution computed tomography scan. Since many lateral skull base CSF leaks have been reported to spontaneously resolve, conservative management can be initiated with or without the addition of a lumbar drain or a ventriculostomy to decompress the leak. Use of prophylactic antibiotics for meningitis remains controversial in the literature. When surgical intervention is implicated, an algorithm for surgical approach and postoperative care should be followed and tailored according to surgeon preference and the size, location, and number of skull base defects.

References

1. Lloyd KM, DelGaudio JM, Hudgins PA. Imaging of skull base cerebrospinal fluid leaks in adults. *Radiology.* 2008;248(3):725–736.
2. Zapalac JS, Marple BF, Schwade ND. Skull base cerebrospinal fluid fistulas: a comprehensive diagnostic algorithm. *Otolaryngol Head Neck Surg.* 2002;126(6):669–676.
3. Zlab MK, Moore GF, Daly DT, Yonkers AJ. Cerebrospinal fluid rhinorrhea: a review of the literature. *Ear Nose Throat J.* 1992;71(7):314–317.
4. Ommaya AK, Di Chiro G, Baldwin M, Pennybacker JB. Non-traumatic cerebrospinal fluid rhinorrhoea. *J Neurol Neurosurg Psychiatry.* 1968;31(3):214–225.
5. Loew F, Pertuiset B, Chaumier EE, Jaksche H. Traumatic, spontaneous and postoperative CSF rhinorrhea. *Adv Tech Stand Neurosurg.* 1984;11:169–207.
6. Prosser JD, Vender JR, Solares CA. Traumatic cerebrospinal fluid leaks. *Otolaryngol Clin.* 2011;44(4):857–873.
7. Rao N, Redleaf M. Spontaneous middle cranial fossa cerebrospinal fluid otorrhea in adults. *Laryngoscope.* 2016;126(2):464–468.
8. Scholsem M, Scholtes F, Collignon F, et al. Surgical management of anterior cranial base fractures with cerebrospinal fluid fistulae: a single-institution experience. *Neurosurgery.* 2008;62(2):463–469. ; discussion 469–471.
9. Yilmazlar S, Arslan E, Kocaeli H, et al. Cerebrospinal fluid leakage complicating skull base fractures: analysis of 81 cases. *Neurosurg Rev.* 2006;29(1):64–71.
10. Mendizabal GR, Moreno BC, Flores CC. Cerebrospinal fluid fistula: frequency in head injuries. *Rev Laryngol Otol Rhinol.* 1992;113(5):423–425.
11. Rangel-Castilla L, Gopinath S, Robertson CS. Management of intracranial hypertension. *Neurol Clin.* 2008;26(2):521–541.
12. Gray ST, Wu AW. Pathophysiology of iatrogenic and traumatic skull base injury. *Adv Oto-Rhino-Laryngol.* 2013;74:12–23.
13. Kral T, Zentner J, Vieweg U, Solymosi L, Schramm J. Diagnosis and treatment of frontobasal skull fractures. *Neurosurg Rev.* 1997;20(1):19–23.
14. Wax MK, Ramadan HH, Ortiz O, Wetmore SJ. Contemporary management of cerebrospinal fluid rhinorrhea. *Otolaryngol Head Neck Surg.* 1997;116(4):442–449.
15. Friedman JA, Ebersold MJ, Quast LM. Post-traumatic cerebrospinal fluid leakage. *World J Surg.* 2001;25(8):1062–1066.
16. Bernal-Sprekelsen M, Bleda-Vazquez C, Carrau RL. Ascending meningitis secondary to traumatic cerebrospinal fluid leaks. *Am J Rhinol.* 2000;14(4):257–259.
17. Brodie HA. *Management of Temporal Bone Trauma.* Cummings Otolaryngology Head & Neck Surgery; 2010:2036–2047.
18. Liao KH, Wang JY, Lin HW, et al. Risk of death in patients with post-traumatic cerebrospinal fluid leakage—analysis of 1773 cases. *J Chin Med Assoc.* 2016;79(2):58–64.
19. Varshneya K, Rodrigues AJ, Medress ZA, et al. Risks, costs, and outcomes of cerebrospinal fluid leaks after pediatric skull fractures: a MarketScan analysis between 2007 and 2015. *Neurosurg Focus.* 2019;47(5):E10.

20. Mourad M, Inman JC, Chan DM, Ducic Y. Contemporary trends in the management of posttraumatic cerebrospinal fluid leaks. *Craniomaxillofacial Trauma Reconstr.* 2018; 11(1):71−77.

21. Brodie HA, Thompson TC. Management of complications from 820 temporal bone fractures. *Am J Otol.* 1997;18(2):188−197.

22. Lobo BC, Baumanis MM, Nelson RF. Surgical repair of spontaneous cerebrospinal fluid (CSF) leaks: a systematic review. *Laryngoscope Investig Otolaryngol.* 2017;2(5): 215−224.

23. Stevens SM, Rizk HG, Golnik K, et al. Idiopathic intracranial hypertension: contemporary review and implications for the otolaryngologist. *Laryngoscope.* 2018;128(1): 248−256.

24. Stucken EZ, Selesnick SH, Brown KD. The role of obesity in spontaneous temporal bone encephaloceles and CSF leak. *Otol Neurotol.* 2012;33(8):1412−1417.

25. Nelson RF, Gantz BJ, Hansen MR. The rising incidence of spontaneous cerebrospinal fluid leaks in the United States and the association with obesity and obstructive sleep apnea. *Otol Neurotol.* 2015;36(3):476−480.

26. LeVay AJ, Kveton JF. Relationship between obesity, obstructive sleep apnea, and spontaneous cerebrospinal fluid otorrhea. *Laryngoscope.* 2008;118(2):275−278.

27. Leonetti JP, Marzo S, Anderson D, Origitano T, Vukas DD. Spontaneous transtemporal CSF leakage: a study of 51 cases. *Ear Nose Throat J.* 2005;84(11), 700, 702−704, 706.

28. Kutz Jr JW, Husain IA, Isaacson B, Roland PS. Management of spontaneous cerebrospinal fluid otorrhea. *Laryngoscope.* 2008;118(12):2195−2199.

29. Brown NE, Grundfast KM, Jabre A, Megerian CA, O'Malley Jr BW, Rosenberg SI. Diagnosis and management of spontaneous cerebrospinal fluid-middle ear effusion and otorrhea. *Laryngoscope.* 2004;114(5):800−805.

30. Naples JG, Shah RR, Ruckenstein MJ. The evolution of presenting signs and symptoms of lateral skull base cerebrospinal fluid leaks. *Curr Opin Otolaryngol Head Neck Surg.* 2019;27(5):344−348.

31. Gacek RR. Arachnoid granulation cerebrospinal fluid otorrhea. *Ann Otol Rhinol Laryngol.* 1990;99(11):854−862.

32. Oakley GM, Alt JA, Schlosser RJ, Harvey RJ, Orlandi RR. Diagnosis of cerebrospinal fluid rhinorrhea: an evidence-based review with recommendations. *Int Forum Allergy Rhinol.* 2016;6(1):8−16.

33. Song SW, Jun BC, Kim H. Clinical features and radiological evaluation of otic capsule sparing temporal bone fractures. *J Laryngol Otol.* 2017;131(3):209−214.

34. Tos M. Prognosis of hearing loss in temporal bone fractures. *J Laryngol Otol.* 1971; 85(11):1147−1159.

35. Schell A, Kitsko D. Audiometric outcomes in pediatric temporal bone trauma. *Otolaryngol Head Neck Surg.* 2016;154(1):175−180.

36. Dedhia RD, Chin OY, Kaufman M, et al. Predicting complications of pediatric temporal bone fractures. *Int J Pediatr Otorhinolaryngol.* 2020;138:110358.

37. Magliulo G, Ciniglio Appiani M, Iannella G, Artico M. Petrous bone fractures violating otic capsule. *Otol Neurotol.* 2012;33(9):1558−1561.

38. Braca 3rd JA, Marzo S, Prabhu VC. Cerebrospinal fluid leakage from tegmen tympani defects repaired via the middle cranial fossa approach. *J Neurol Surg B Skull Base.* 2013;74(2):103−107.

39. Warnecke A, Averbeck T, Wurster U, Harmening M, Lenarz T, Stover T. Diagnostic relevance of beta2-transferrin for the detection of cerebrospinal fluid fistulas. *Arch Otolaryngol Head Neck Surg.* 2004;130(10):1178−1184.

40. Lin DT, Lin AC. Surgical treatment of traumatic injuries of the cranial base. *Otolaryngol Clin.* 2013;46(5):749−757.

41. Shetty PG, Shroff MM, Sahani DV, Kirtane MV. Evaluation of high-resolution CT and MR cisternography in the diagnosis of cerebrospinal fluid fistula. *AJNR Am J Neuroradiol.* 1998;19(4):633−639.

42. Eljazzar R, Loewenstern J, Dai JB, Shrivastava RK, Iloreta Jr AM. Detection of cerebrospinal fluid leaks: is there a radiologic standard of care? A systematic review. *World Neurosurg.* 2019;127:307−315.

43. Lipschitz N, Hazenfield JM, Breen JT, Samy RN. Laboratory testing and imaging in the evaluation of cranial cerebrospinal fluid leaks and encephaloceles. *Curr Opin Otolaryngol Head Neck Surg.* 2019;27(5):339−343.

44. Stone JA, Castillo M, Neelon B, Mukherji SK. Evaluation of CSF leaks: high-resolution CT compared with contrast-enhanced CT and radionuclide cisternography. *AJNR Am J Neuroradiol.* 1999;20(4):706−712.

45. Phang SY, Whitehouse K, Lee L, Khalil H, McArdle P, Whitfield PC. Management of CSF leak in base of skull fractures in adults. *Br J Neurosurg.* 2016;30(6):596−604.

46. Keerl R, Weber RK, Draf W, Wienke A, Schaefer SD. Use of sodium fluorescein solution for detection of cerebrospinal fluid fistulas: an analysis of 420 administrations and reported complications in Europe and the United States. *Laryngoscope.* 2004;114(2):266−272.

47. Raza SM, Banu MA, Donaldson A, Patel KS, Anand VK, Schwartz TH. Sensitivity and specificity of intrathecal fluorescein and white light excitation for detecting intraoperative cerebrospinal fluid leak in endoscopic skull base surgery: a prospective study. *J Neurosurg.* 2016;124(3):621−626.

48. Seth R, Rajasekaran K, Benninger MS, Batra PS. The utility of intrathecal fluorescein in cerebrospinal fluid leak repair. *Otolaryngol Head Neck Surg.* 2010;143(5):626−632.

49. Friedman RA, Cullen RD, Ulis J, Brackmann DE. Management of cerebrospinal fluid leaks after acoustic tumor removal. *Neurosurgery.* 2007;61(3 Suppl):35−39. ; discussion 39−40.

50. Khan R, Sajjad M, Khan AA, et al. Comparison of lumbar drain insertion and conservative management in the treatment of traumatic CSF rhinorrhoea. *J Ayub Med Coll Abbottabad.* 2019;31(3):441−444.

51. Bell RB, Dierks EJ, Homer L, Potter BE. Management of cerebrospinal fluid leak associated with craniomaxillofacial trauma. *J Oral Maxillofac Surg.* 2004;62(6):676−684.

52. Carrion E, Hertzog JH, Medlock MD, Hauser GJ, Dalton HJ. Use of acetazolamide to decrease cerebrospinal fluid production in chronically ventilated patients with ventriculopleural shunts. *Arch Dis Child.* 2001;84(1):68−71.

53. Chaaban MR, Illing E, Riley KO, Woodworth BA. Acetazolamide for high intracranial pressure cerebrospinal fluid leaks. *Int Forum Allergy Rhinol.* 2013;3(9):718−721.

54. Nelson RF, Roche JP, Gantz BJ, Hansen MR. Middle cranial fossa (MCF) approach without the use of lumbar drain for the management of spontaneous cerebral spinal fluid (CSF) leaks. *Otol Neurotol.* 2016;37(10):1625−1629.

55. Lai LT, Danesh-Meyer HV, Kaye AH. Visual outcomes and headache following interventions for idiopathic intracranial hypertension. *J Clin Neurosci.* 2014;21(10):1670−1678.

56. McGirt MJ, Woodworth G, Thomas G, Miller N, Williams M, Rigamonti D. Cerebrospinal fluid shunt placement for pseudotumor cerebri-associated intractable headache: predictors of treatment response and an analysis of long-term outcomes. *J Neurosurg.* 2004;101(4):627−632.

57. Stevens SM, Smith CJ, Lawton M. Postoperative management of patients with spontaneous cerebrospinal fluid leak. *Curr Opin Otolaryngol Head Neck Surg.* 2019;27(5):361−368.

58. Ratilal BO, Costa J, Pappamikail L, Sampaio C. Antibiotic prophylaxis for preventing meningitis in patients with basilar skull fractures. *Cochrane Database Syst Rev.* 2015;4:CD004884.

59. Klastersky J, Sadeghi M, Brihaye J. Antimicrobial prophylaxis in patients with rhinorrhea or otorrhea: a double-blind study. *Surg Neurol.* 1976;6(2):111−114.

60. MacGee EE, Cauthen JC, Brackett CE. Meningitis following acute traumatic cerebrospinal fluid fistula. *J Neurosurg.* 1970;33(3):312−316.

61. Brodie HA. Prophylactic antibiotics for posttraumatic cerebrospinal fluid fistulae. A meta-analysis. *Arch Otolaryngol Head Neck Surg.* 1997;123(7):749−752.

62. Gonen L, Handzel O, Shimony N, Fliss DM, Margalit N. Surgical management of spontaneous cerebrospinal fluid leakage through temporal bone defects−case series and review of the literature. *Neurosurg Rev.* 2016;39(1):141−150. ; discussion 150.

63. Tolisano AM, Kutz Jr JW. Middle fossa approach for spontaneous cerebrospinal fluid fistula and encephaloceles. *Curr Opin Otolaryngol Head Neck Surg.* 2019;27(5):356−360.

64. Oliaei S, Mahboubi H, Djalilian HR. Transmastoid approach to temporal bone cerebrospinal fluid leaks. *Am J Otolaryngol.* 2012;33(5):556−561.

65. Kari E, Mattox DE. Transtemporal management of temporal bone encephaloceles and CSF leaks: review of 56 consecutive patients. *Acta Otolaryngol.* 2011;131(4):391−394.

66. Son HJ, Karkas A, Buchanan P, et al. Spontaneous cerebrospinal fluid effusion of the temporal bone: repair, audiological outcomes, and obesity. *Laryngoscope.* 2014;124(5):1204−1208.

67. McNulty B, Schutt CA, Bojrab D, Babu S. Middle cranial fossa encephalocele and cerebrospinal fluid leakage: etiology, approach, outcomes. *J Neurol Surg B Skull Base.* 2020;81(3):268−274.

68. Stevens SM, Rizk HG, McIlwain WR, Lambert PR, Meyer TA. Association between lateral skull base thickness and surgical outcomes in spontaneous CSF otorrhea. *Otolaryngol Head Neck Surg.* 2016;154(4):707−714.

69. Perez E, Carlton D, Alfarano M, Smouha E. Transmastoid repair of spontaneous cerebrospinal fluid leaks. *J Neurol Surg B Skull Base.* 2018;79(5):451−457.

70. Kim L, Wisely CE, Dodson EE. Transmastoid approach to spontaneous temporal bone cerebrospinal fluid leaks: hearing improvement and success of repair. *Otolaryngol Head Neck Surg.* 2014;150(3):472−478.

71. Gioacchini FM, Cassandro E, Alicandri-Ciufelli M, et al. Surgical outcomes in the treatment of temporal bone cerebrospinal fluid leak: a systematic review. *Auris Nasus Larynx.* 2018;45(5):903−910.

72. Stevens SM, Crane R, Pensak ML, Samy RN. Middle ear obliteration with blind-sac closure of the external auditory canal for spontaneous CSF otorrhea. *Otolaryngol Head Neck Surg.* 2017;156(3):534−542.

73. Kveton JF. Obliteration of mastoid and middle ear for severe trauma to the temporal bone. *Laryngoscope.* 1987;97(12):1385−1387.

74. Hamilton JW, Foy PM, Lesser TH. Subtotal petrosectomy in the treatment of cerebrospinal fluid fistulae of the lateral skull base. *Br J Neurosurg.* 1997;11(6):496−500.

75. Cheng E, Grande D, Leonetti J. Management of spontaneous temporal bone cerebrospinal fluid leak: a 30-year experience. *Am J Otolaryngol.* 2019;40(1):97−100.

76. Kutz Jr JW, Johnson AK, Wick CC. Surgical management of spontaneous cerebrospinal fistulas and encephaloceles of the temporal bone. *Laryngoscope*. 2018;128(9): 2170−2177.

77. Adkins WY, Osguthorpe JD. Mini-craniotomy for management of CSF otorrhea from tegmen defects. *Laryngoscope*. 1983;93(8):1038−1040.

78. Stenzel M, Preuss S, Orloff L, Jecker P, Mann W. Cerebrospinal fluid leaks of temporal bone origin: etiology and management. *ORL J Otorhinolaryngol Relat Spec*. 2005;67(1): 51−55.

79. Carlson ML, Copeland 3rd WR, Driscoll CL, et al. Temporal bone encephalocele and cerebrospinal fluid fistula repair utilizing the middle cranial fossa or combined mastoid-middle cranial fossa approach. *J Neurosurg*. 2013;119(5):1314−1322.

80. Savva A, Taylor MJ, Beatty CW. Management of cerebrospinal fluid leaks involving the temporal bone: report on 92 patients. *Laryngoscope*. 2003;113(1):50−56.

81. Selesnick SH, Liu JC, Jen A, Carew JF. Management options for cerebrospinal fluid leak after vestibular schwannoma surgery and introduction of an innovative treatment. *Otol Neurotol*. 2004;25(4):580−586.

82. Pitkanen A, Bolkvadze T. Head trauma and epilepsy. In: Noebels JL, Avoli M, Rogawski MA, Olsen RW, Delgado-Escueta AV, eds. *Jasper's Basic Mechanisms of the Epilepsies. Bethesda, MD*. 2012.

83. Thomsen J, Stougaard M, Becker B, Tos M, Jennum P. Middle fossa approach in vestibular schwannoma surgery. Postoperative hearing preservation and EEG changes. *Acta Otolaryngol*. 2000;120(4):517−522.

84. Temkin NR, Dikmen SS, Wilensky AJ, Keihm J, Chabal S, Winn HR. A randomized, double-blind study of phenytoin for the prevention of post-traumatic seizures. *N Engl J Med*. 1990;323(8):497−502.

85. Zampella B, Patchana T, Wiginton JG, et al. Seizure prophylaxis in traumatic brain injury: a comparative study of levetiracetam and phenytoin cerebrospinal fluid levels in trauma patients with signs of increased intracranial pressure requiring ventriculostomy. *Cureus*. 2019;11(9):e5784.

86. Perez MA, Bialer OY, Bruce BB, Newman NJ, Biousse V. Primary spontaneous cerebrospinal fluid leaks and idiopathic intracranial hypertension. *J Neuro Ophthalmol*. 2013; 33(4):330−337.

Medical and surgical management of otic barotrauma

Matthew J. Wu, MD [1,2], **Elliott D. Kozin, MD** [1,3]

[1]*Department of Otolaryngology, Massachusetts Eye and Ear, Boston, MA, United States;*
[2]*Department of Otolaryngology-Head and Neck Surgery, Washington University School of Medicine in St Louis, St Louis, MO, United States;* [3]*Department of Otolaryngology, Harvard Medical School, Boston, MA, United States*

Overview

Otic barotrauma (OBT) is traumatic injury of the middle ear and tympanic membrane resulting from a high-pressure differential existing between the middle ear and external environment. In common daily activities (e.g., driving to different elevations, air travel), individuals may experience slight changes in pressure of the middle ear, which results in mild, self-limiting otologic symptoms (e.g., slight aural discomfort). However, it is possible for these same activities to cause OBT, which is an increasingly encountered issue by otolaryngologists and otologists given the wide adoption of air travel; Over the past 50 years, the number of passengers has increased from 310 million to 3.7 billion annually, with approximately 1 million passengers flying at any given moment[1,2] and this number will likely continue to grow. Estimating the overall prevalence of OBT though varies considerably by types of activities that individuals participate in (e.g., scuba diving) and risk factors such as history of otitis media[3] and head and neck cancers.[4] To help address this clinical issue, this chapter will provide an overview of the pathophysiology, diagnosis, and medical and surgical management of OBT.

Eustachian tube and middle ear function

As described previously, the pathophysiology of OBT is related to an imbalance of pressures between the air-filled space of the middle ear and the external environment, which are separated by the tympanic membrane. Normally, the Eustachian tube, which connects the middle ear and the nasopharynx, will open briefly while yawning or swallowing to equalize middle ear pressure via the levator and tensor veli palatini muscles. Eustachian tube dysfunction (ETD), which reduces the ability for the Eustachian tube to open, may arise from several reasons such as increased mass near the Eustachian tube's nasopharyngeal opening (e.g., tumor,[4] enlarged adenoids) or swelling due to infections (e.g., acute otitis media).[3] In addition, the middle ear mucosa and underlying vessels promote equalization of middle ear pressure via gas exchange.[5] These intact physiologic processes are required to accommodate for ambient pressure changes that follow Boyle's law, which states that as the volume of a gas increases, the pressure decreases proportionally, and vice versa.[6] If the middle ear compartment's pressure is not able to equalize properly, OBT can occur through a variety of mechanisms that are described below.

Pathophysiologic mechanisms
Air travel

Flying is the most common etiology of barotrauma[7,8] and can occur during both ascent and descent. As the aircraft ascends, the ambient cabin pressure gradually decreases, and the middle ear pressure must equilibrate through swallowing and passive Eustachian tube ventilation.[9] If the middle ear gas volume remains elevated, the relatively positive pressure of this compartment will cause lateral movement of the tympanic membrane. During aircraft descent, the middle ear pressure conversely must reduce. Unlike ascent, the Eustachian tube cannot passively diffuse air from the middle ear, which may be related to the increase prevalence of OBT during descent.[9] If compensations are not adequate, the tympanic membrane may bruise, bleed, or rupture, and the middle ear may produce fluid exudates.

Diving

OBT that occurs due to diving has a similar mechanism to flying, but pressure changes are of much greater magnitude, which rely on height and fluid density.[10] Given water's greater density than air and a diver's relatively uncompensated state compared to a passenger in a dynamically-pressurized plane cabin, a minor change in water depth leads to a relatively greater increase in pressure where OBT has been observed to occur most often near the surface of the water.[10] During descent, external pressure from the surrounding water moves the tympanic membrane medially and reduces middle ear space gas volume. Without performing a Valsalva maneuver, the pressure differential between the middle ear and external environment will continue to grow, leading to subsequent hemotympanum, middle ear edema, or tympanic membrane rupture. If the diver attempts to perform a Valsalva maneuver but the descent occurs too rapidly or has a blocked Eustachian tube, this may lead to inner ear barotrauma.[11] Inner ear barotrauma may also occur during descent due to external water pressure pushing the tympanic membrane and stapes into the oval window. Within the labyrinth, perilymph and endolymph are not compressible, and the increased intracranial pressure may lead to rupture of the oval or round windows[11,12] and formation of a perilymphatic fistula.[13] The presence of a perilymphatic fistula then allows for gases in the middle ear to enter in the inner ear, which may lead to permanent hearing loss. While ascending, OBT can also occur if middle ear gas does not pass through the Eustachian tube, leading to relatively a positive pressure gradient in the middle ear compartment.

Hyperbaric oxygen therapy

It is important to recognize that patients receiving hyperbaric oxygen therapy (HBOT) such as in settings to promote wound healing from burns and infections[14] and improve flap circulation[15] may experience OBT, which is one of the most common complications following HBOT.[16] While receiving treatment in either a monoplace or a multiplace chamber, the supine positioning increases venous congestion and hinders the ability to increase pressure in the middle ear space. Given the middle ear's relatively lower pressure compared with the ambient environment, medial movement of the tympanic membrane occurs with transudation of fluid in the middle ear space and OBT.[17]

Blast injuries

Following an explosion, the creation of air pressure waves leads to a rapid increase in the ambient air pressure. In turn, the lack of time to equalize pressure between the middle and external ear results in OBT.[18,19] A more in-depth discussion is provided in Chapters 2 and 5.

Diagnosis

History

When evaluating a patient with suspected OBT, a history should be focused on understanding possible exposures to changes in ambient pressure through mechanisms such as those previously described. Patients with minor OBT may have mild symptoms including aural fullness and ear discomfort. It is important to note that ear pain is not a reliable indicator of OBT; in a study of repeated dives, 82% of dives were asymptomatic and did not report ear pain.[20] For patients with more severe OBT, they may describe hearing loss due to transudative effusions in the middle ear space, hemotympanum,[21] or tympanic membrane rupture. Often, patients with tympanic membrane rupture may report improvement of their pain and discomfort involving the affected ear. If patients describe may describe vestibular symptoms (e.g., vertigo, nausea)[13,22] or auditory symptoms (e.g., tinnitus, hyperacusis, and hearing loss),[22] inner ear barotrauma may have occurred with possible development of a perilymphatic fistula.

Additional history should also be directed toward eliciting if the Eustachian tube's ability to ventilate air may be compromised or if ETD is present. Specifically, history should be gathered for the presence of structures that impede the Eustachian tube's ventilation function externally (e.g., adenoid hypertrophy or nasopharyngeal cancer[4]) or internally via polyps. Inflammation of the nasopharynx from several conditions such as gastroesophageal reflux disease,[23] allergies,[24] or viral infections[25] may also decrease the ability for the Eustachian tube to open adequately.

Physical examination and evaluation

The physical examination for suspected OBT begins with examining the external auditory canal, which may reveal cerumen or exostoses that may prevent visualization of the tympanic membrane and be removed if possible. An otoscope should be used to examine the tympanic membrane for signs of hemotympanum, perforation, or effusions in the middle ear space. The Teed classification of middle ear barotrauma can be used to document the appearance of the tympanic membrane.[26] While it may be challenging to obtain otoscopic examination prior to air travel or diving, the Teed classification can be used to monitor for the development of OBT following HOBT. There are six grades: 0 (normal tympanic membrane), 1 (erythema and retraction of the tympanic membrane), 2 (erythema of the entire tympanic membrane with slight hemorrhage), 3 (erythema of the entire tympanic membrane with gross hemorrhage), 4 (air–fluid level with gross blood), and 5 (tympanic membrane perforation) (Fig. 13.1).[26,27] Periodic documentation with this classification

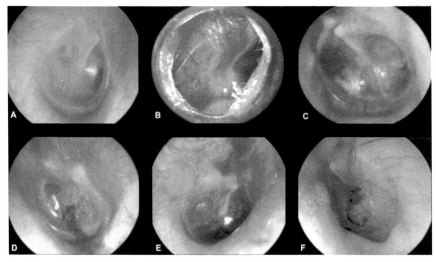

FIGURE 13.1

Teed classification of middle ear barotrauma in increasing severity from grade 0 to 5 (A–F).

Adapted from Hamilton–Farrell and Bhattacharyya (2003). https://doi.org/10.1016/j.injury.2003.08.020.

system allows to track the resolution of OBT injury. Additionally, in severe cases of barotrauma, facial nerve weakness may be present, which is reversible.[28]

If hearing loss is present, examination with a tuning fork and audiometric evaluation should be performed, which may reveal a conductive (e.g., hemotympanum, effusion) or sensorineural (e.g., inner ear barotrauma or perilymphatic fistula) hearing loss. If patients present with vestibular symptoms, patients should be examined for a positive Hennebert's sign (positional nystagmus when the involved ear is moved into the dependent position)[29] or gait instability.

Management

Acute management

In the acute setting, if symptoms of OBT are recognized, individuals should attempt to reverse the underlying etiology causing the ambient pressure change. If OBT begins during HOBT, additional pressurization should not occur to provide time for pressures in the middle ear space to equilibrate. If symptoms persist or continue to worsen during HOBT, emergent intervention via myringotomy or tympanostomy tubes may be performed.[30] To minimize the risk of injury to middle and inner ear structures, these procedures should be performed in the anterior inferior quadrant of the tympanic membrane.[30] If individuals suspect OBT while diving, they should move in the opposite direction that caused symptoms to emerge (e.g., more shallow water after moving to a greater depth). In certain scenarios, however, individuals such as those operating aircrafts, it may not be appropriate to rapidly change altitudes.

If tympanic membrane rupture occurs, smaller defects will generally heal in several weeks,[31] whereas larger defects and those that are not resolving will require surgical repair. Antibiotics are generally not needed unless if signs of infection develop. Ototoxic antibiotics such as gentamicin, neomycin sulfate, or tobramycin should not be used to prevent causing sensorineural hearing loss.[32] At present, there is also no evidence to support the use of corticosteroids to promote tympanic membrane healing.

If inner ear barotrauma is suspected, patients should receive prompt conservative management to decrease intracranial pressure by remaining supine with head elevation for 1 week, use stool softeners, and avoid the Valsalva maneuver[12,33] while monitoring for resolution of audiovestibular symptoms. In most cases, these symptoms will improve in several days.

At present, there is no standardized approach to diagnose perilymphatic fistula. Historically, middle ear exploration was performed to directly visualize perilymph leakage, but the limited volume of perilymph in the inner ear is approximately equal to three drops of water,[34,35] and intermittent perilymphatic fluid flow raises the question if this diagnostic method is reliable. If surgical exploration is pursued, it may be difficult to discern if fluid in the middle ear may be present from middle ear mucosa or local anesthetic.[36] Transudates in the middle ear space may also increase in volume due to heat from surgical instruments or manipulation of the middle ear mucosa. Recent studies suggest that improved resolution and availability of high-resolution computed tomography (HRCT) and magnetic resonance imaging (MRI) may adequately diagnose perilymphatic fistulas.[37,38] The presence of pneumolabyrinth or air in the inner ear[37] or fluid in the round and oval windows[38] on HRCT may suggest a perilymphatic fistula, which are repaired surgically.[22] MRI may be used to visualize for the presence of congenital conditions such as Mondini dysplasia,[39] which may raise suspicion for perilymphatic fistula as it increases the risk of formation; in these scenarios, the otolaryngologist may be more likely to pursue surgical management as the risk of meningitis is increased if left untreated.[40,41]

Prevention

After addressing OBT in the acute setting, any predisposing factors for future development of OBT should be identified. Underlying causes of ETD that may prevent pressure equalization of the middle ear space should be addressed during the history and physical exam.[42] If patients can anticipate when they will be in settings that may increase the risk of OBT, prophylactically using medications such as decongestants before diving[43] or flying[44] may improve ETD and reduce the probability of developing OBT. At present, however, limited evidence exists to support the use of decongestants to prevent OBT in children. For healthcare providers administering HBOT, evidence exists to support that a slow, linear increase in pressurization may decrease the risk of developing OBT.[45]

Prophylactic myringotomy and/or tympanotomy tube placement can be used in select settings if patients experience recurrent OBT. In settings where the middle ear will remain dry, such as prior to HBOT and flying, these procedures do not significantly increase the risk of infection. However, this should not be performed to prevent OBT secondary to diving as this will increase the risk of otitis media.

Providing patient education plays an important role to prevent future OBT. Teaching patients how to perform techniques to promote pressure equilibrium between the external and middle ear can reduce the risk of developing OBT in settings with changes in ambient pressure such as the Valsalva maneuver (forced exhalation against a closed mouth and nose to open the Eustachian tube), Toynbee maneuver (swallowing air while pinching the nose to open the Eustachian tube), or yawning or swallowing.[46] During HBOT sessions, using devices, such as the EarPopper, may help increase air pressure in a relatively negative middle ear space,[47,48] which uses a modified Politzer Maneuver[49] (constant stream of air into the Eustachian tube),[48,50] to help improve middle ear ventilation.[51] Additionally, if patients have an upper respiratory infection, which temporarily increases congestion and reduces Eustachian tube functioning, they may consider postponing activities that have increased risk for OBT until it resolves.[8]

References

1. Rodrigue J-P. *The Geography of Transport Systems*. New York: Routledge; 2020. https://transportgeography.org.

2. Bank TW. *International Civil Aviation Organization, Civil Aviation Statistics of the World and ICAO Staff Estimates*; 2021. https://data.worldbank.org/indicator/IS.AIR.PSGR.

3. Cohn JE, Pfeiffer M, Patel N, Sataloff RT, McKinnon BJ. Identifying Eustachian tube dysfunction prior to hyperbaric oxygen therapy: who is at risk for intolerance? *Am J Otolaryngol*. 2018;39(1):14−19.

4. Daniel A, Fasunla AJ. Nasopharyngeal cancer mimicking otitic barotrauma in a resource-challenged center: a case report. *J Med Case Rep*. 2011;5:532.

5. Hamada Y, Utahashi H, Aoki K. Physiological gas exchange in the middle ear cavity. *Int J Pediatr Otorhinolaryngol*. 2002;64(1):41−49.

6. West JB. The original presentation of Boyle's law. *J Appl Physiol*. 1999;87(4):1543−1545.

7. Brown TP. Middle ear symptoms while flying. Ways to prevent a severe outcome. *Postgrad Med*. 1994;96(2):135−137, 141−142.

8. Rosenkvist L, Klokker M, Katholm M. Upper respiratory infections and barotraumas in commercial pilots: a retrospective survey. *Aviat Space Environ Med*. 2008;79(10):960−963.

9. Mirza S, Richardson H. Otic barotrauma from air travel. *J Laryngol Otol*. 2005;119(5):366−370.

10. Lynch JH, Deaton TG. Barotrauma with extreme pressures in sport: from scuba to skydiving. *Curr Sports Med Rep*. 2014;13(2):107−112.

11. Klingmann C, Praetorius M, Baumann I, Plinkert PK. Barotrauma and decompression illness of the inner ear: 46 cases during treatment and follow-up. *Otol Neurotol*. 2007;28(4):447−454.

12. Parell GJ, Becker GD. Conservative management of inner ear barotrauma resulting from scuba diving. *Otolaryngol Head Neck Surg*. 1985;93(3):393−397.

13. Pullen 2nd FW. Perilymphatic fistula induced by barotrauma. *Am J Otol*. 1992;13(3):270−272.

14. Feldmeier JJ, Hopf HW, Warriner 3rd RA, Fife CE, Gesell LB, Bennett M. UHMS position statement: topical oxygen for chronic wounds. *Undersea Hyperb Med*. 2005;32(3):157−168.

15. Francis A, Baynosa RC. Hyperbaric oxygen therapy for the compromised graft or flap. *Adv Wound Care*. 2017;6(1):23−32.

16. Nasole E, Zanon V, Marcolin P, Bosco G. Middle ear barotrauma during hyperbaric oxygen therapy; a review of occurrences in 5962 patients. *Undersea Hyperb Med*. 2019;46(2):101−106.

17. Shupak A, Attias J, Aviv J, Melamed Y. Oxygen diving-induced middle ear underaeration. *Acta Otolaryngol*. 1995;115(3):422−426.

18. Darley DS, Kellman RM. Otologic considerations of blast injury. *Disaster Med Public Health Prep*. 2010;4(2):145−152.

19. Ritenour AE, Wickley A, Ritenour JS, et al. Tympanic membrane perforation and hearing loss from blast overpressure in Operation Enduring Freedom and Operation Iraqi Freedom wounded. *J Trauma*. 2008;64(2 Suppl):S174−S178, discussion S178.

20. Jansen S, Meyer MF, Boor M, et al. Prevalence of barotrauma in recreational scuba divers after repetitive saltwater dives. *Otol Neurotol.* 2016;37(9):1325−1331.
21. Kim CH, Shin JE. Hemorrhage within the tympanic membrane without perforation. *J Otolaryngol Head Neck Surg.* 2018;47(1):66.
22. Park GY, Byun H, Moon IJ, Hong SH, Cho YS, Chung WH. Effects of early surgical exploration in suspected barotraumatic perilymph fistulas. *Clin Exp Otorhinolaryngol.* 2012;5(2):74−80.
23. Yan S, Wei Y, Zhan X, et al. Gastroesophageal reflux disease: a cause for Eustachian tube dysfunction in obstructive sleep apnea. *Ear Nose Throat J.* 2020.
24. Juszczak HM, Loftus PA. Role of allergy in Eustachian tube dysfunction. *Curr Allergy Asthma Rep.* 2020;20(10):54.
25. Fireman P. Otitis media and Eustachian tube dysfunction: connection to allergic rhinitis. *J Allergy Clin Immunol.* 1997;99(2):S787−S797.
26. Beuerlein M, Nelson RN, Welling DB. Inner and middle ear hyperbaric oxygen-induced barotrauma. *Laryngoscope.* 1997;107(10):1350−1356.
27. Hamilton-Farrell M, Bhattacharyya A. Barotrauma. *Injury.* 2004;35(4):359−370.
28. Molvaer OI, Eidsvik S. Facial baroparesis: a review. *Undersea Biomed Res.* 1987;14(3): 277−295.
29. Kohut RI, Hinojosa R, Thompson JN, Ryu JH. Idiopathic perilymphatic fistulas. A temporal bone histopathologic study with clinical, surgical, and histopathologic correlations. *Arch Otolaryngol Head Neck Surg.* 1995;121(4):412−420.
30. Capes JP, Tomaszewski C. Prophylaxis against middle ear barotrauma in US hyperbaric oxygen therapy centers. *Am J Emerg Med.* 1996;14(7):645−648.
31. Orji FT, Agu CC. Determinants of spontaneous healing in traumatic perforations of the tympanic membrane. *Clin Otolaryngol.* 2008;33(5):420−426.
32. Matz GJ. Aminoglycoside cochlear ototoxicity. *Otolaryngol Clin.* 1993;26(5):705−712.
33. Becker GD, Parell GJ. Barotrauma of the ears and sinuses after scuba diving. *Eur Arch Oto-Rhino-Laryngol.* 2001;258(4):159−163.
34. Hornibrook J. Perilymph fistula: fifty years of controversy. *ISRN Otolaryngol.* 2012; 2012:281248.
35. Maitland CG. Perilymphatic fistula. *Curr Neurol Neurosci Rep.* 2001;1(5):486−491.
36. Gibson WP. Spontaneous perilymphatic fistula: electrophysiologic findings in animals and man. *Am J Otol.* 1993;14(3):273−277.
37. Mafee MF, Valvassori GE, Kumar A, Yannias DA, Marcus RE. Pneumolabyrinth: a new radiologic sign for fracture of the stapes footplate. *Am J Otol.* 1984;5(5):374−375.
38. Venkatasamy A, Al Ohraini Z, Karol A, et al. CT and MRI for the diagnosis of perilymphatic fistula: a study of 17 surgically confirmed patients. *Eur Arch Oto-Rhino-Laryngol.* 2020;277(4):1045−1051.
39. Gupta SS, Maheshwari SR, Kirtane MV, Shrivastav N. Pictorial review of MRI/CT scan in congenital temporal bone anomalies, in patients for cochlear implant. *Indian J Radiol Imag.* 2009;19(2):99−106.
40. Schuknecht HF. Mondini dysplasia; a clinical and pathological study. *Ann Otol Rhinol Laryngol Suppl.* 1980;89(1 Pt 2):1−23.
41. Burton EM, Keith JW, Linden BE, Lazar RH. CSF fistula in a patient with Mondini deformity: demonstration by CT cisternography. *AJNR Am J Neuroradiol.* 1990;11(1): 205−207.

42. Gates GA, Avery CA, Prihoda TJ, Cooper Jr JC. Effectiveness of adenoidectomy and tympanostomy tubes in the treatment of chronic otitis media with effusion. *N Engl J Med*. 1987;317(23):1444−1451.

43. Brown M, Jones J, Krohmer J. Pseudoephedrine for the prevention of barotitis media: a controlled clinical trial in underwater divers. *Ann Emerg Med*. 1992;21(7):849−852.

44. Csortan E, Jones J, Haan M, Brown M. Efficacy of pseudoephedrine for the prevention of barotrauma during air travel. *Ann Emerg Med*. 1994;23(6):1324−1327.

45. Varughese L, O'Neill OJ, Marker J, Smykowski E, Dayya D. The effect of compression rate and slope on the incidence of symptomatic Eustachian tube dysfunction leading to middle ear barotrauma: a Phase I prospective study. *Undersea Hyperb Med*. 2019;46(2):95−100.

46. Bhattacharya S, Singh A, Marzo RR. "Airplane ear"-A neglected yet preventable problem. *AIMS Public Health*. 2019;6(3):320−325.

47. O'Neill OJ, Smykowski E, Marker JA, Perez L, Gurash S, Sullivan J. Proof of concept study using a modified Politzer inflation device as a rescue modality for treating Eustachian tube dysfunction during hyperbaric oxygen treatment in a multiplace (Class A) chamber. *Undersea Hyperb Med*. 2019;46(1):55−61.

48. Tham T, Rahman L, Costantino P. Efficacy of a non-invasive middle ear aeration device in children with recurrent otitis media: a randomized controlled trial protocol. *Contemp Clin Trials Commun*. 2018;12:92−97.

49. Casale M, Rinaldi V, Setola R, Salvinelli F. The old-fashioned Politzer maneuver: a video clip demonstration. *Laryngoscope*. 2007;117(11):2002.

50. Silman S, Arick D. Efficacy of a modified politzer apparatus in management of Eustachian tube dysfunction in adults. *J Am Acad Audiol*. 1999;10(9):496−501.

51. O'Neill MP, Gopalan PD. Endotracheal tube cuff pressure change: proof of concept for a novel approach to objective cough assessment in intubated critically ill patients. *Heart Lung*. 2020;49(2):181−185.

Adult vestibular dysfunction following head injury: diagnosis and management

14

Matthew Gordon Crowson, MD, MPA, MASc, FRCSC

Department of Otolaryngology-Head and Neck Surgery, Massachusetts Eye and Ear, Boston, MA, United States

Introduction

A patient's sense of "balance" is a complex, dynamic phenomenon that integrates information from the visual, peripheral vestibular, and somatosensory systems. The vestibular system is comprised of both peripheral sensory organs and central structures within the brainstem, cerebellum, and cerebrum. Chiefly, the peripheral portion consists of the semicircular canal system and otolith organs of the ear. These peripheral components of the vestibular system continuously collect and relay information about motion and position to the central vestibular system. The circuitry of the central vestibular system then integrates these sensory data into the sense of balance and sensory—motor control.[1] Appropriate function is crucial to maintaining the compensatory movements involved with postural control and gaze stabilization in the face of both internally produced and external forces. Damage to either the peripheral and/or central vestibular symptoms can produce debilitating symptoms. Such signs and symptoms may include objective nystagmus, unsteady gait, subjective vertigo, disorientation, postural instability, and imbalance. Given the possibility and symptomatic overlap of both peripheral and central vestibular dysfunction, proper screening and evaluation following identification of vestibular impairments are crucial both to diagnose the causative agent and to tailor intervention.[2,3]

Approximately 35% of Americans aged 40 or older have experienced some form of vestibular dysfunction.[4] This figure rises rapidly with age, with 85% of Americans age 80 or older having evidence of vestibular dysfunction.[4] Among individuals who have suffered a traumatic brain injury, nearly half will experience some form of vestibular dysfunction.[5] Other subpopulations that report high incidences of vestibular dysfunction after head injury include individuals with diabetes mellitus and military veterans.[6,7] Patients' postural instability, imbalance, and gaze instability can have a significant and deleterious impact on quality of life and balance confidence, underscoring the need for proper management.[8]

Otologic and Lateral Skull Base Trauma. https://doi.org/10.1016/B978-0-323-87482-3.00014-0

Diagnosis

As introduced previously, "normal" vestibular function arises from the interplay between the peripheral organs of the inner ear's vestibular organs, associated nerves, and signal relay centers within the central nervous system. Since damage at any of these constituent components may result in dysfunction, diagnosis of vestibular dysfunction begins by acknowledging that symptoms may manifest from a wide variety of conditions and processes that primarily affect the inner ear and regions of the central nervous system.[9] As such, there is a diverse array of recognized vestibular disorders (i.e., more than 25). These disorders may be discerned via features that can be identified through a patient's history, physical exam, and diagnostic testing. Analysis of history and the results from physical exams can establish whether further diagnostic testing is required.[10]

Generally, vestibular disorders can be classified as either peripheral or central. The most frequent peripheral vestibular disorders include paroxysmal positional vertigo (BPPV), vestibular neuritis, labyrinthitis, and Ménière's disease. Common causes of central vestibular dysfunction are more varied and can include demyelinating diseases that affect the vestibular tracts, cerebellum, and brainstem, acute or hemorrhagic ischemic stroke of the vestibular nerve tracts, cerebellum, or brainstem, vertebrobasilar transient ischemic events, and brain injury of the cerebellum and brainstem. Head trauma can result in either peripheral or central dysfunction, thus heightening the importance of correct and precise assessment. Before objective testing is deployed, patient history and a physical exam can begin to narrow the origins of vestibular dysfunction.[11–13]

History

Clinicians can begin assessing subjective patient symptoms of imbalance through a directed history. Validated survey instruments, such as the Dizziness Handicap Inventory (DHI) and the Veritgo Symptom Scale (VSS), can also assist in itemizing and quantifying vestibular symptoms and their impact.[29,30] Scores from these assessments and discussion of patient symptoms, such as gait instability and nausea, can indicate the severity of the patient's vestibular dysfunction and impact on quality a life.[31,32]

The duration of symptomatic episodes with or without auditory features can be helpful in identifying the type and localization of the physiologic insult (Table 14.1). Acute peripheral vestibular dysfunction is often defined by constant or multiply recurrent and rapid symptom episodes, whereas chronic vestibular dysfunction manifests with less severe or infrequent episodes owing to a process of central compensation in the brain. For example, short bursts of vertigo that last less than a couple of minutes, usually induced by the adoption of certain positions such as lying down, can be suggestive of benign paroxysmal positional vertigo (BPPV). Head trauma is a common catalyst for such brief events such as BPPV or perilymphatic fistula.[34] Longer-duration events that may span hours that occur frequently may indicate

Table 14.1 Common peripheral and central disorders, symptom duration, and association with auditory features (i.e., hearing loss, tinnitus).[33]

Disorder	Symptom episode duration	Auditory symptoms	Incidence (per 100,000)	Etiology
Benign paroxysmal positional vertigo[14]	Seconds	No	107	Peripheral
Perilymphatic fistula[15]	Seconds	Yes	1.5	Peripheral
Vascular ischemia: transient ischemic attack[16]	Seconds to hours	Typically no	29–61	Central or peripheral
Ménière's disease[17]	Minutes to hours	Yes	3.5–513	Peripheral
Syphilis[18]	Hours	Yes	2.3–16.9	Peripheral
Vertiginous migraine[19]	Hoursddays	Yes	11,900	Peripheral
Labyrinthine concussion	Days	Yes	Unknown	Peripheral
Labyrinthitis[20]	Days	Yes	3.5	Peripheral
Vascular ischemia: stroke[21]	Days	Typically no	37	Central or peripheral
Vestibular neuronitis[22]	Days	No	3.5	Peripheral
Anxiety disorder[23]	Variable	Typically no	24,900	Unspecified
Acoustic neuroma[24]	Months	Yes	0.3–1	Peripheral
Cerebellar degeneration[25]	Months	No	20	Central
Cerebellar tumor[26]	Months	No	14.1	Central
Multiple sclerosis[27]	Months	No	309.2	Central
Vestibular ototoxicity[28]	Months	Yes	Unknown	Peripheral

Ménière's disease. In addition, the presence of vertigo alongside "central signs" such as diplopia, weakness, and dysarthria can suggest central nervous system conditions such as multiple sclerosis or acute ischemic stroke.[35,36]

The patient's medical history can also aid in a diagnosis. Vascular risk factors including hypertension, diabetes mellitus, and smoking can increase the probability of stroke. Cardiovascular symptoms such as chest pain/angina, sweating, and palpitations may occur in tandem with dysfunction of the vestibuloautonomic pathway; failure to recognize the interplay of these systems can lead to an incorrect diagnosis.[3] Medications including aminoglycosides and chemotherapeutic treatments can result in vestibular toxicity and symptoms of sustained peripheral vestibular dysfunction. Additionally, a history of using seizure medications may result in the patient experiencing symptoms, such as ataxia, which are commonly attributed to pathology of the cerebellum.[37]

Physical examination

In addition to patient history and discussion of symptoms, physical examination can provide complementary insight.[38] The clinician should perform a complete otologic examination, which includes bed side tests such as a tuning fork exam (i.e., Rinne and Weber), the Dix-Hallpike maneuver to assess for positional vertigo and the HINTS examination (horizontal head impulse testing [**H**ead **I**mpulse]; direction-changing nystagmus in eccentric gaze [**N**ystagmus]; and vertical skew [**T**est of **S**kew]) to gain the information required for a proper diagnosis.[39] The rationale for these tests and investigations is elaborated in the following.

Due to the proximity between auditory and vestibular systems, hearing loss, either conductive or sensorineural, can coincide with certain vestibular disorders. The clinician can employ the Rinne and Weber tests to quickly screen if either sensorineural or conductive hearing deficits are present.[1] A formal audiogram should follow.

For the Weber test, the clinician oscillates a 512-Hz tuning fork. The oscillating fork is placed on top of the patient's head in the midline, usually at the forehead, and the patient is asked about the location of the sound. In a patient with normal hearing, the sound is heard in the center of the head or is interpreted as being heard equally in both ears. If the patient has a sensorineural hearing loss, then the perceived sound should lateralize to the normal ear. In the presence of conductive hearing loss, the sound should lateralize to the affected ear.[40]

For the Rinne test, the clinician can further examine whether conductive hearing loss is present. The examiner oscillates a 512-Hz tuning fork, and the patient indicates when the sound is no longer heard. The tuning fork is then repositioned to be adjacent to the auricula, and the patient is again asked if now audible. In a normal test, air conduction (the second tuning fork position) is louder than bone conduction (the first fork position on the mastoid). With conductive loss present, the reverse will be true. Typically, bone conduction is less effective than air conduction. As a result, the patient should hear a louder sound when the fork is placed on the mastoid when a conductive hearing deficit afflicts him or her. Conversely, a patient with sensorineural deficits should have both air and bone conduction loss.[41] The identification of unilateral sensorineural hearing loss helps to define the vestibular dysfunction as possessing a peripheral etiology. For instance, Ménière's disease manifests with at least a low- to medium-frequency hearing loss and fluctuating aural symptoms such as tinnitus, and sensorineural hearing loss induced by trauma may be associated with a perilymphatic fistula.[42]

In addition to using hearing to identify etiology, assessment of the visual and oculomotor function is prudent.

Bedside vestibular examination

A key component of the bedside vestibular evaluation is the assessment of the vestibuloocular reflex (VOR). Assessing the VOR at the bedside involves observing for the presence of pathologic nystagmus—involuntary "jerky" movements of the eyes—in response to a directed examination that involves specific tasks and patient positioning. as the characteristics of the nystagmus are also important as specific features can suggest a peripheral or central lesion.[43] While a full review of nystagmus and its correlates is beyond the scope of this chapter, peripheral nystagmus is characterized by a horizontal vector, unidirectional, fatiguability, and suppresses with fixation. In contrast, central vestibular dysfunction may manifest as a vertical vector nystagmus, direction changing, and does not suppress with fixation[44]

In the remainder of this section, we review several common bedside examinations that can be helpful in screening for peripheral or central vestibular dysfunction.

Positioning maneuvers

Positioning maneuvers such as the Dix-Hallpike maneuver (DHM) should be deployed to assess for benign paroxysmal positional vertigo—one of the most common causes of peripheral vertigo after a traumatic brain injury. The DHM begins with the patient sitting upright on an exam table with legs stretched out and head facing 45 degrees toward the ear that is being tested. After the clinician leans the patient back into a supine position, the clinician observes the patient's eyes for the presence of nystagmus. If BPPV is present and affecting the posterior canal, the most common site for BPPV, the clinician may observe torsional and upbeat nystagmus.[45,46] The clinician waits for the nystagmus to extinguish prior to testing the opposite ear. Alternatively, the clinician may elect to proceed with the Epley maneuver. The Dix-Hallpike test has an estimated sensitivity of 79% and a specificity of 75%. Testing of each ear enables localization of the disorder.[47]

Head impulse test

The head impulse test (HIT) allows the clinician to gain insight into the patient's angular vestibuloocular reflex (aVOR) function.[48] The clinician begins the HIT examination by having a sitting patient focus on a target object at midline. As the patient maintains their gaze, the clinician rotates the head approximately 10−15 degrees on the horizontal plane relative to the original position and then returns to the original position via an unpredictable and quick motion. As the clinician performs this maneuver, he or she maintains observation of the patient's eyes. Typically, the eyes of the patient will track the observed target while the patient's head is in motion; a positive, abnormal response involves the patient's eyes "slipping" off of the target following the head thrust, followed by a rapid correction of the eyes back to the target—a response known as a "catch-up" saccade. For detecting vestibular hypofunction, the test has greater sensitivity than specificity. These values are estimated at 82%−100% and 34%−39%, respectively. The test's sensitivity increases to 71%−84% by modifying the angle of rotation to go to 30 degrees. The use of the HIT at the bedside can aid in screening for a peripheral vestibular dysfunction. In contrast, patients with central lesions tend to have negative results (i.e., no "catch-up" saccade), except for central disorders that also involve the inner ear or eighth cranial nerve pathways. One consideration before performing the HIT test is to consider the possibility of neck trauma. A history of neck trauma may be a contraindication to the HIT test.[49–51]

Skew deviation

Examination for skew deviation can evaluate for the possibility of a central vestibular lesion. Skew deviation refers to the degree of relative vertical misalignment of the visual axes. The clinician can assess for skew via the alternate cover test while the patient is fixating on a visual target. The patient is instructed to fixate on a stationary target while the examiner covers one of the patient's eyes. Then, the examiner quickly moves their hand to cover the patient's other eye. During this process, the examiner is observing the uncovered eye for a corrective movement.[27,52]

Head-shaking nystagmus

The head shake test can be useful for screening for a unilateral vestibular lesion. The examiner beings by tilting the patient's head 30 degrees downward and oscillates the head for 20–30 revolutions at a gentle velocity of 1–2 Hz. At the end of the oscillation, the examiner observes for the presence or absence of nystagmus. In patients with symmetrical vestibular loss, the test should not elicit nystagmus. Conversely, patients with a unilateral lesion, such as with unilateral vestibular neuritis, typically have nystagmus—usually, the fast phase of the nystagmus is directed away from the lesioned ear. The test has a sensitivity of 46% and a specificity of 75%; in patients with vestibular neuritis, between 85% and 100% display head-shaking nystagmus.[53] The rare presence of pure vertical nystagmus may indicate central etiology, most likely arising from a lateral medullary lesion.[53,54]

Dynamic visual acuity

Vestibular dysfunction may be present in a patient who has degradation in visual acuity with active head movements. The corresponding test, dynamic visual acuity (DVA), involves assessing for changes in acuity before and during oscillatory head movements. The clinician begins by establishing a baseline of visual acuity by having the patient read from a Snellen chart. The examiner clasps the patients head and begins oscillating at a gentle frequency of 1–2 Hz while the patient attempts to read the visual acuity chart. A significant decline in visual acuity suggests a peripheral vestibular loss.[3]

The Romberg

The sharpened, or tandem, Romberg test is a practical test for global balance function. Balance function is dependent on the sensory inputs via vision, somatosensory, and the peripheral vestibular system. Isolation of the peripheral vestibular system can be realized by selectively removing the influence of the visual and somatosensory sensory inputs. The Romberg simulates this isolation by placing an emphasis on the vestibular system. To achieve this result, the patient closes his or her eyes, puts their feet in a tandem arrangement, and crosses their arms. If the patient consistently falls or sways to one side, then there is an indication of a balance dysfunction that may be related to a vestibular deficit.[55–57]

Objective vestibular testing

In some cases, additional objective vestibular function training may provide additional data to support a diagnosis. A modern battery of studies includes electronystagmography (ENG), videonystagmography (VNG), and rotary chair testing. The increased objectivity of the laboratory testing can enable more impartial and sensitive information, from which patient etiology can be diagnosed.[58]

ENG (or more appropriately VNG in today's modern vestibular laboratories) comprises noninvasive techniques that assess the vestibular function.[59] During ENG, the patient wears small electrodes placed at various locations along the skin. These electrical sensors monitor eye movement by measuring the corneoretinal potential—a DC potential naturally present between the cornea and the retina. More recently, the development of VNG can conduct the same battery of tests without the use of skin surface electrodes. VNG systems include a pair of goggles with infrared cameras that track and record eye movements during testing.

The modern vestibular test battery consists of several assessments: oculomotor and optokinetic testing, positional testing, caloric testing, and rotational studies.

Oculomotor involves examining the eyes' ability to track a target as it moves between various locations. Typically, a red light is employed as the target. Optokinetic testing is a variant of target tracking but involves tracking a moving range, typically a field of alternating and contrasting stripes. Abnormalities in oculomotor or optokinetic function may indicate a neurological problem, potentially in the central nervous system or the pathway between the peripheral vestibular system and the brain.[60]

The positional tests assess the presence or absence of nystagmus within different head positions and changes in head position. The patient is instructed to maintain a steady gaze while moving their head and body, such as in the DHM. While the patient is guided through these positions, the electrodes in an ENG or cameras in a VNG goggle measure the velocity, frequency, amplitude, and latency of any nystagmus present.

Caloric testing examines the horizontal semicircular canal of each ear, independently, in addition to offering information on the responsiveness of these pathways and the relative functionality between the left and right. The efficacy of caloric testing arises from how a density change brought about by a temperature differential in the endolymph of the lateral semicircular canal induces nystagmus. Caloric testing can isolate peripheral vestibular dysfunction.[61,62]

Complementing the test battery of ENG/VNG, rotary chair testing can assist in assessing for a bilateral vestibular disorder. Rotary chair testing protocols typically employ a chair capable of rotation in a dark room coupled with VNG goggles to track eye movement. The head is held steady by a security head strap, and a seatbelt secures the body. Lab-specific protocols can vary, but in general three tests are performed including varying the velocity and acceleration of the patient, optokinetic tests, and fixation tests. Using regiments with different chair velocities and acceleration, information regarding the presence or absence of unilateral or bilateral vestibular loss is observed. The optokinetic and fixation tests are helpful in assessing for the presence of central vestibular dysfunction.

Imaging

In some cases where a central process is suspected or needs to be ruled out, magnetic resonance imaging (MRI) of the brain is useful for the identification of central nervous system tumors or masses, cerebrovascular accidents (i.e., stroke), and other soft tissue abnormalities that may account for a patient's presentation.[4,63] Computed tomography (CT) scans provide excellent detail on the bony anatomy of the temporal bone. Abnormalities such as temporal bone fractures can be readily assessed.[64]

Treatment

Treatments for vestibular dysfunction following traumatic brain injury depend on, in part, on the identification of a specific vestibular disorder. As such, the treatment of vestibular dysfunction should address the identified conditions in the given patient.[4]

Most treatment plans should utilize medication for symptomatic management. Medications that mitigate the vegetative symptoms of vestibular dysfunction include antiemetics to reduce nausea, and vestibular suppressants (e.g., benzodiazepines) to minimize the debilitating effects of acute vertiginous events. One potential concern with the sustained use of vestibular suppressants, however, is that their overuse may prolong the period of vestibular compensation.[65]

BPPV is among the most common vestibular disorders after traumatic brain injury. In response, canalith repositioning maneuvers such as the Epley maneuver in the case of posterior canalithiasis are helpful. BPPV arises from the presence of broken calcium carbonate crystals (otoconia) from the utricle in the endolymph of the semicircular canals. Changes in head position can produce the movement of the otoconia in the canals, which leads to vertiginous symptoms.[66] The Epley maneuver aims to resolve BPPV by ushering the otoconia out of the posterior canal and into the vestibule. In the case of BPPV of the right posterior canal, the Epley maneuver begins with the patient rotating their head 45 degrees to the right while sitting upright on the end table. After at least 30 s, the clinician reclines the patient back over the end of the table just lower than the horizontal. After another period of at least 30 s, the patient's head is to be rotated 90 degrees to the left. After the duration of this position for at least 30 s, the patient adopts a left lateral position with the head facing 135 degrees from supine. Last, the patient should return to a sitting position. Throughout these maneuvers, the examiner observes for the presence or absence of nystagmus. The Epley maneuver can be repeated if necessary. The stated directions should be reversed if BPPV is present in the left ear. The Epley maneuver has a significant probability of success if BPPV is present.[67] Other treatment variants for BPPV include Brandt-Daroff exercise, foster maneuver, half-somersault, and Semont maneuver.[1]

Trauma to the cochlea or vestibular system may be a precipitating factor for Ménière's disease. Although a full discussion on the treatment for Ménière's disease is beyond the scope of this chapter, the treatment algorithm typically employs escalating symptom management in response to the frequency and severity of a patient's symptoms. For example, the prescription of motion sickness and antiemetic medications can help alleviate acute vertiginous symptoms during discrete episodes. Lifestyle changes, such as reducing salt intake to less than two or 3 grams per day, may also help with the frequency and severity of attacks. Patients with Ménière's disease may also benefit from vestibular rehabilitation for persistent disequilibrium. In addition, audiologist referral for services, including hearing aid fitting, should be done to reduce or eliminate hearing loss and tinnitus.[68]

More invasive surgical options may become necessary for some patients with vestibular hypofunction and unrelenting vestibular symptoms. Broadly speaking, surgical options for peripheral vestibular disorders are classified as either being ablative (i.e., destructive) or nonablative. Such surgical procedures for severe or unrelenting peripheral vestibular symptoms include endolymphatic sac decompression, labyrinthectomy, and vestibular nerve sectioning.[69]

In addition to medication and surgery, many patients suffering from vestibular dysfunction after a traumatic brain injury will benefit from vestibular rehabilitation therapy (VRT) due to the presumed effects on neuroplasticity of brain regions involved with balance (i.e., so-called "central compensation"). Even in extreme cases of compete unilateral vestibular loss, central adaptation can and does occur with the input of intact visual and proprioceptive pathways. Through VRT exercises, the vestibular system compensates for deficits by sensory reweighting. While this compensation occurs progressively in patients not enrolled in a VRT program, VRT may expedite and assist recovery. The primary goals of VRT are to reduce the primary and secondary impairments found in a patient's diagnosis, such as vertigo, dizziness, gaze instability, and imbalance. Individuals with peripheral vestibular dysfunction are more likely to make a more significant recovery than those with central vestibular dysfunction due to the role of pathological involvement in limiting compensation in the latter.[70]

Patient utilization of VRT depends on a problem-oriented approach with a specialty-trained vestibular physical therapist. A comprehensive initial assessment comprising balance, gait, visual stability, and positional assessments helps determine patients' vestibular dysfunction functional deficits. In response to this assessment, the therapist prescribes habituation, gaze stabilization, and balance training exercises in an outpatient setting. Habituation exercises focus on reducing vertiginous symptoms brought about by rapid head or body position changes. Gaze stabilization exercises target proper coordination of eye movements to ensure stable vision throughout dynamic head and bodily motion. Balance training exercises work to reduce the patient's risk of falling and balance confidence. Additionally,

VRT should be contextualized in a wider rehabilitation program focused on addressing and reducing the other neurological sequelae that can be present after a traumatic brain injury.[71,72]

Future research

Further work is needed to understand the pathophysiology and optimal treatment programs for patients suffering from vestibular dysfunction after a traumatic brain injury. Other important questions pertain to how vestibular dysfunction presents in diverse patient populations. For example, recent military conflicts have heightened the need to investigate the relationship between traumatic brain injury and vestibular dysfunction.[7] Another line of investigation with limited literature is that of the impact of age on vestibular dysfunction. Among geriatric patient populations, work involving the topic of presbyvertigo—akin to the hearing loss that is attributable to age (presbycusis)—has yet to see significant investigation.

A secondary and important domain for future research involves developing efficacious diagnostic and treatments. Several studies have attempted to use autonomous algorithms, such as machine learning, to process the vast amounts of vestibular laboratory data for accurate diagnostic prediction. Still, more work is needed to improve the sensitivity and specificity of these algorithms.[73,74] For treatments, the literature offers a limited perspective on the effectiveness beyond different forms of vestibular rehabilitation therapy, especially in context of significant head trauma. More research is needed to standardize and best target rehabilitation exercises for this specific patient populations.

Conclusion

Vestibular dysfunction after traumatic brain injury is common and requires a comprehensive diagnostic and management approach. Accurate clinical knowledge of specific end-organ sources of vestibular dysfunction is important for proper workup and management. Perhaps most importantly, the diagnostic and treatment journey typically involves collaboration among several specialists including otolaryngology, audiology, neurology, and physical therapy.

References

1. Dougherty JM, Carney M, Emmady PD. *Vestibular Dysfunction* [Updated 2021 Jul 7]. In: StatPearls [Internet]. Treasure Island (FL): StatPearls Publishing; 2021 Jan. Available from: https://www.ncbi.nlm.nih.gov/books/NBK558926/.
2. Bisdorff A, Von Brevern M, Lempert T, Newman-Toker DE. Classification of vestibular symptoms: towards an international classification of vestibular disorders. *J Vestib Res.* 2009;19(1,2):1−13. https://doi.org/10.3233/ves-2009-0343.

3. Renga V. Clinical evaluation of patients with vestibular dysfunction. *Neurol Res Int.* 2019;2019:8. https://doi.org/10.1155/2019/3931548. Article ID 3931548.

4. Agrawal Y, Ward BK, Minor LB. Vestibular dysfunction: prevalence, impact and need for targeted treatment. *J Vestib Res.* 2013;23(3):113−117. https://doi.org/10.3233/VES-130498.

5. Marcus HJ, Paine H, Sargeant M, et al. Vestibular dysfunction in acute traumatic brain injury. *J Neurol.* 2019;266(10):2430−2433. https://doi.org/10.1007/s00415-019-09403-z.

6. Agrawal Y, Carey JP, Della Santina CC, Schubert MC, Minor LB. Diabetes, vestibular dysfunction, and falls: analyses from the national health and nutrition examination survey. *Otol Neurotol: Off Publ Am Otol Soc Am Neurotol Soc [and] Eur Acad Otol Neurotol.* December 2010;31(9):1445−1450. https://doi.org/10.1097/MAO.0b013e3181f2f035.

7. Swan AA, Jeremy TN, Pogoda TK, et al. Association of traumatic brain injury with vestibular dysfunction and dizziness in post-9/11 veterans. *J Head Trauma Rehabil.* June 2020;35(3):E253−E265. https://doi.org/10.1097/HTR.0000000000000513.

8. Fife TD, Blum D, Fisher RS. Measuring the effects of antiepileptic medications on balance in older people. *Epilepsy Res.* 2006;70(2−3):103−109. https://doi.org/10.1016/j.eplepsyres.2006.03.004.

9. Choi JY, Kim JS. Nystagmus and central vestibular disorders. *Curr Opin Neurol.* 2017;30(1):98−106. https://doi.org/10.1097/WCO.0000000000000416.

10. Ward PH. XX the histopathology of auditory and vestibular disorders in head trauma. *Ann Otol Rhinol Laryngol.* 1969;78(2):227−238. https://doi.org/10.1177/000348946907800203.

11. Scherer M, Burrows H, Pinto R, Somrack E. Characterizing self-reported dizziness and otovestibular impairment among blast-injured traumatic amputees: a pilot study. *Mil Med.* 2007;172(7):731−737. https://doi.org/10.7205/milmed.172.7.731.

12. Kolev OI, Sergeeva M. Vestibular disorders following different types of head and neck trauma. *Funct Neurol.* 2016;31(2):75−80. https://doi.org/10.11138/fneur/2016.31.2.075.

13. Hoffer ME, Balaban C, Gottshall K, Balough BJ, Maddox MR, Penta JR. Blast exposure: vestibular consequences and associated characteristics. *Otol Neurotol: Off Publ Am Otol Soc Am Neurotol Soc [and] Eur Acad Otol Neurotol.* 2010;31(2):232−236. https://doi.org/10.1097/MAO.0b013e3181c993c3.

14. Brevern M von, Radtke A, Lezius F, et al. Epidemiology of benign paroxysmal positional vertigo: a population based study. *J Neurol Neurosurg Psychiatry.* July 2007;78(7):710−715. https://doi.org/10.1136/jnnp.2006.100420.

15. Sarna B, Abouzari M, Merna C, et al. Perilymphatic fistula: a review of classification, etiology, diagnosis, and treatment. *Front Neurol.* September 15, 2020;11:1046. https://doi.org/10.3389/fneur.2020.01046.

16. Degan D, Ornello R, Tiseo C, et al. Epidemiology of transient ischemic attacks using time- or tissue-based definitions. *Stroke.* March 1, 2017;48(3):530−536. https://doi.org/10.1161/STROKEAHA.116.015417.

17. Koenen L, Andaloro C. Meniere disease. In: *StatPearls.* Treasure Island (FL): StatPearls Publishing; 2021. http://www.ncbi.nlm.nih.gov/books/NBK536955/.

18. Schmidt R, Carson PJ, Jansen RJ. Resurgence of syphilis in the United States: an assessment of contributing factors. *Infectious Diseases.* October 16, 2019;12. https://doi.org/10.1177/1178633719883282, 1178633719883282.

19. Formeister EJ, Rizk HG, Kohn MA, Sharon JD. The epidemiology of vestibular migraine: a population-based survey study. *Otol Neurotol,* September 2018;39(8):1037−1044, https://doi.org/10.1097/MAO.0000000000001900.

20. Jeong S-H, Kim H-J, Kim J-S. Vestibular neuritis. *Semin Neurol*. July 2013;33(3): 185−194. https://doi.org/10.1055/s-0033-1354598.

21. Duloquin G, Graber M, Garnier L, et al. Incidence of acute ischemic stroke with visible arterial occlusion. *Stroke*. July 1, 2020;51(7):2122−2130. https://doi.org/10.1161/STROKEAHA.120.029949.

22. Strupp M, Brandt T. Vestibular neuritis. *Semin Neurol*. November 2009;29(5):509−519. https://doi.org/10.1055/s-0029-1241040.

23. Bandelow B, Michaelis S. Epidemiology of anxiety disorders in the 21st century. *Dialogues Clin Neurosci*. September 2015;17(3):327−335.

24. The Prevalence of 'Incidental' Acoustic Neuroma | Neurology | JAMA Otolaryngology−Head & Neck Surgery | JAMA Network." Accessed October 9, 2021. https://jamanetwork.com/journals/jamaotolaryngology/fullarticle/648807.

25. Louis ED, Faust PL. Essential tremor: the most common form of cerebellar degeneration? *Cerebellum & Ataxias*. August 14, 2020;7(1):12. https://doi.org/10.1186/s40673-020-00121-1.

26. Bondy ML, Scheurer ME, Malmer B, et al. Brain tumor epidemiology: consensus from the brain tumor epidemiology consortium (BTEC). *Cancer*. October 1, 2008;113(7 Suppl.):1953−1968. https://doi.org/10.1002/cncr.23741.

27. Wallin MT, Culpepper WJ, Campbell JD, et al. The prevalence of ms in the United States: a population-based estimate using health claims data. *Neurology*. March 5, 2019;92(10):e1029−e1040. https://doi.org/10.1212/WNL.0000000000007035.

28. Ganesan P, Schmiedge J, Manchaiah V, Swapna S, Dhandayutham S, Kothandaraman PP. Ototoxicity: a challenge in diagnosis and treatment. *J Audiol Otol*. April 2018;22(2): 59−68. https://doi.org/10.7874/jao.2017.00360.

29. Symptoms, Anxiety and Handicap in Dizzy Patients: Development of the Vertigo Symptom Scale—ScienceDirect." Accessed October 9, 2021. https://www.sciencedirect.com/science/article/abs/pii/002239999290131K?via%3Dihub.

30. Mutlu B, Serbetcioglu B. Discussion of the dizziness handicap inventory. *J Vestib Res: Equilib Orient*. 2013;23(6):271−277. https://doi.org/10.3233/VES-130488.

31. Kondo M, Kiyomizu K, Goto F, et al. Analysis of vestibular-balance symptoms according to symptom duration: dimensionality of the vertigo symptom scale-short form. *Health Qual Life Outcome*. 2015;13(4). https://doi.org/10.1186/s12955-015-0207-7. Published 2015 Jan 22.

32. Weightman MM, Bolgla R, McCulloch KL. Physical therapy recommendations for service members with mild traumatic brain injury. *J Head Trauma Rehabil*. 2010;25: 206−218.

33. Swartz R, Longwell P. Treatment of vertigo. *Am Fam Physician*. 2005;71(6):1115−1122.

34. Naguib MB, Madian Y, Refaat M, Mohsen O, El Tabakh M, Abo-Setta A. Characterisation and objective monitoring of balance disorders following head trauma, using videonystagmography. *J Laryngol Otol*. 2012;126(1):26−33. https://doi.org/10.1017/S002221511100291X.

35. Kerber KA, Baloh RW. The evaluation of a patient with dizziness. *Neurol Clin Pract*. December 2011;1(1):24−33.

36. Newman-Toker DE, Hsieh YH, Camargo CA, Pelletier AJ, Butchy GT, Edlow JA. Spectrum of dizziness visits to US emergency departments: cross-sectional analysis from a nationally representative sample. *Mayo Clin Proc*. July 2008;83(7):765−775.

37. Bladin PF. History of "epileptic vertigo": its medical, social, and forensic problems. *Epilepsia*. 1998;39(4):442−447.

38. Kaufman KR, Brey RH, Chou LS, Rabatin A, Brown AW, Basford JR. Comparison of subjective and objective measurements of balance disorders following traumatic brain injury. *Med Eng Phys*. 2006;28(3):234−239.

39. Cohn B. Can bedside oculomotor (HINTS) testing differentiate central from peripheral causes of vertigo? *Ann Emerg Med*. September 1, 2014;64(3):265−268. https://doi.org/10.1016/j.annemergmed.2014.01.010.

40. Wahid NWB, Hogan CJ, Attia M. *Weber Test* [Updated 2021 Feb 9]. In: StatPearls [Internet]. Treasure Island (FL): StatPearls Publishing; January 2021. Available from: https://www.ncbi.nlm.nih.gov/books/NBK526135/.

41. Chole RA, Cook GB. The Rinne test for conductive deafness: a critical reappraisal. *Arch Otolaryngol Head Neck Surg*. 1988;114(4):399−403. https://doi.org/10.1001/archotol.1988.01860160043018.

42. Shea JJ. Classification of Menière's disease. *Am J Otol*. May 1993;14(3):224−229.

43. Whitney SL, Sparto PJ. Eye movements, dizziness, and mild traumatic brain injury (mTBI): a topical review of emerging evidence and screening measures. *J Neurol Phys Ther: J Neurol Phys Ther*. 2019;43(Suppl. 2):S31−S36. https://doi.org/10.1097/NPT.0000000000000272.

44. Sekhon RK, Rocha Cabrero F, Deibel JP. *Nystagmus Types* [Updated 2020 Nov 9]. In: StatPearls [Internet]. Treasure Island (FL): StatPearls Publishing; 2021 Jan. Available from: https://www.ncbi.nlm.nih.gov/books/NBK539711/.

45. Johns P, Quinn J. Clinical diagnosis of benign paroxysmal positional vertigo and vestibular neuritis. *CMAJ (Can Med Assoc J)*. 2020;192(8):E182−E186. https://doi.org/10.1503/cmaj.190334.

46. Talmud JD, Coffey R, Edemekong PF. *Dix Hallpike Maneuver* [Updated 2021 Jul 1]. In: StatPearls [Internet]. Treasure Island (FL): StatPearls Publishing; January 2021. Available from: https://www.ncbi.nlm.nih.gov/books/NBK459307/.

47. Halker RB, Barrs DM, Wellik KE, Wingerchuk DM, Demaerschalk BM. Establishing a diagnosis of benign paroxysmal positional vertigo through the dix-hallpike and side-lying maneuvers: a critically appraised topic. *Neurol*. 2008;14(3):201−204. https://doi.org/10.1097/NRL.0b013e31816f2820.

48. Weber KP, Aw ST, Todd MJ, McGarvie LA, Curthoys IS, Head GMH. Impulse test in unilateral vestibular loss: vestibulo-ocular reflex and catch-up saccades. *Neurology*. February 5, 2008;70(6):454−463. https://doi.org/10.1212/01.wnl.0000299117.48935.2e.

49. MacDougall HG, Weber KP, McGarvie LA, Halmagyi GM, Curthoys IS. The video head impulse test: diagnostic accuracy in peripheral vestibulopathy. *Neurology*. 2009;73(14):1134−1141. https://doi.org/10.1212/WNL.0b013e3181bacf85.

50. Beynon GJ, Jani P, Baguley DM. A clinical evaluation of head impulse testing. *Clin Otolaryngol Allied Sci*. 1998;23(2):117−122. https://doi.org/10.1046/j.1365-2273.1998.00112.

51. Hammond S, Harro CC. Vestibular evaluation in individuals with mild brain injury. *J Neurol Phys Ther*. 2006;29(4):209.

52. Traccis S, Zoroddu GF, Zecca MT, Cau T, Solinas MA, Masuri R. Evaluating patients with vertigo: bedside examination. *Neurol Sci*. March 2004;25(Suppl 1):S16−S19.

53. Choi KD, Kim JS. Head-shaking nystagmus in central vestibulopathies. *Ann N Y Acad Sci*. May 2009;1164:338−343.

54. Takahashi S, Fetter M, Koenig E, Dichgans J. The clinical significance of head-shaking nystagmus in the dizzy patient. *Acta Otolaryngol*. 1990;109(1−2):8−14. https://doi.org/10.3109/00016489009107409.

55. Cohen HS, Mulavara AP, Peters BT, et al. Sharpening the tandem walking test for screening peripheral neuropathy. *South Med J.* 2013;106(10):565−569. https://doi.org/10.1097/SMJ.0000000000000009.

56. Fitzgerald B. A review of the sharpened Romberg test in diving medicine. *SPUMS J (South Pacific Underw Med Soc).* 1996;26(3):142−146.

57. Forbes J, Cronovich H. *Romberg Test* [Updated 2020 Sep 23]. In: StatPearls [Internet]. Treasure Island (FL): StatPearls Publishing; 2021 Jan. Available from: https://www.ncbi.nlm.nih.gov/books/NBK563187/.

58. Zhou G, Brodsky JR. Objective vestibular testing of children with dizziness and balance complaints following sports-related concussions. *Otolaryngol Head Neck Surg.* 2015;152:1133−1139.

59. Littlefield PD, Pinto RL, Burrows HL, Brungart DS. The vestibular effects of repeated low-level blasts. *J Neurotrauma.* 2016;33(1):71−81. https://doi.org/10.1089/neu.2014.3824.

60. Nicholson M, King J, Smith PF, Darlington CL. Vestibulo-ocular, optokinetic and postural function in diabetes mellitus. *Neuroreport.* January 21, 2002;13(1):153−157.

61. Formby C, Carter RL, Hansen CA, Kuntz LA. Measurement, analysis and modeling of the caloric response. 1. A descriptive mathematical model of the caloric response over time. *Acta Otolaryngol.* 1992;(Suppl. 498):4−18.

62. Gupta SK, Mundra RK. Electronystagmography a very useful diagnostic tool in cases of vertigo. *Indian J Otolaryngol Head Neck Surg.* 2015;67(4):370−374. https://doi.org/10.1007/s12070-015-0859-y.

63. Mostafa BE, Kahky AO, Kader HM, Rizk M. Central vestibular dysfunction in an otorhinolaryngological vestibular unit: incidence and diagnostic strategy. *Int Arch Otorhinolaryngol.* 2014;18(3):235−238. https://doi.org/10.1055/s-0034-1370884.

64. Kerber KA, Schweigler L, West BT, Fendrick AM, Morgenstern LB. Value of computed tomography scans in ED dizziness visits: analysis from a nationally representative sample. *Am J Emerg Med.* 2010;28(9):1030−1036. https://doi.org/10.1016/j.ajem.2009.06.007.

65. Soto E, Vega R. Neuropharmacology of vestibular system disorders. *Curr Neuropharmacol.* 2010;8(1):26−40. https://doi.org/10.2174/157015910790909511. Swartz R, Longwell P. Treatment of vertigo. Am Family Phys 2005;71(6):1115−1122.

66. You P, Instrum R, Parnes L. Benign paroxysmal positional vertigo. *Laryngoscope Investig Otolaryngol.* 2018;4(1):116−123. https://doi.org/10.1002/lio2.230. Published 2018 Dec 14.

67. Nguyen CT, Basso M. *Epley Maneuver* [Updated 2020 Oct 1]. In: StatPearls [Internet]. Treasure Island (FL): StatPearls Publishing; January 2021. Available from: https://www.ncbi.nlm.nih.gov/books/NBK563287/.

68. Morrison AW. Anticipation in Ménière's disease. *J Laryngol Otol.* June 1995;109(6):499−502. Foster CA. Optimal management of Ménière's disease. Ther Clin Risk Manag 2015;11:301−307. Published 2015 Feb 25. doi:10.2147/TCRM.S59023.

69. Volkenstein S, Dazert S. Recent surgical options for vestibular vertigo. *GMS Curr Top Otorhinolaryngol, Head Neck Surg.* 2017;16:Doc01. https://doi.org/10.3205/cto000140. Published 2017 Dec 18.

70. Shepard NT, Telian SA, Smith-Wheelock M, Raj A. Vestibular and balance rehabilitation therapy. *Ann Otol Rhinol Laryngol.* 1993;102(3 Pt 1):198−205.

71. Alsalaheen BA, Mucha A, Morris LO, et al. Vestibular rehabilitation for dizziness and balance disorders after concussion. *J Neurol Phys Ther: J Neurol Phys Ther.* 2010;34(2):87−93. https://doi.org/10.1097/NPT.0b013e3181dde568.

72. Han BI, Song HS, Kim JS. Vestibular rehabilitation therapy: review of indications, mechanisms, and key exercises. *J Clin Neurol*. 2011;7(4):184−196. https://doi.org/10.3988/jcn.2011.7.4.184.

73. Master CL, Master SR, Wiebe DJ, et al. Vision and vestibular system dysfunction predicts prolonged concussion recovery in children. *Clin J Sport Med*. 2018;28(2):139−145.

74. Kamogashira T, Fujimoto C, Kinoshita M, Kikkawa Y, Yamasoba T, Iwasaki S. Prediction of vestibular dysfunction by applying machine learning algorithms to postural instability. Published 2020 Feb 5 *Front Neurol*. 2020;11:7. https://doi.org/10.3389/fneur.2020.00007. Yeh S-C, Huang M-C, Wang P-C, et al. Machine learning-based assessment tool for imbalance and vestibular dysfunction with virtual reality rehabilitation system. Comput Methods Prog Biomed 2014;116(3):311−318. doi:10.1016/j.cmpb.2014.04.014.

Vestibular rehabilitation following head injury

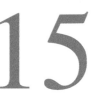

Kathryn C. MacDonald[1], Seth Herman[2], Leanna W. Katz[3]

[1]*Wentworth-Douglass Hospital, Dover, NH, United States;* [2]*California Rehabilitation Institute, Cedars Sinai Medical Center, Los Angeles, CA, United States;* [3]*Boston University, Boston, MA, United States*

H.R. is a 53-year-old male who fell on ice, resulting in traumatic brain injury (TBI) characterized by a subdural hematoma. He returned to work within 2 months, as a computer programmer, working 6 −8 h per day. He was referred to outpatient physical therapy, with a chief complaint of cervical pain. During the examination of the cervical spine, the patient moved from a sitting to supine position and reported vertigo. Through further subjective history, the patient noted vertigo with positional changes when laying down or sitting up, since the fall, lasting approximately 10 s. He also notes imbalance when walking and descending stairs. Given this history, an oculomotor and vestibular assessment was completed. The exam was unremarkable, except for observation of brief upbeat, left torsional nystagmus, with subsequent complaints of vertigo, when in a left Dix-Hallpike position. The patient was treated for a left posterior canal canalithiasis with two canalith repositioning maneuvers (CRMs). One week later, upon reassessment, there were no signs or symptoms, suggesting resolution of benign paroxysmal positional vertigo (BPPV) and treatment continued with the cervical spine.[1−3]

Introduction

Traumatic brain injury (TBI) is a disruption in the normal function of the brain that can be caused by a direct blow or jolt to the head, penetration through the skull into the brain tissue and/or forces such as rotational or acceleration and deceleration forces. TBI is characterized by a change in brain function notable for one of the following: loss or decreased consciousness, amnesia of the event before or after the injury, focal neurological deficits such as weakness, vision, cognition, and language, and slowed thinking or processing. The symptoms can range from mild to severe depending on the amount of injury to the brain. Severe cases may result in extended periods of unconsciousness, coma, or even death.

TBI is a major healthcare problem. In 2014, there were about 2.87 million cases of TBI in the United States alone.[4] It is a leading cause of death and disability with an estimated 13.5 million individuals living with TBI-associated deficits. The cost of TBI is about $76.5 billion directly and indirectly. There are about 288,000

Otologic and Lateral Skull Base Trauma. https://doi.org/10.1016/...

hospitalizations for TBI every year. Males represent 78.8% of all reported TBIs with higher rates of TBI among males (959 per 100,000) than females (811 per 100,000). The highest rates of TBI are observed in older adults (≥75 years; 2232 per 100,000 population), very young (0–4 years; 1591 per 100,000), and young adults (15–24 years; 1081 per 100,000). The leading causes of TBI-related deaths are due to motor vehicle crashes, suicides, and falls. The leading causes of nonfatal TBI in the United States occur from falls (35%), motor vehicle-related injuries (17%), and strikes or blows to the head from or against an object (17%), such as sports injuries.[4]

TBI results in complex body system and structure deficits that interact across several domains including physical, sensory, cognitive, behavioral, and emotional. Vestibular dysfunction and associated balance, ocular, and auditory dysfunction are important issues that affect the function and quality-of-life of TBI survivors. Since TBI is characterized by sudden and often violent causes, trauma to the vestibular system is common. As noted, TBI affects a wide spectrum of ages and has multiple causes such as falls, motor vehicle accidents, sports-related injuries, and military blast wave exposures among other causes. Patients often report problems with dizziness and or lightheadedness or other issues related to the auditory or vestibular system. Such complaints warrant further investigation into the vestibular system including balance testing. Clinicians must be aware of the potential problems associated with trauma including the need to consider not only TBI but other problems such as benign positional vertigo, cervicogenic headache and dizziness, visual deficits, ototoxic side effects of medications, and other vestibular pathology. It is beyond the scope of this chapter to review the full differential diagnoses. Nonetheless, assessment that includes cervical, oculomotor, postural stability, and gait is important to further delineate the potential causes in order to provide physical therapist who performs the bulk of the evaluation and rehabilitative treatment with guidance for diagnosis. The goal of this chapter is to describe the rehabilitative approach to ameliorating the deficits and restoring function and quality of life.

Vestibular anatomy and physiology

The vestibular system (Table 15.1 and 15.2) assists with understanding body position and motion. It uses spatial orientation and stabilizes vision to maintain balance, especially with movement. The vestibular end organs sense angular and linear acceleration and transduce these forces to signals that can be interpreted by the central nervous system (CNS). The CNS integrates this information from the vestibular system to stabilize gaze during head movement through the vestibulocular reflex (VOR), in addition to modulating muscle tone through the vestibulocollic (VCR) and vestibulospinal (VSR) reflexes (Table 15.3a and 15.3b).

Sensory inputs include vestibular, proprioception, and vision (Table 15.3c). The sensory inputs are integrated by the central processors, known as the vestibular

Table 15.1 Peripheral anatomy of the vestibular system.[5]

Peripheral apparatus	Function
Semicircular canals	Provide sensory information about the velocity of the head, which enables the VOR to generate a proportional eye movement, by responding to angular velocity. The eyes therefore remain stationary, during head motion, maintaining clear vision.
Otoliths	Determine forces related to linear acceleration, by responding to both linear head motion and static tilt with respect to the gravitational axis.
Vestibular nerve (CN VIII)	Transmits afferent signals from the labyrinth through the internal auditory canal (IAC). The IAC also contains the cochlear nerve (hearing), the facial nerve, the nervus intermedius, and the labyrinth artery. The IAC travels through the dense petrous portion of the temporal bone and opens into the posterior fossa at the level of the pons. The vestibular nerve enters the brainstem at the pontomedullary junction.
Vascular supply	The labyrinthine artery supplies the peripheral vestibular system. It is often a branch of the anterior–inferior cerebellar artery (AICA), though occasionally it is a direct branch of the basilar artery. The labyrinthine artery divides into the anterior vestibular artery and the common cochlear artery. The anterior vestibular artery supplies the vestibular nerve, most of the utricle, and the ampullae of the lateral and anterior SCC. The common cochlear artery divides into the main cochlear artery, which supplies the cochlea, and the vestibulocochlear artery, which supplies part of the cochlea, the ampulla of the posterior semicircular canal, and the inferior portion of the saccule.

Table 15.2 Central anatomy of the vestibular system.[5]

Central apparatus	Function
Vestibular nucleus	Consists of four major nuclei: superior, medial, lateral, and descending and at least seven minor nuclei. The structure is located within the pons, though it extends to the medulla. The superior and medial vestibular nucleus are relays for the VOR. The medial vestibular nucleus is involved in the vestibulospinal reflexes and manages head and eye movements that occur together. The lateral vestibular nucleus is the primary nucleus for the vestibulospinal reflex. The descending nucleus is connected to the other nuclei and the cerebellum, though it has no outflow of its own.
Vascular supply	The vertebral–basilar arterial system supplies blood to the peripheral and central nervous system. The posterior–inferior cerebellar arteries (PICAs) branch off the vertebral artery. The PICAs are the most important arteries for the CNS. They supply the inferior portions of the cerebellar hemispheres and the dorsolateral medulla, which includes aspects of the vestibular nuclear complex. The basilar artery supplies central vestibular structures via perforator branches. The AICA is the sole blood supply for the peripheral vestibular system via the labyrinthine artery. The AICA also supplies blood to a portion of the cerebellum and pons.
Cerebellum	The recipient of outflow from the vestibular nucleus complex. It is not required for vestibular reflexes, though those reflexes become uncalibrated and ineffective when the cerebellum is removed.

Table 15.3a Motor outputs and vestibular reflexes.[5]

Reflex	Function
Vestibulocular reflex (VOR)	The motor neurons of the ocular motor nuclei, drive the extraocular eye muscles, which are the output neurons of the VOR. The VOR maintains stable vision during head motion. The VOR has two components: the angular VOR, compensates for rotation, mediated by the SCC, and the linear VOR, compensates for translation, mediated by the otoliths. The linear VOR is important in circumstances in which the target is near with relatively high frequency of head movement.
Vestibulospinal reflex (VSR)	The anterior horn cells of the spinal cord gray matter, drive skeletal muscle, which is the output neuron of the VSR. The purpose of the VSR is to stabilize the body, though it consists of several reflexes named according to the timing (static vs. dynamic) and sensory input (canal vs. otolith).
Vestibulocollic reflex (VCR)	Entails the cervical muscles to stabilize the head. The head movement counteracts the movement sensed by the otolithic or semicircular canal organs. The precise pathway of this reflex has yet to be detailed.

Table 15.3b Cervical reflexes.[5]

Reflex	Function
Cervicoocular reflex (COR)	The COR interacts with the VOR. The COR entails eye movements, driven by cervical proprioceptors that supplement the VOR under certain conditions. When the vestibular apparatus is injured, the COR is facilitated.[6]
Cervicospinal reflex (CSR)	Defined as changes in limb position driven by cervical afferent activity. The CSR supplements the VSR by altering muscle tone in the body.[7]
Cervicocollic reflex (CCR)	Stabilizes the head on the body. The afferent sensory changes caused by an alteration in cervical position create opposition to the stretch through reflexive contractions of appropriate cervical muscles.[8] The degree to which the CCR contributes to head stabilization in humans is uncertain.

Table 15.3c Other reflexes.[5]

Reflex	Function
Visual reflexes	The visual system influences vestibular central circuitry and drives following visual responses (i.e., smooth pursuit) and postural reactions. Visual tracking responses may be facilitated following vestibular loss.
Somatosensory reflexes	Somatosensory mechanics are involved in postural stability. Individuals with bilateral vestibular loss use somatosensory information to a greater extent than those with all balance systems intact.[9]

nuclear complex, which creates motor outputs to activate the eyes and body. To maintain the accuracy of the vestibular system, the cerebellum monitors and calibrates the system.

History and clinical examination

The management of a patient with dizziness is dependent on history, bedside clinical examination, and laboratory testing. An accurate history is essential to determine the onset of symptoms, the description of symptoms, and how the symptoms affect the individual's lifestyle. The bedside examination is used to distinguish peripheral from central problems, how acute the problem may be, and the extent of the loss. Laboratory testing confirms the diagnosis based on history and clinical examination, quantifies the degree of loss, provides evidence of central compensation, and shows evidence of a physiological component.

The subjective history is the most informative part of evaluation. Although this can be tedious, many patients present with vague complaints of dizziness and symptoms. This can also be complicated by anxiety-provoked symptoms. Elements that assist with the diagnosis include the temporal course, the symptoms and what the patient means by "dizziness," and the circumstance of the symptoms. Furthermore, auditory involvement is important to consider (Fig. 15.1).

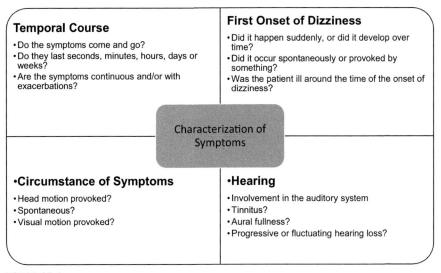

Temporal Course
- Do the symptoms come and go?
- Do they last seconds, minutes, hours, days or weeks?
- Are the symptoms continuous and/or with exacerbations?

First Onset of Dizziness
- Did it happen suddenly, or did it develop over time?
- Did it occur spontaneously or provoked by something?
- Was the patient ill around the time of the onset of dizziness?

Characterization of Symptoms

•Circumstance of Symptoms
- Head motion provoked?
- Spontaneous?
- Visual motion provoked?

•Hearing
- Involvement in the auditory system
- Tinnitus?
- Aural fullness?
- Progressive or fluctuating hearing loss?

FIGURE 15.1

Characterization of symptoms.

Additional elements of dizziness

How is the dizziness affecting an individual's life?

It is important to note that there may be a different response, even when two patients have the same diagnosis. For example, one individual may state that the dizziness is not affecting them, though they want to be assured that nothing is seriously wrong. No extensive evaluation is indicated. A second individual may state that they may have no difficulties with day-to-day activities, including walking, though they are no longer able to participate in recreational activities, such as tennis or golf. This individual would benefit from a referral to physical therapy, to address high-level balance impairments. A third individual may state they are devastated by their dizziness and may not leave their home or participate in any social activities. In addition to a physical therapy referral, this individual may need a referral for psychological counseling for improved coping strategies of the symptoms.

To complete a thorough evaluation of the effects of dizziness on an individual's daily routine, it is best to assess the individual completing various daily tasks and activities that involve different head positions and body positions. For example, reaching down to tie shoelaces while dressing or turning head to check a blind spot while driving can cause dizziness in someone with a vestibular injury. Furthermore, any activity that involves dynamic standing balance, such as meal preparation or showering, may also be a challenge for this individual. Any activity that requires rapid head movement or repositioning and/or dynamic standing balance may be problematic for someone experiencing significant dizziness. This can greatly impact one's quality of life when something as simple as washing feet in the shower or reaching for a pan in a cupboard can turn devastating and lead to poor health-related quality of life and decreased independence.[10]

It is also important to obtain a complete list of prescription and over-the-counter medications. Several medications can cause dizziness, some of which are used to also treat dizziness.

What does the individual believe is causing the dizziness?

Finally, it is important to ask the individual if they have a specific concern of what is causing the dizziness, which may not be addressed routinely by a healthcare provider. If the concern is not addressed, the patient may leave the clinic unsatisfied (Fig. 15.2).

Epidemiology

Symptoms associated with mTBI

Dizziness is a common symptom after head injury, present generally in 23%–81% of cases within the first few days after injury.[11–14] Athletes reports dizziness 55% of time following a concussion.[15] Military personnel who have undergone a blast injury report dizziness as the most common postinjury symptom.[16]

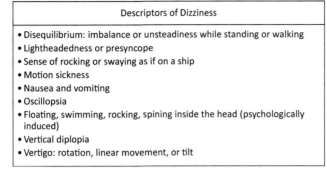

Descriptors of Dizziness
• Disequilibrium: imbalance or unsteadiness while standing or walking
• Lightheadedness or presyncope
• Sense of rocking or swaying as if on a ship
• Motion sickness
• Nausea and vomiting
• Oscillopsia
• Floating, swimming, rocking, spining inside the head (psychologically induced)
• Vertical diplopia
• Vertigo: rotation, linear movement, or tilt

FIGURE 15.2

Possible descriptors of dizziness, each of which has a different mechanism, including through not limited to loss of vestibulospinal, proprioception, visual and/or motor function, loss of vestibular—ocular reflex, visuovestibular mismatch, imbalance of tonic neural activity to vestibular cerebral cortex, skew eye deviation, psychological factors, and decreased blood flow to the brain.

The etiology of dizziness following head injury is diverse. It is important to keep in mind dizziness is diverse and can have multiple meanings (Fig.15.2). Possible causes of dizziness can be from labyrinthine concussion, temporal bone fractures, benign paroxysmal positional vertigo (BPPV), central lesions, vascular lesions, and perilymphatic fistula.[17,18] There are sequelae of a head injury that can also cause dizziness including anxiety-related dizziness, migraine-associated dizziness, autonomic dysregulation, and cervicogenic dizziness.

Anxiety-related dizziness

The pathophysiology of anxiety-related dizziness is thought to be caused by central pathways in the brainstem that perceive dizziness and vertigo, which also control anxiety.[19,20] Stress management, which may be situational, with a recent head injury, though may be a result of preinjury factors, is an important part of recovery. Increased symptoms, decreased speed of processing, and memory deficits are greater in individuals with an mTBI as compared with noninjured individuals.[21] It is important to discuss relaxation and stress management retraining, through meditation and mindfulness, using online resources, including apps and podcasts as part of the rehabilitation. However, a referral to a specialist may be indicated for improved management.

Posttraumatic headaches

Migrainous and nonmigrainous are common posttraumatic headaches following a traumatic brain injury. In addition to phono- and photophobia, nausea and visual changes, dizziness, and vertigo are common symptoms, occurring in 25%–30% of individuals.[22] These symptoms may occur with or without the headache. The pathophysiology is not well understood, though it may be a result of neuroanatomical connections between the trigeminal and vestibular nuclei.[22] Medical management of the migraine is important to allow for progress during rehabilitation.

Autonomic dysregulation

Dizziness with position changes, including sit to stand, bending over to pick something up off the floor, and negotiation of stairs, are often reported in those who have autonomic dysregulation. At times, there may be evidence of orthostatic hypotension, which should be ruled out. Given autonomic symptoms can mimic motion intolerance, including the report of dizziness with walking, running, or any aerobic activity that causes an increase in heart rate, assessment may be indicated. It is theorized that there are central and physiological regulatory dysfunctions that cause symptoms with exertion following an mTBI.[23] The Buffalo Concussion Treadmill Test (BCTT) assesses exercise tolerance in individuals who have suffered from an mTBI. The heart rate at which concussion symptoms are exacerbated is referred to as symptom threshold.[24–26] The Buffalo Concussion Bike Test (BCBT) has been developed, which requires further research to determine its clinical value.[27] However, preliminary data does demonstrate beneficial results as compared to the BCTT. [28]

Postural instability

Sensory organization dysfunction and vestibulospinal reflex impairments cause impaired balance reactions and postural instability. Abnormal central processing input from the peripheral end organ and, in the case of peripheral lesions, impairments of the end organ cause sensory organization impairments.

Cognitive symptoms

The hallmark signs of an mTBI include somatic and cognitive symptoms. Individuals may report fogginess, poor attention, impaired recall (immediate and delayed), limited cognitive endurance, and slowed cognitive processing. Novel learning is difficult due to a decrease in metabolism and increased energy demands.[29]

Sleep disturbance

Sleep complicates other functions and is often impaired following a brain injury. Individuals may have challenges with initiating sleep, maintaining sleep, or hypersomnia.[30] Inadequate sleep causes an exacerbation of symptoms, including anxiety, depression, irritability, decreased attention and concentration, delayed reaction time, decreased energy, and fatigue.[31]

Emotional symptoms

Symptoms such as irritability, anxiety, depression, and emotional lability are commonly described after a head injury. It is important to monitor these symptoms and have them addressed by a multidisciplinary team if these symptoms are limiting progress with rehabilitation.[32,33]

Subjective symptom scales

Self-report measures that are focused on global symptoms following an mTBI and not solely focused on vestibular symptoms include the Postconcussion Symptom Scale (PCSS),[34] Rivermead Post Concussion Questionnaire,[35] Concussion Symptom Inventory,[36] and Graded Symptom Checklist.[36] These assessments vary from 12 to 22 items and use either a five- or seven-point Likert scale. The Dizziness Handicap Inventory (DHI) can be a useful tool to clarify symptoms in relation to functional abilities.[37] Items relate to functional, physical, and emotional problems. The DHI has high test–retest reliability; therefore, it can be used to track changes over time.[38] The DHI correlates to the Activities-specific Balance Confidence (ABC) Scale, in those with vestibular disorders.[39] The ABC quantifies balance confidence with progressively more challenging functional activities from mobility in the home to walking on icy sidewalks.[40] Caution is advised with management decisions based only on subjective symptoms, as symptoms may be under- or overreported.[41,42]

Peripheral and central vestibular disorders

There are several peripheral and central vestibular disorders that involve some type of dizziness. It is important to be able to determine what type of dizziness the individual is having as temporal course, symptoms, and circumstance vary with each disorder (Fig. 15.3).

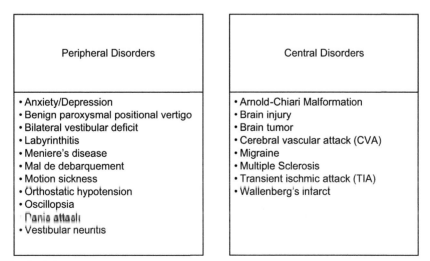

Peripheral Disorders	Central Disorders
• Anxiety/Depression • Benign paroxysmal positional vertigo • Bilateral vestibular deficit • Labyrinthitis • Meniere's disease • Mal de debarquement • Motion sickness • Orthostatic hypotension • Oscillopsia Panic attack • Vestibular neuritis	• Arnold-Chiari Malformation • Brain injury • Brain tumor • Cerebral vascular attack (CVA) • Migraine • Multiple Sclerosis • Transient ischmic attack (TIA) • Wallenberg's infarct

FIGURE 15.3

Peripheral and central vestibular disorders.

Assessments

A variety of oculomotor impairments can be seen in individuals due to a TBI. Some findings may be related to loss of vestibular function, deficits of the central oculomotor pathways, or damage to the extraocular eye muscles. A thorough oculomotor and vestibular examination is critical in the assessment of these individuals (Fig. 15.4).[37]

When assessing ocular alignment, it is important to consider skew deviation, ocular tilt response, tropias, and phorias. In respect to visual acuity, it is important to look at both static and dynamic visual acuity as this provides evidence for impairment of gaze stabilization. Further static visual acuity is important, given the influence of vision on the postural control system. Impairments with smooth pursuit and saccades, and VOR cancellation are indicative of a central lesion. Impairments with the head impulse test and visual acuity are indicative of peripheral lesions. If spontaneous and gaze evoked nystagmus are present, these can be indicative of a central or peripheral lesion, dependent on the direction of the nystagmus (Table 15.4).

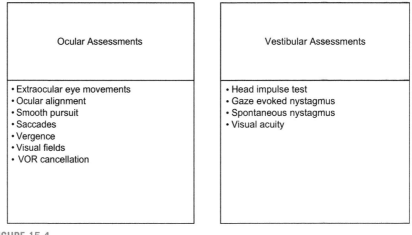

FIGURE 15.4

Ocular and vestibular assessments.

Table 15.4 Possible impaired ocular assessments following TBI.

Assessment	Subjective report
Smooth pursuit	Difficulty reading, tracking people of objects in environment, visual scanning[43,44]
Saccades	Difficulty reading, tracking people of objects in environment, visual scanning[43,44]
Vergence	Dizziness caused by blurred vision or diplopia, headache, fatigue, loss of concentration[45]

In individuals who have suffered from a sports related concussion, the Vestibular Ocular Motor Screening (VOMS) should be used to detect signs and symptoms of a concussion. It assesses the systems that integrate balance, vision, and movement. Abnormal findings or provocation of symptoms during the assessments may indicate a dysfunction, subsequently guiding appropriate referrals to vision therapy and vestibular rehabilitation. Additional research is evolving regarding its use in combination with the SCAT3 for collegiate athletes to improve diagnostic value. The vestibular ocular system is the most accurate predictor of long-term outcomes from sports-related concussions.[46]

Additional clinical examination

Postural assessment

Generally, posture is not altered in an individual with a peripheral vestibular disorder. However, it may be present with central vestibular disorders. It is important to assess predisposed postural deviations, including orthopedic conditions, as this can influence rehabilitation.

Coordination

Assessment of coordination is important, most especially in those who have suffered a severe TBI, in which the cerebellum is involved. Rapid alternating movements, heel-to-shin and finger-to-nose, can be a quick screen of coordination. Depending on results, further coordination assessment may be indicated. Vestibular deficits generally do not cause poor coordination or limb ataxia.

Positional assessment

Benign paroxysmal positional vertigo (BPPV) should be ruled out in all individuals who have suffered from head trauma—from minor injuries such as whiplash to move severe injuries.[37,47] Some individuals may not be aware of positional symptoms following head trauma as they are cautious and moving slowly. Therefore, they may not report dizziness with positional changes. There are several characteristics that are known to describe positional vertigo, including (1) nystagmus is provoked by positional changes against gravity, resulting in vertigo, (2) while maintaining the provocative position, the nystagmus and vertigo are of a brief duration, and (3) nystagmus and vertigo fatigues with repetition of exposure to provocative positioning.[48] There are two proposed mechanisms to explain the presentation of BPPV, named cupulolithiasis and canalithiasis. Cupololithiasis was termed with the thought that otoconia is adhered to the cuplia.[49] Therefore, it is characterized by (1) immediate onset of vertigo when moved into the provoking position, (2) presence of nystagmus, consistent with the latency of vertigo, and (3) persistence of vertigo and nystagmus while the individuals head remains in the provoking position. Conversely, canalithiasis is theorized as debris from the utricle is floating in the long arm of the semicircular canal.[50] The intensity of nystagmus and vertigo are consistent with the degree of deflection of the cupula.

Table 15.5 Benign paroxysmal positional vertigo.

Canal affected	Assessment	Nystagmus	Treatment
Posterior	Dix-Hallpike	Upbeating and torsional toward affected ear	Canalith repositioning procedure (CRP) Liberatory
Horizontal canalithiasis	Roll test and bow and lean test	Geotropic (right beating in head right position, left beating in head left position) Canalithiasis: beats toward affected ear during bow Cupulolithiasis: beats toward affected ear in lean	Bar-B-Que Roll Appiani maneuver Forced prolonged positioning
Horizontal cupulolithiasis	Roll test and bow and lean test	Apogeotropic (left beating in head right position, right beating in head left position)	Casani (Gufoni) maneuver
Anterior	Head hang	Downbeating and torsional toward the affected ear	CR

Canalithiasis is characterized by (1) a latency of onset of vertigo, once the individual is placed in the provoking position, (2) nystagmus consistent with the report of vertigo, and (3) an increase, followed by a decrease in vertigo and nystagmus, ceasing within 60 s.

Table 15.5 discusses assessments and treatments for each canal with the resulting nystagmus and vertigo.

Prevalence of BPPV:[51]

- Posterior: 85%
- Horizontal: 5%–13.6%
- Anterior: 1.2%–13%

Postural control

Postural demands vary across individuals due to age, lifestyle demands, and activity levels. For those who have suffered a brain injury, postural stability can be complicated due to the diffuse injuries. In addition to having challenges with sensory cues to maintain balance, they may also have difficulty with autonomic postural responses and anticipatory postural reactions. With the role, the vestibular system plays in postural control; generally, more than one postural control assessment is indicated (Tables 15.6 and 15.7).[37]

The mini-BESTest may be considered to assess balance as it categorizes balance impairments into four categories—anticipatory, reactive, sensory orientation, and dynamic,[63] therefore assisting with making interventions more specific to the needs

Table 15.6 Static balance assessments.

Assessment	Purpose	Comments
Modified Clinical Test for Sensory Interaction and Balance (mCTSIB)[52,53]	Assesses the influence of visual, somatosensory, and vestibular inputs	Four conditions, tested for 30 s: 1. Solid ground, Romberg stance, eyes open 2. Solid ground, Romberg stance, eyes closed 3. Compliant surface, Romberg stance, eyes open 4. Compliant surface, Romberg stance, eyes closed In condition 4 where the somatosensory inputs are altered and vision is eliminated, the vestibular system therefore acts to provide information on postural control.
Balance Error Scoring System (BESS)[54,55]	Designed for the mTBI population to assess static postural control	Six conditions, tested for 20 s, eyes closed, barefoot: 1. Romberg stance—firm and compliant surface 2. Single limb stance (nondominant foot)—firm and compliant surface 3. Tandem stance (nondominant foot in back)—firm and compliant surface

Table 15.7 Dynamic balance assessments.

Assessment	Purpose	Comments
Dynamic Gait Index (DGI)[56–58]	Assesses gait, balance, and risk of falls, in the presence of external demands	
Functional Gait Assessment (FGA)[59]	Assesses the ability to complete motor tasks while walking	Modification of DGI to improve reliability and reduce ceiling effect
Timed Up and Go (TUG)[60]	Assesses mobility, balance, walking ability, and fall risk	
Modified TUG[60–62] — Cognitive — Manual	Assesses the ability to allocate attention on balance and walking ability	Not validated for use in those with vestibular deficits, though it adds a component to balance assessment—the effect of cognition on balance

of the individual. However, it is not one that is recommend in the physical therapy clinical practice guidelines for assessment of those with mTBI.

Balance assessments are used to guide treatment.

Gait

An observational gait analysis can be completed to provide a functional aspect of the individual's postural control. Gait speed correlates with functional ability, balance, confidence, and fall risk, which can be assessed through the 10 Meter Walk Test.[64] Gait should be assessed in variable situations, including a crowded hallway and quiet hallway and at various speeds - fast, normal, and slow. It is important to document the individual's movement strategy, gait deviations, and any report of symptoms, such as an abnormal sensation of movement, while ambulating.

Sensation

It is important to evaluate sensation to rule out concurrent pathologies and assist with treatment plan. Proprioception and kinesthesia are likely the most important assessments as they influence postural control. However, profound loss of light touch and pressure also affect postural control and increase the risk of falls.[65,66]

Range of motion and strength

Range of motion and strength assessment is not indicated for all individuals. However, those who present following an mTBI or report cervical impairments warrant cervical assessment.[36] Those individuals who have an exacerbation of symptoms with head movements may restrict active range of motion of the cervical spine, causing eventual loss of range of motion. Furthermore, upper cervical spine instability can be a consequence of a head injury.[67]

Cervical proprioception and vestibular information converge throughout the spinal cord, brainstem, cerebral cortex, and cerebellum.[68] In addition to postural neck reflexes, upper cervical spine proprioception is theorized to be responsible for the cervicoocular reflex (COR), which compliments the VOR, at decreased frequency of movement.[69] Therefore, upper cervical spine proprioception may play a role in postural control and influence the vestibular function. The smooth pursuit neck torsion test (SPNT) is a laboratory test that is proposed to identify cases of cervicogenic dizziness, though it is not currently validated. With the lack of definitive assessments for cervicogenic dizziness, the diagnosis is one of exclusion and based on symptoms and the absence of neurologic and otologic findings.[70] Individuals generally present with disequilibrium, lightheadedness, cervical pain, unsteadiness, and limited range of motion. Head movements frequently aggravate symptoms. However, other disease processes manifest with similar symptoms; therefore, these symptoms do not conclusively indicate cervicogenic dizziness.

A clinical assessment to differentiate between a cervical and vestibular cause of dizziness is the Head–Neck Differentiation test, focusing on provocation of symptoms, rather than neck torsion nystagmus test, which assesses for nystagmus.[71–73] To assess the cervical spine in isolation, the body needs to be moved under a stable head. Symptom provocation in this position may indicate a cervical component to dizziness. To assess the vestibular system in isolation, the head and body must move en bloc. Provocation of symptoms may indicate a vestibular component to dizziness. Cervical kinesthesia has been performed in the laboratory, though it can also be performed clinically.[74] Altered proprioceptive signals may be caused by miscommunication among the vestibular, visual, and cervical inputs. These clinical findings can guide treatment.

Treatment
Mild traumatic brain injury

Exercises will likely provoke symptoms, though dizziness should be monitored through numerical rating scale or visual analog scale. Resulting dizziness from exercises should not exceed a 3 or 4 out of 10 and symptoms should return to a baseline level within a few minutes after the completion of an exercise (Table 15.8 and Fig. 15.5).

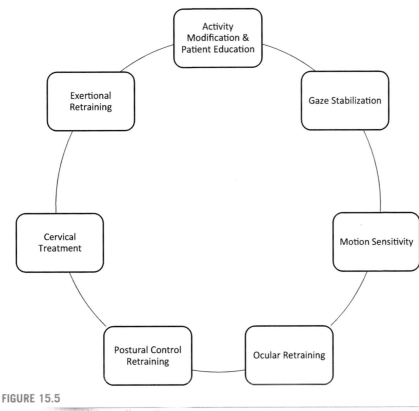

FIGURE 15.5

Problem oriented interventions.[??]

Table 15.8 Treatment following mTBI.

Interventions	Deficits	Treatment
Activity modification and patient education	Exacerbation of symptoms with school/work, day-to-day activities.	Education regarding the importance of pacing of activity; minimizing significant exacerbation of symptoms.
Gaze stabilization	Caused by peripheral vestibular loss, focal central lesion, or mixed central and peripheral deficits. During head movement, the vestibular–ocular reflex (VOR) primarily stabilizes gaze by moving the eyes at the exact same time as the head. When there is a delay in eye movement, individuals will experience a visual blur or the feeling of disequilibrium.	The goal is to promote change in the system and adaptation of the VOR. VOR ×1: Head moving while visually fixating on a stationary target. VOR ×2: Head moving while visually fixating on a moving target.
Motion sensitivity	Decreased tolerance to complex visual environments and visual motion.	Based on principles of habituation. Frequent, daily exposure, with duration of exposure set within individual's tolerance and slowly increased. Gradual introduction of head motion retraining to minimize sensitivity of movement. Begin in a seated position and progress to a standing position.[75]
Ocular retraining	May report headaches, blurred vision diplopia, and poor concentration with reading.	Convergence retraining through use of brock string, convergence dot card, and pencil pushups. Consider vision therapy if symptoms are not improving.
Cervical treatment	Cervicogenic dizziness may be identified as an impairment once involved in therapy and there is increased activity (movement of head). May report headaches, disequilibrium, lightheadedness, cervical pain, and unsteadiness. May note dizziness aggravated by head movement.	Cervical spine mobilization, including upper cervical spine (occipitoatlas distraction), thoracic spine mobilization, cervical and postural strengthening, cervical proprioception, soft tissue mobilization, range of motion, pain management. To address symptoms of disequilibrium or motion sensitivity, head movement exercises, habituation exercises, and postural control exercises can be completed, as deemed appropriate.[76–79]

Table 15.8 Treatment following mTBI.—*cont'd*

Interventions	Deficits	Treatment
Exertional retraining	Theorized that there is a central and physiological regulatory dysfunction, causing symptoms with exertion, including headache, dizziness, poor balance, sadness, irritability, fatigue, and concentration/memory impairments.[25]	Aerobic program at a subsymptom threshold. Following BCTT, exertion level as noted through heart rate can be identified. Exercise begins at 80% of symptom threshold, 5–6 days a week. Exertional level and duration are gradually increased, with symptoms remaining under control. Eventual return to sport-specific or recreational activities.[26]
Postural control retraining	May report difficulty with balance on uneven terrain, walking with head turns, or walking in a dark environment. Also needs to be considered for the return to recreational activities and sports.	Integrate static and dynamic balance exercises with head rotations to alter visual input, increasing amplitude of head movement, integrating VOR with pursuits and saccades. Advance to eyes closed. Consider decreasing the base of support and changing the somatosensory input beginning on solid ground and advancing to various compliant surfaces - equilibrium board, inclines, etc. For dynamic balance retraining, also consider changing gait speed, changing directions, stepping over or weaving around obstacles. Static and dynamic balance, incorporating dual task is beneficial. Determine meaningful activities for the individual. Consider alternative means to postural control retraining including Tai Chi, yoga, golf, tennis, etc. Be mindful of the needs of the individual with respect to postural demands with daily and sport specific activity, in addition to work.

Table 15.9 Progression for gaze stabilization.

Background	Plain → complex (i.e., checkerboard)
Position	Sitting → standing → walking
Surface	Solid ground → compliant surface
Distance	Close (3 feet) → far (8–10 feet)

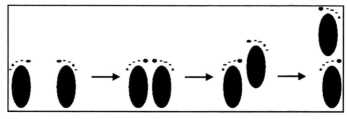

FIGURE 15.6

Standing progression for gaze stabilization and static balance on solid ground and compliant surface.

To progress gaze stabilization exercises, the following should be considered (Table 15.9 and Fig. 15.6).

Technology

There is limited evidence to support the use of virtual reality therapy and video game therapy when treating vestibular injuries. In one recent systematic review, it was reported that virtual reality therapy and video game therapy were no more superior to traditional rehabilitation interventions.[80] Although there exists in the literature some support for virtual reality (VR) to address symptoms of vertigo and other vestibular injuries, few trials were compared with traditional vestibular rehabilitation and thus remain inconclusive regarding efficacy in comparison with standard vestibular rehabilitation.[81] However, if a patient is motivated by the use of technology, this may be an appropriate treatment approach to target gaze stability, postural control, and subsequently quality of life. Most VR treatments involve a headset with a head-mounted display that provides input through the auditory, visual, and touch pathways with the therapist's ability to provide some control over the input provided with the plan for gradual habituation in mind. Easily accessible technology, such as the WiiFit balance platform, has been proven to improve balance function and quality of life in one pilot study.[82] Furthermore, there exists high-tech equipment that some patients may come across in some clinics, which includes the Man&Tel Vestibular Trainer (which assess center of gravity movement) and the Bioness BITS (which is similar to the WiiFit in that it uses dual-task training to improve gaze stability and overall balance).[83] Generally, there may be some benefit for using virtual reality and video game training to treat vestibular symptoms when in conjunction with traditional vestibular rehabilitation.

Other considerations

Cognition and degree of agitation need to be accounted for when initiating exercises. Symptom provocation may not be tolerated well. In individuals with extensive dizziness, motion sensitivity, and agitation, ×1 viewing may provoke too many symptoms. Therefore, it is recommended to begin with habituation exercises, to tolerance. Once these exercises have decreased dizziness and motion sensitivity, ×1 viewing may be initiated, if needed.

As the status of the patient improves, including agitation, the intensity of habituation or adaptation exercises can be increased. This will cause a greater provocation of symptoms, though this will be beneficial for the ongoing recovery. Generally, if symptoms last for longer than 15−30 min after the completion of the exercises, the duration, speed, or stimulus should be reduced. Exercises should be performed to challenge the system, to allow the error signals to be generated. If not, adaptation will not occur. CNS depressants (such as meclizine), used to treat symptoms of dizziness, are thought to delay adaptation.

Conclusion

In conclusion, brain injuries include a complex sequelae of symptoms. The etiology of dizziness may be vestibular or nonvestibular in nature. It is important to refer to a vestibular therapist if dizziness is consistent with a vestibular disorder. If the individual has suffered a concussion and has the postconcussion symptom cluster or has suffered from a whiplash injury, a vestibular therapist is likely able to assist with management of symptoms. Furthermore, individuals who have dizziness related to multiple sclerosis or any acquired brain injury should be referred to a vestibular therapy. Management of the whole patient, using a multidisciplinary approach, appears to be the most appropriate to effective rehabilitation.

Rehabilitation for mild brain injury continues to be researched, and there is more to learn about recovery from vestibular dysfunction. Vestibular rehabilitation is also known to be beneficial for those with unexplained dizziness. It is important to remember that individuals may present with a wide range of symptoms and assessments should include, though not limited to, a thorough history, outcome measures, and balance confidence. A daily, challenging, home exercise program addressing the impairments is imperative.

The goals of the clinician in vestibular rehabilitation are to minimize symptom severity, maximize safety and independence with functional mobility, and subsequently improve the quality of life. Ongoing research focusing on the efficacy of vestibular rehabilitation following a traumatic brain injury is needed, most especially those injuries not associated with athletics or the military.

Supplemental 1

Case 1

The patient is a 20-year-old collegiate diver, enrolled in her senior year. During diving practice, while on the 3-meter board, she entered the water headfirst, without her arms breaking the water. She did not suffer a loss of consciousness, though she did have immediate head pain. She sat on the edge of the pool, due to head pain, but was exhorted by her coaches to get back onto the diving board and continue her warmup. On her next dive, she again struck the water headfirst. She experienced immediate dizziness, tinnitus, and worsening head pain. She pulled herself from practice, reported her head was spinning, and subsequently vomited. She was assessed by the athletic trainer, who completed an unspecified evaluation. She was advised not to compete that day and saw the team physician later that day. Results of this evaluation could not be recalled, though she was advised not to practice for 1 week. She was seen by the athletic trainer daily thereafter for repeated assessments. She reported her initial symptoms were headache, dizziness, fogginess, blurred vision, neck pain, and poor sleep. The team physician prescribed amitriptyline 10 mg at bedtime, which helped her headache, though not significantly. The dose was increased to 25 mg, which assisted in restoring her sleep hygiene, though it did not improve the headache.

The patient presented to physical therapy for vestibular therapy evaluation 19 days after injury. Her chief complaints at that time included daily headaches, dizziness with head motion and bed mobility; blurred vision; imbalance; spatial disorientation, which increased in the dark; and inability to complete aerobic exercise for 4 min without provocation of dizziness and headache.

She lives in a house with roommates, close to campus. She had been practicing or competing 6 days a week and was a full-time student with a 3.6 GPA. Her medical history included one prior concussion at age 15, as a competitive gymnast, resulting in postconcussive symptoms, which lasted 3 months. Her current head injury occurred 6 weeks prior to the completion of the semester. The University transitioned most of her in-person classes to remote learning due to the ongoing exacerbation of headache and fatigue, related to busy environments, noise, and fluorescent lights. The University provided her extra time for assignments and test completion, but her primary difficulties were around assimilation of novel information, application of it, and problem-solving. By the end of the semester, her workload eased, and she felt less stressed. Although her headache improved minimally, it persisted. Her tinnitus eased within a week of the concussion, and the dizziness largely remitted within a month though balance and spatial orientation challenges remained. She has had several near falls but has been able to "catch herself."

At the time of the evaluation, the patient reported the following activities exacerbated her headache, dizziness, and unsteadiness: rolling to the right side in bed, walking with head turns, most especially in a busy environment, headache originating in the posterior skull, referring to the superior aspect of skull and eventually to the frontal region, reading/computer work, aerobic exercise greater than 4 min, visual motion, standing with a narrow base of support or walking, further exacerbated when in a dak environment. She also noted poor concentration and limited sleep.

She rated her headache as follows: rest: 3/10, with daily activities: 5/10 and at worst: 8/10. Her dizziness was rated as follows: rest: 0/10; with daily activities: 4/10 and at worst: 7/10.

The clinical oculomotor and vestibular examination, completed through the VOMS, can be seen in Table 15.10.

Dizziness resolved within 5 min, though headache remained elevated throughout the evaluation.

Results for subjective and objective balance and cervical tests can be found in Table 15.11 There were no impairments related to sensation range of motion of her extremities and trunk, strength, or coordination. She had limitations of the cervical spine.

The following impairments were identified based on patient's report and clinical examination:

- Positional vertigo
- Gaze stability
- Convergence insufficiency
- Head motion sensitivity
- Visual dependence for balance
- Visual motion intolerance
- Cervicogenic headaches and dizziness
- Exertion-provoked symptoms

Plan of care

The patient verbalized the following goals: alleviation of symptoms to return to prior level of function and begin a new job. She did not express a desire to return to diving. The following short- and long-term goals were established:

Short-term goals (4 weeks):

- Resolution of positional vertigo
- Tolerate gaze stabilization ×1 viewing for 30 s with complex background while standing with a narrow base of support, with symptom provocation of less than 3/10
- Improve FGA to 24/30
- Improve condition 4 of mCTSIB to 30 s
- Tolerate watching motion induced videos for 10 min, with provocation of dizziness to less than 5/10

Table 15.10 VOMS.

	NT	Headache 0–10	Dizziness 0–10	Nausea 0–10	Fogginess 0–10	Comments
Baseline		3	0	0	0	
Smooth pursuit		3	3	0	0	Intact
Saccades horizontal		4	4	0	0	Hypometric
Saccades vertical		4	4	0	0	Intact
Convergence (near point)		5	3	0	0	(Near point in cm) 1. 15 2. 18 3. 20
VOR horizontal		5	3	0	0	Intact
VOR vertical		5	3	0	0	Intact
Visual motion sensitivity test		5	4	2	0	Intact

Table 15.11 Subjective and objective measures.

Measure	Initial visit	10 Weeks
DHI[a]	68/100, indicating severe dizziness	12/100, indicating mild dizziness
VVAS[a]	5/10	1.8/10
Dizziness severity	0 to 7/10, with daily tasks	0 to 2/10, intermittently with head movements in busier environments
FGA[a]	20/30	29/30 (WNL)
mCTSIB	**1.** Eyes open, firm: 30 s **2.** Eyes closed, firm: 30 s **3.** Eyes open, compliant: 30 s **4.** Eyes closed, compliant: 24 s	**1.** Eyes open, firm: 30 s **2.** Eyes closed, firm: 30 s **3.** Eyes open, compliant: 30 s **4.** Eyes closed, compliant: 30 s
Positional assessments (BPPV)	Right posterior canalithiasis	Resolved
Cervical range of motion	Flexion: 60° Extension: 55° Left rotation: 55° Right rotation: 68°	WNL
Upper cervical range of motion	Left rotation: significantly limited Right rotation: WNL	WNL, bilaterally
Cervical endurance test	4.3 s	18 s
Cervical motor control	Poor	Good
Joint position error	Left rotation: 0/3 accurate Right rotation: 0/3 accurate Flexion: 1/3 accurate Extension: 1/3 accurate	Left rotation: 3/3 accurate Right rotation: 3/3 accurate Flexion: 3/3 accurate Extension: 3/3 accurate

[a] *Measures and abbreviations:* DHI, *Dizziness Handicap Inventory (0–100, 100 = worst);* FGA, *Functional Gait Assessment (0–30, <22 = fall risk);* VVAS, *Visual Vertigo Analog Scale (0–10, 10 = worst);* WNL, *Within normal limits. Cervical endurance test: Normative data for women 29.4 s.*

- Tolerate 15 min of aerobic exercise without an exacerbation of symptoms
- Tolerate 30 min of sitting at desk with improved posture

Long-term goals (10 weeks):

- Tolerate gaze stabilization ×1 viewing for 60 s with complex background while walking, with symptom provocation of less than 1/10
- Tolerate 30 min of complex visual and auditory environments, without an increase in headache or dizziness
- Successfully begin a new job in a complex environment, without exacerbation of symptoms

- Tolerate 30 min of aerobic exercise without an exacerbation of symptoms
- Improve cervical endurance test by greater than 10 s
- Improve joint position error to 3/3 accurate repetitions in all directions
- Improve FGA to 30/30

Intervention

Patient was scheduled to receive vestibular physical therapy twice a week for 6 weeks, followed by one time per week for 4 weeks. Therapy sessions were 45–60 min. She attended 16 sessions total.

The initial visits included patient education regarding rationale for vestibular rehabilitation and pacing of activity to manage symptoms. Further education was provided on the importance and benefits of a walking program. Written handouts were provided for all education materials. She was referred to occupational therapy to address visual-related symptoms.

A 10-point verbal rating scale was used to assess headache, dizziness, and cervical pain at the initiation and completion of each session. It was also intermittently used throughout the session to monitor tolerance to symptom-exacerbating tasks. Interventions are as follows:

To improve positional vertigo:

- CRMs for the right posterior canal were completed two times per session for two sessions. There was an 80% resolution of symptoms following the initial CRM.

To improve gaze stability:

- ×1 and ×2 viewing: Initiated standing with feet separated shoulder width on a plain background. Progressed by narrowing the base of support and then adding a dynamic component of walking. The plain background was progressed to a complex background. Increasing the velocity of head movement and performing the exercises in a complex visual and auditory environment were added as tolerated.

To address convergence insufficiency:

- Exercise was performed with a Brock string in the clinic and pencil pushups for home. Progressed with increasing the time she participated in the exercise.

To improve static and dynamic balance:

- Decreasing the base of support on firm and compliant surfaces. Progressed with eliminating vision.
- Head motion exercises were incorporated via habituation with progressively more challenging and complex movements, including gait with head turns, 180 and 360° turns, combined head and eye movements in standing, and progressing to walking. Agility drills and rapid direction changes were added to walking activities. Eventually began more sport-specific training that included hopping, jumping, and more rapid turns.

To improve motion sensitivity:

- Head motion exercises were incorporated via habituation, initially watching videos of individuals merging onto highways, walking through a grocery store. Progressed to walking through a hotel on multicolored and patterned carpet busier urban environments. Started at 3 min and progressed to 10 min. Once the patient tolerated visual motion, progressed to walking through a grocery store, attending her graduation ceremony, and riding the subway to get to work.

To manage cervicogenic headache and dizziness:

- Focus on posture and ergonomics when sitting at her desk.
- Manual therapy to the upper cervical spine and cervical–thoracic junction to improve hypomobility.
- Stretching of the suboccipitals, levator scapulae, and upper trapezius muscles bilaterally.
- Progressive strengthening of paraspinals, periscapular, and core musculature.
- Joint position error and motor control training with use of a head laser.

To improve aerobic conditioning and decrease exertion-provoked symptoms:

- Walking program: 20 min daily in a quieter environment. Provided as part of initial home exercise program.
- Stationary bicycle: Initially 10 min and progressed the duration when the patient rated dizziness less than 3/10, which lasted for less than 10 min following the completion of the exercise.
- Elliptical: Added at 3 weeks of the plan of care. Progressed by increasing speed and duration, following the same guidelines as used for the stationary bike.
- Jogging on treadmill: Added at 5 weeks of plan of care. Progressed by increasing speed and duration, following the same guidelines as used for the stationary bike.

Outcomes

After 10 weeks of vestibular therapy, the patient met all goals. Her symptoms of dizziness had almost completely resolved, though she remained with a mild headache in the frontal region that increased as the day progressed. Her greatest challenges remained being in a busier environment and agility moves. Being on the computer and reading no longer provoked her symptoms. She started a job as a rehabilitation aide in a hospital-based outpatient therapy clinic, which caused a slight provocation of symptoms. Her work entails assisting physical and occupational therapists in a distraction-intensive environment with multiple auditory and visual inputs and direct and indirect light and is generally task-oriented requiring sustained concentration and the ability to shift attention on demand. Her sleep hygiene improved significantly, and after a month at her new job, her cognitive symptoms resolved. Given two significant concussions within 5 years, she was advised to avoid diving. However, she accepted a second job as a recreational diving coach for her local town (Table 15.11).

Supplemental 2
Case 2

The patient is a 30-year-old female who fell 130 feet while hiking, resulting in left cerebellar lobe, left pontine and bifrontal contusions, and extradural pontine and extradural occipital hematoma. Additional injuries included right malleolar fracture and occipital temporal skull fractures involving petrous, extra labyrinthine, bilateral, and luxation of ossicular bones of left ear. Initial GCS on admission was 13, but condition rapidly declined. She required evacuation of clot resulting in occipital craniectomy. Once medically stable, she was transferred to acute rehabilitation, for 3 weeks, with focus on functional mobility, to return home with the support of her parents. She received home health services, and approximately 2 months after the fall, she presented to outpatient physical therapy.

Objective

Oculomotor and vestibular assessments demonstrate central and peripheral vestibular dysfunction (Table 15.12). She also demonstrates a risk of falls as noted through balance assesments (Table 15.13).

Table 15.12 Oculomotor and vestibular assessments at initial evaluation.

Assessment	Initial visit
Alignment	Left esotropia
EOM	CN VI palsy
Smooth pursuit	Saccadic breakdown
Gaze evoked nystagmus	Direction changing
Saccades	Hypermetric
Head impulse test	(+) bilaterally

Report of significant dizziness with assessments.

Table 15.13 Objective assessments.

Measure	Initial visit	6 months
FGA[a]	Unable to complete	29/30 (WNL)
mCTSIB	1. Eyes open, firm: 20 s 2. Eyes closed, firm: 8 s[a] 3. Eyes open, compliant: unable 4. Eyes closed, compliant: unable	1. Eyes open, firm: 30 s 2. Eyes closed, firm: 30 s 3. Eyes open, compliant: 30 s 4. Eyes closed, compliant: 30 s
	[a]Trucal ataxia noted	
Gait	Ambulating with a rolling walker, with an ataxic gait, absent head movement, and turns en bloc	No assistive device, unremarkable gait pattern

[a] *Measures and abbreviations: FGA, Functional Gait Assessment (0–30, <22 = fall risk); WNL, within normal limits.*

Intervention

While in acute rehabilitation, it was too soon to begin vestibular rehabilitation. The focus was on independence with functional mobility, while minimizing provocation of symptoms. Therefore, strategies were provided to maintain visual fixation on a stable object with all functional (i.e., rolling, supine <-> sit, sit <-> stand, walking, etc.)

Once in the outpatient setting, the impairments addressed were dizziness, balance, gait, and ataxia. To remain in the scope of this chapter, the dizziness and balance components of treatment are only discussed.

To improve gaze stability:

- ×1 viewing: Initiated in supported sitting, in a quiet environment on a plain background. Progressed to sitting unsupported, then standing with feet separated and narrowing the base of support. Progressed to a compliant surface for additional postural control retraining. Once appropriate, focused on performing the exercise on a visually complex background, in addition to a busier environment, as tolerated.

To improve static and dynamic balance:

- Decreasing the base of support on firm and compliant surfaces. Progressed with eliminating vision.
- Head motion exercises were incorporated via habituation with progressively more challenging and complex movements, including gait with head turns, 180 and 360° turns, combined head and eye movements in standing and progressing to walking. Agility drills and rapid direction changes were added to walking activities. Eventually began more recreational-specific training that included hopping, jumping, and increasing speed of activities.

Outcome

After 6 months of outpatient physical therapy, including vestibular rehabilitation, the patient met all rehabilitation goals. She returned to being an independent community ambulator and was able to return to graduate school to complete her PhD. She was also able to return to recreational activities, including running and hiking.

References

1. Baloh RW, Honrubia V, Jacobson K. Benign positional vertigo: clinical and oculographic features in 240 cases. *Neurology*. 1987;37(3):371–378. https://doi.org/10.1212/wnl.37.3.371.
2. Prokopakis E, Vlastos IM, Tsagournisakis M, Christodoulou P, Kawauchi H, Velegrakis G. Canalith repositioning procedures among 965 patients with benign paroxysmal positional vertigo. *Audiol Neuro Otol*. 2013;18(2):83–88. https://doi.org/10.1159/000343911.

3. Kansu L, Avci S, Yilmaz I, Ozluoglu LN. Long-term follow-up of patients with posterior canal benign paroxysmal positional vertigo. *Acta Otolaryngol*. 2010;130(9):1009−1012. https://doi.org/10.3109/00016481003629333.

4. Centers for Disease Control and Prevention (CDC). *Traumatic brain injury (TBI): incidence and distribution, 2014. Introduction to Brain Injury − Facts and Stats*. February 2000.

5. Herdman SJ, Clendaniel RA, Waltner P, O'Brien C. *Vestibular Rehabilitation*. 4th ed. F. A. Davis Company; 2014.

6. Botros G. The tonic oculomotor function of the cervical joint and muscle receptors. *Adv Oto-Rhino-Laryngol*. 1979;25:214−220. https://doi.org/10.1159/000402945.

7. Pompeiano O. The tonic neck reflex: supraspinal control. In: Peterson BW, Richmond FJ, eds. *Control of Head Movement*. Oxford University Press; 1988:108−119.

8. Peterson BW. Cervicocollic and cervico-ocular reflexes. In: Peterson BW, Richmond FJ, eds. *Control of Head Movement*. Oxford University Press; 1988:90−99.

9. Bles W, de Jong JM, de Wit G. Somatosensory compensation for loss of labyrinthine function. *Acta Otolaryngol*. 1984;97(3−4):213−221. https://doi.org/10.3109/00016488409130982.

10. Cohen H. Vestibular rehabilitation improves daily life function. *Am J Occup Ther*. 1994;48(10):919−925.

11. Kisilevski V, Podoshin L, Ben-David J, et al. Results of oto-vestibular tests in mild head injuries. *Int Tinnitus J*. 2001;7(2):118−121.

12. Maskell F, Chiarelli P, Isles R. Dizziness after traumatic brain injury: overview and measurement in the clinical setting. *Brain Inj*. 2006;20(3):293−305. https://doi.org/10.1080/02699050500488041.

13. Maskell F, Chiarelli P, Isles R. Dizziness after traumatic brain injury: results from an interview study. *Brain Inj*. 2007;21(7):741−752. https://doi.org/10.1080/02699050701472109.

14. Terrio H, Brenner LA, Ivins BJ, et al. Traumatic brain injury screening: preliminary findings in a US army brigade combat team. *J Head Trauma Rehabil*. 2009;24(1):14−23. https://doi.org/10.1097/HTR.0b013e31819581d8.

15. Lovell M, Collins M, Bradley J. Return to play following sports-related concussion. *Clin Sports Med*. 2004;23(3):421−441. https://doi.org/10.1016/j.csm.2004.04.001.

16. Hoffer ME, Balaban C, Gottshall K, Balough BJ, Maddox MR, Penta JR. Blast exposure: vestibular consequences and associated characteristics. *Otol Neurotol*. 2010;31(2):232−236. https://doi.org/10.1097/MAO.0b013e3181c993c3.

17. Herdman SJ. Treatment of vestibular disorders in traumatically brain-injured patients. *J Head Trauma Rehabil*. 1990;5(4):63−76. https://doi.org/10.1097/00001199-199012000-00008.

18. Furman JM, Whitney SL. Central causes of dizziness. *Phys Ther*. 2000;80(2):179−187.

19. Balaban CD, Jacob RG. Background and history of the interface between anxiety and vertigo. *J Anxiety Disord*. 2001;15(1−2):27−51. https://doi.org/10.1016/s0887-6185(00)00041-4.

20. Balaban CD. Neural substrates linking balance control and anxiety. *Physiol Behav*. 2002;77(4−5):469−475. https://doi.org/10.1016/s0031-9384(02)00935-6.

21. Hanna-Pladdy B, Berry ZM, Bennett T, Phillips HL, Gouvier WD. Stress as a diagnostic challenge for postconcussive symptoms: sequelae of mild traumatic brain injury or physiological stress response. *Clin Neuropsychol*. 2001;15(3):289−304. https://doi.org/10.1076/clin.15.3.289.10272.

22. Furman JM, Balaban CD, Jacob RG, Marcus DA. Migraine-anxiety related dizziness (MARD): a new disorder? *J Neurol Neurosurg Psychiatr.* 2005;76(1):1−8. https://doi.org/10.1136/jnnp.2004.048926.

23. Leddy JJ, Kozlowski K, Donnelly JP, Pendergast DR, Epstein LH, Willer B. A preliminary study of subsymptom threshold exercise training for refractory post-concussion syndrome. *Clin J Sport Med Off J Can Acad Sport Med.* 2010;20(1): 21−27. https://doi.org/10.1097/JSM.0b013e3181c6c22c.

24. Esterov D, Greenwald BD. Autonomic dysfunction after mild traumatic brain injury. *Brain Sci.* 2017;7(8):100. https://doi.org/10.3390/brainsci7080100.

25. Leddy JJ, Willer B. Use of graded exercise testing in concussion and return-to-activity management. *Curr Sports Med Rep.* 2013;12(6):370−376. https://doi.org/10.1249/JSR.0000000000000008.

26. Leddy J, Baker JG, Haider MN, Hinds A, Willer B. A physiological approach to prolonged recovery from sport-related concussion. *J Athl Train.* 2017;52(3):299−308. https://doi.org/10.4085/1062-6050-51.11.08.

27. Janssen A, Pope R, Rando N. Clinical application of the Buffalo Concussion Treadmill Test and the Buffalo Concussion Bike Test: a systematic review. *J. Concussion.* 2022.

28. Haider MN, Johnson SL, Mannix R, et al. The Buffalo Concussion Bike Test for concussion assessment in adolescents. *Sports Health.* 2019;11(6):492−497. https://doi.org/10.1177/1941738119870189.

29. Lau B, Lovell MR, Collins MW, Pardini J. Neurocognitive and symptom predictors of recovery in high school athletes. *Clin J Sport Med Off J Can Acad Sport Med.* 2009; 19(3):216−221. https://doi.org/10.1097/JSM.0b013e31819d6edb.

30. Leddy JJ, Kozlowski K, Fung M, Pendergast DR, Willer B. Regulatory and autoregulatory physiological dysfunction as a primary characteristic of post concussion syndrome: implications for treatment. *NeuroRehabilitation.* 2007;22(3):199−205.

31. Williams L. *Sleep Deprivation: Global Prevalence, Dangers and Impacts on Cognitive Performance.* Nova Science Publishers, Inc; 2017.

32. Moore EL, Terryberry-Spohr L, Hope DA. Mild traumatic brain injury and anxiety sequelae: a review of the literature. *Brain Inj.* 2006;20(2):117−132. https://doi.org/10.1080/02699050500443558.

33. Jacob RG, Furman JM. Psychiatric consequences of vestibular dysfunction. *Curr Opin Neurol.* 2001;14(1):41−46. https://doi.org/10.1097/00019052-200102000-00007.

34. Randolph C, Millis S, Barr WB, et al. Concussion symptom inventory: an empirically derived scale for monitoring resolution of symptoms following sport-related concussion. *Arch Clin Neuropsychol Off J Natl Acad Neuropsychologists.* 2009;24(3): 219−229. https://doi.org/10.1093/arclin/acp025.

35. King NS, Crawford S, Wenden FJ, Moss NE, Wade DT. The Rivermead Post Concussion Symptoms Questionnaire: a measure of symptoms commonly experienced after head injury and its reliability. *J Neurol.* 1995;242(9):587−592. https://doi.org/10.1007/BF00868811.

36. McCrea M, Kelly JP, Randolph C, et al. Standardized Assessment of Concussion (SAC): on-site mental status evaluation of the athlete. *J Head Trauma Rehabil.* 1998;13(2): 27−35. https://doi.org/10.1097/00001199-199804000-00005.

37. Quatman-Yates CC, Shimamura KK, Alsalaheen BA, et al. Physical therapy evaluation and treatment after concussion/mild traumatic brain injury. *J Orthop Sports Phys Ther.* 2020;50(4):CPG1−CPG73. https://doi.org/10.2519/jospt.2020.0301.

38. Jacobson GP, Newman CW. The development of the dizziness handicap inventory. *Arch Otolaryngol Head Neck Surg.* 1990;116(4):424−427.

39. Whitney SL, Hudak MT, Marchetti GF. The activities-specific balance confidence scale and the dizziness handicap inventory: a comparison. *J Vestib Res Equilibrium Orientation.* 1999;9(4):253−259.

40. Powell LE, Myers AM. The activities-specific balance confidence (ABC) scale. *J Gerontol Ser A Biol Sci Med Sci.* 1995;50A(1):M28−M34.

41. Williamson IJ, Goodman D. Converging evidence for the under-reporting of concussions in youth ice hockey. *Br J Sports Med.* 2006;40(2):128−132. https://doi.org/10.1136/bjsm.2005.021832.

42. McCrea M, Hammeke T, Olsen G, Leo P, Guskiewicz K. Unreported concussion in high school football players: implications for prevention. *Clin J Sport Med Off J Can Acad Sport Med.* 2004;14(1):13−17. https://doi.org/10.1097/00042752-200401000-00003.

43. Heitger MH, Jones RD, Macleod AD, Snell DL, Frampton CM, Anderson TJ. Impaired eye movements in post-concussion syndrome indicate suboptimal brain function beyond the influence of depression, malingering or intellectual ability. *Brain J Neurol.* 2009;132(Pt 10):2850−2870. https://doi.org/10.1093/brain/awp181.

44. Ciuffreda KJ, Han Y, Kapoor N, Ficarra AP. Oculomotor rehabilitation for reading in acquired brain injury. *NeuroRehabilitation.* 2006;21(1):9−21. https://doi.org/10.3233/NRE-2006-21103.

45. Adler P. Efficacy of treatment for convergence insufficiency using vision therapy. *Ophthalmic Physiol Opt J Br Coll Ophthalmic Opticians (Optometrists).* 2002;22(6):565−571. https://doi.org/10.1046/j.1475-1313.2002.00080.x.

46. Mucha A, Collins MW, Elbin RJ, et al. A brief vestibular/ocular motor screening (VOMS) assessment to evaluate concussions: preliminary findings. *Am J Sports Med.* 2014;42(10):2479−2486. https://doi.org/10.1177/0363546514543775.

47. Katsarkas A. Benign paroxysmal positional vertigo (BPPV): idiopathic versus posttraumatic. *Acta Otolaryngol.* 1999;119(7):745−749. https://doi.org/10.1080/00016489950180360.

48. Lanska DJ, Remler B. Benign paroxysmal positioning vertigo: classic descriptions, origins of the provocative positioning technique, and conceptual developments. *Neurology.* 1997;48(5):1167−1177. https://doi.org/10.1212/wnl.48.5.1167.

49. Schuknecht HF. Positional vertigo: clinical and experimental observations. *Transact Am Acad Ophthalmol Otolaryngol.* 1962;66:319−332.

50. Hall SF, Ruby RR, McClure JA. The mechanics of benign paroxysmal vertigo. *J Otolaryngol.* 1979;8(2):151−158.

51. Cakir BO, Ercan I, Cakir ZA, Civelek S, Sayin I, Turgut S. What is the true incidence of horizontal semicircular canal benign paroxysmal positional vertigo? *Otolaryngology-Head Neck Surg (Tokyo).* 2006;134(3):451−454. https://doi.org/10.1016/j.otohns.2005.07.045.

52. Shumway-Cook A, Horak FB. Assessing the influence of sensory interaction on balance: suggestion from the field. *Phys Ther.* 1986;66(10):1548−1550.

53. Cohen H, Blatchly CA, Gombash LL. A study of the clinical test of sensory interaction and balance. *Phys Ther.* 1993;73(6):346−351.

54. Riemann BL, Guskiewicz KM, Shields EW. Relationship between clinical and forceplate measures of postural stability. *J Sport Rehabil.* 1999;8(2):71.

55. Riemann BL, Guskiewicz KM. Effects of mild head injury on postural stability as measured through clinical balance testing. *J Athl Train.* 2000;35(1):19.

56. Shumway-Cook A, Woollacott MH. *Motor Control: Theory and Practical Applications.* Williams & Wilkins; 1995.

57. Whitney SL, Hudak MT, Marchetti GF. The dynamic gait index relates to self-reported fall history in individuals with vestibular dysfunction. *J Vestib Res Equilibrium Orientation.* 2000;10(2):99−105.

58. Whitney SL, Marchetti GF, Schade A, Wrisley DM. The sensitivity and specificity of the Timed "Up & Go" and the dynamic gait index for self-reported falls in persons with vestibular disorders. *J Vestib Res Equilibrium Orientation.* 2004;14(5):397−409.

59. Wrisley DM, Marchetti GF, Kuharsky DK, Whitney SL. Reliability, internal consistency, and validity of data obtained with the Functional Gait Assessment. *Phys Ther.* 2004; 84(10):906−918.

60. Shumway-Cook A, Brauer S, Woollacott M. Predicting the probability for falls in community-dwelling older adults using the timed up & go test. *Phys Ther.* 2000; 80(9):896−903.

61. Lundin OL, Nyberg L, Gustafson Y. Attention, frailty, and falls: the effect of a manual task on basic mobility. *J Am Geriatr Soc.* 1998;46(6):758−761.

62. Giné-Garriga M, Guerra M, Marí-Dell'Olmo M, Martin C, Unnithan VB. Sensitivity of a modified version of the 'timed get up and go' test to predict fall risk in the elderly a pilot study. *Arch Gerontol Geriatr.* 2009;49(1):e60−e66.

63. Godi M, Franchignoni F, Caligari M, Giordano A, Turcato AM, Nardone A. Comparison of reliability, validity, and responsiveness of the mini-BESTest and Berg Balance Scale in patients with balance disorders. *Phys Ther.* 2013;93(2):158−167. https://doi.org/ 10.2522/ptj.20120171.

64. Fritz S, Lusardi M. White paper: "walking speed: the sixth vital sign". *J Geriatr Phys Ther.* 2009;32(2):46−49.

65. Richardson JK, Hurvitz EA. Peripheral neuropathy: a true risk factor for falls. *J Gerontol Ser A Biol Sci Med Sci.* 1995;50(4):M211−M215. https://doi.org/10.1093/gerona/ 50a.4.m211.

66. Richardson JK, Ashton-Miller JA, Lee SG, Jacobs K. Moderate peripheral neuropathy impairs weight transfer and unipedal balance in the elderly. *Arch Phys Med Rehabil.* 1996;77(11):1152−1156. https://doi.org/10.1016/s0003-9993(96)90139-2.

67. Mathers KS, Schneider M, Timko M. Occult hypermobility of the craniocervical junction: a case report and review. *J Orthop Sports Phys Ther.* 2011;41(6):444−457. https://doi.org/10.2519/jospt.2011.3305.

68. Mergner T, Becker W, Deecke L. Canal-neck interaction in vestibular neurons of the cat's cerebral cortex. *Exp Brain Res.* 1985;61(1):94−108.

69. Barnes GR, Forbat LN. Cervical and vestibular afferent control of oculomotor response in man. *Acta Otolaryngol.* 1979;88(1−2):79−87. https://doi.org/10.3109/ 00016487909137143.

70. Reiley AS, Vickory FM, et al. How to diagnose cervicogenic dizziness. *Ach Physiotherapy.* 2017;7:12.

71. Philipszoon AJ, Bos JH. Neck torsion nystagmus. *Prac Otorhinolaryngol (Basel).* 1963; 25:339.

72. Fitz-Ritson D. Assessment of cervicogenic vertigo. *J Manipulative Physiol Therapeut.* 1991;14(3):193−198.

73. Norré ME. Cervical vertigo. Diagnostic and semiological problem with special emphasis upon "cervical nystagmus. *Acta Oto-Rhino-Laryngol Belg.* 1987;41(3):436−452.

74. Revel M, Andre-Deshays C, Minguet M. Cervicocephalic kinesthetic sensibility in patients with cervical pain. *Arch Phys Med Rehabil.* 1991;72(5):288−291.

75. Pavlou M. The use of optokinetic stimulation in vestibular rehabilitation. *J Neurol Phys Ther.* 2010;34(2):105−110.

76. Treleaven J, Jull G, Sterling M. Dizziness and unsteadiness following whiplash injury: characteristic features with cervical joint position error. *J Rehabil Med.* 2003;35(1): 36−43.

77. Kristjansson E, Treleaven J. Sensorimotor function and dizziness in neck pain: implications for assessment and management. *J Orthop Sports Phys Ther.* 2009;39(5):364−377.

78. Reid SA, Rivett DA. Manual therapy treatment of cervicogenic dizziness: a systematic review. *Man Ther.* 2005;10(1):4−13.

79. Lystad Reidar P, Bell G, Bonnevie-Svendsen M, Carter Catherine V. Manual therapy with and without vestibular rehabilitation for cervicogenic dizziness: a systematic review. *Chiropr Man Ther.* 2011;19(1):21.

80. Alashram AR, Annino G, Raju M, Padua E. Effects of physical therapy interventions on balance ability in people with traumatic brain injury: a systematic review. *NeuroRehabilitation.* 2020;46(4):455−466. https://doi.org/10.3233/NRE-203047.

81. Xie M, Zhou K, Patro N, et al. Virtual reality for vestibular rehabilitation: a systematic review. *Otol Neurotol.* 2021;42:967−977.

82. Phillips JS, Fitzgerald J, Phillis D, Underwood A, Nunney I, Bath A. Vestibular rehabilitation using video gaming in adults with dizziness: a pilot study. *J Laryngol Otol.* 2018; 132(3):202−206.

83. Davis J, Donaldson M, Ashe M, Khan K. The role of balance and agility training in fall reduction: a comprehensive review [Abstract]. *Eura Medicophys.* 2004;40(3):211−221.

Management of pediatric otologic trauma

16

Evette A. Ronner, MD[1]**, Michael S. Cohen, MD**[2]

[1]*Department of Otolaryngology-Head and Neck Surgery, Boston University Medical Center, Boston, MA, United States;* [2]*Department of Otolaryngology-Head and Neck Surgery, Massachusetts Eye and Ear, Harvard Medical School, Boston, MA, United States*

Overview

There are a variety of injuries to the ear that can be seen in the pediatric population. These vary from minor lacerations of the external ear to more severe cases of traumatic injury such as temporal bone fractures. Children with ear injuries may present in the outpatient setting, such as a pediatrician or otolaryngologist's office, or in the emergency department, depending on the nature of the otologic trauma as well as other concurring injuries. While there are many articles that summarize the management of otologic injuries in adults, few discuss the management of ear trauma specifically in children.

External ear trauma

Trauma to the external ear most commonly results from blunt force. Less often, injury is caused by penetrating trauma, nonaccidental trauma, or self-injury. These injuries often involve the external ear, including the auricle and external auditory canal only; however, some severe injuries may also involve the middle and inner ear structures. Comprehensive history and physical exam is important to determine the extent of the injury, and in some cases, diagnostic testing with audiogram or imaging may be necessary to evaluate for injuries extending beyond the external ear.

The ears are particularly susceptible to trauma given their protrusion from the face overlying a bony surface.[1] Auricular lacerations can either be simple or complex depending on whether the injury extends into the cartilage. Simple lacerations can often be repaired using sutures with a local anesthetic, whereas complex lacerations that expose cartilage require careful reapproximation. Patients who present within 24 h of the injury should undergo repair. If the injury occurred over 24 h prior, or if there are signs of active infection, then delayed closure may be optimal. Another common laceration is a split earlobe, which can be caused by pulling at an earring through the piercing hole. Repair by a surgical subspecialist may be warranted, as there are a variety of cosmetic techniques that can be used to repair these

Otologic and Lateral Skull Base Trauma. https://doi.org/10.1016/B978-0-323-87482-3.00007-7

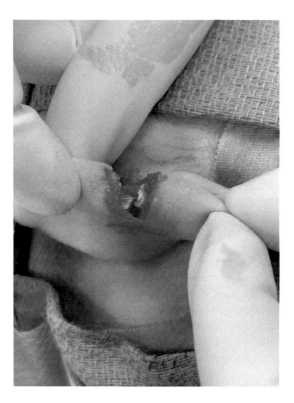

FIGURE 16.1

Full-thickness auricular laceration in a pediatric patient.

lacerations. For all auricular laceration repairs, the contralateral ear should be used as a guide to optimize symmetry between the two ears Fig. 16.1.

Auricular hematoma is a collection of blood between the perichondrium and cartilage of the ear. This is commonly seen in the pediatric setting of trauma, often as sports injuries. Damage to the vasculature and separation of perichondrium from the underlying cartilage can result in the development of a potential space, thereby allowing for the accumulation of blood. Auricular hematomas are diagnosed clinically from obtaining a thorough history and performing a physical exam. Diagnostic imaging is not required and typically only utilized to rule out other diagnoses. Significant pain, erythema, and swelling may be suggestive of cellulitis rather than auricular hematoma. Ultrasound can be helpful to exclude auricular abscess. Hearing is not typically affected in the setting of an isolated auricular hematoma; hearing loss in this setting should prompt imaging with either CT or MRI to evaluate for concurrent damage to middle or inner ear structures.[2] In pediatric patients, or when the mechanism of injury is unclear, nonaccidental trauma should be considered and appropriate protocols should be employed to determine if the patient is at further risk for harm Fig. 16.2.

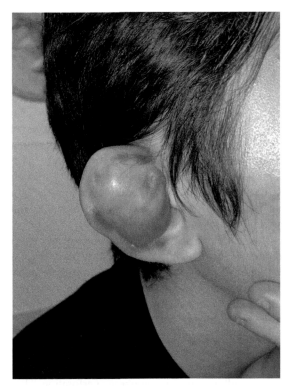

FIGURE 16.2

Auricular hematoma in a pediatric patient.

Treatment for auricular hematoma includes drainage with needle aspiration, incision and drainage, or drainage with placement of bolster, depending on the size and duration of the hematoma. The procedure can be performed at the bedside or in the operating room depending on provider and patient comfort. Drainage should occur as soon as possible after the injury. Untreated or repeated auricular hematomas allow for persistent fluid accumulation within the perichondrium and can result in a swollen and misfolded appearance of the auricle, commonly referred to as "cauliflower ear."[3] In persistent or severe cases, surgical reconstruction with otoplasty may be warranted to improve the cosmetic appearance of the ear.

Injury to the external auditory canal may be seen in isolation or in conjunction with other traumatic injuries. In children, isolated external auditory canal injury is often seen in the setting of a foreign body or use of a cotton swab causing damage to the ear canal skin. Complications may include otitis externa, and with risk of subsequent development of canal stenosis. In the context of a patient presenting with facial trauma, blood in the external auditory canal is suggestive of underlying temporal bone or mandibular fracture.[4] Treatment is variable depending on the mechanism of injury but involves managing risk of infection in the canal, repairing underlying fractures when indicated, and preventing stenosis of the canal during the healing process.

Traumatic tympanic membrane perforation

Perforation of the tympanic membrane can be caused by several mechanisms, including infection, mechanical injury, blast, and barotrauma. Mechanical trauma to the tympanic membrane occurs due to insertion of a foreign body or instrument into the ear canal and is most commonly caused by use of a cotton swab. Although manufacturers and physicians advise against the use of cotton swabs in the ear canal, cotton swab use remains the most common cause of accidental penetrating trauma to the ear.[5] Each year in the United States, over 12,000 children are treated in the emergency room for injury to the ear due to use of a cotton swab.[6] These injuries most often occur at home, in young children, and in the setting of attempting to clean the ear canal. Use of cotton swabs is associated with a number of otologic complications, including tympanic membrane perforation, ossicular injury, conductive hearing loss, cerumen impaction, and otitis externa.

Blast trauma to the ear can also result in tympanic membrane perforation. This injury is more commonly seen in adult patients, particularly those who have served in the military. However, these injuries in children are likely underreported in the literature, especially from regions where access to otolaryngologists is limited.[7] These injuries can occur in the context of warfare, domestic terrorism events,[8] or recreational activities, including the use of fireworks. Blast injuries can cause damage to not only the middle ear but also the inner ear, and they can cause a temporary or permanent sensorineural hearing loss, as well as tinnitus or hyperacusis.[8]

Inadequate pressure equalization between the middle ear space and the external environment can also result in tympanic membrane perforation. The Eustachian tube connects the nasopharynx with the middle ear space; when functional, it allows for exchange of air and subsequently equalizes the pressure between the two spaces. However, when pressure changes are sudden or extreme, or when Eustachian tube function is reduced or absent, traumatic perforation of the tympanic membrane can occur. Approximately 100 kPa of pressure is required to rupture the tympanic membrane.[9] In children, otic barotrauma is most commonly seen in the setting of air travel or diving underwater, where significant changes in pressure occur over a short period of time.

The diagnosis of traumatic tympanic membrane perforation is made clinically. The perforation is often visible on otoscopic examination; however, tympanometry can be used to diagnose perforations which are small, partially healed, or anatomically positioned outside the range of otoscopic visualization. Audiometric evaluation may also be indicated to determine the degree of any hearing loss from the injury and can also be helpful as a baseline measurement to monitor for changes in hearing over time.

Management of tympanic perforations is dependent on the size of the perforation, degree of hearing loss, or development of complications, such as chronic otitis media, cholesteatoma, and mastoiditis.[10] All patients should be instructed to keep the affected ear dry to decrease the risk of infection. Perforations that are small in size and cause minimal hearing loss may be managed conservatively with symptomatic care only, as most small traumatic perforations will heal spontaneously. For large or complicated perforations, surgical repair may be required. Tympanoplasty can be performed either via a transcanal or postauricular approach. Transcanal repair can be performed with use of either a microscope or an endoscope, which can offer a minimally invasive repair in children where transcanal surgery is not otherwise facile. A postauricular incision may be utilized if canalplasty is required for successful repair. Autologous grafts are often used in repair, including temporalis fascia, tragal or conchal cartilage or perichondrium, and split-thickness skin grafts. Cadaveric or sterile, acellular allografts can also be used. Irrespective of surgical approach or graft material, the majority of tympanoplasties result in successful closure of the perforation and improvement in hearing outcomes.[1] In blast injuries, otolaryngologists should have a high index of suspicion for implantation-type cholesteatoma.[8]

Ossicular injury

Injury to the ossicular chain can result directly from trauma or secondarily as a surgical complication. Primary injury to the ossicles can occur via direct pressure waves from a blast or penetrating foreign body. Indirect forces can also cause ossicular chain disruption, such as acceleration—deceleration events or blunt trauma to the head.[11] Fig. 16.3 shows CT imaging of an incus displaced into mastoid antrum in a pediatric patient due to a motor vehicle accident. Ossicular injury is a risk when performing any middle ear surgery, which can result in either disruption of the ossicular chain or accidental removal of the ossicles. There is increased risk when removing a foreign body from the outer or middle ear space, as the object can obstruct visualization of critical structures.

Ossicular injury should be suspected in the setting of a recent trauma or ear procedure accompanied by new hearing loss, vertigo, or tinnitus. Though some cases will be identified close to the time of injury, many will not be identified until weeks

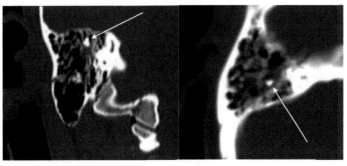

FIGURE 16.3

CT coronal (*left*) and axial (*right*) images of incus displaced into the antrum in a pediatric patient due to a motor vehicle accident.

to months after the traumatic event. Surgical repair of the ossicular chain can be performed with use of the microscope, endoscope, or combination of both. Studies have shown that endoscopic surgery has similar hearing outcomes and rates of complications compared with a microscopic approach and that use of an endoscope can result in fewer postauricular incisions.[12,13] If all three ossicles are present but there is discontinuity or erosion of the long or lenticular process of the incus, incus interposition or hydroxylapatite bone cement may be used. Alternatively, a variety of prostheses can be used depending on the nature of the injury, such as a titanium, Teflon, or hydroxylapatite partial and total ossicular prostheses. All patients with ossicular injury, regardless of whether surgical intervention is performed, should be followed with regular audiograms to monitor for changes in hearing over time.

Perilymph fistula

Trauma can also result in an abnormal connection between the inner ear and middle ear space, mastoid, or intracranial cavity, allowing for passage of perilymph fluid between the spaces, also known as a perilymph fistula. In children, perilymph fistulas can be congenital, seen in approximately 6% of cases of pediatric idiopathic sensorineural hearing loss, or acquired, more commonly seen in the setting of trauma to the ear.[14] Fistulas can form due to blunt or penetrating trauma; however, the injury does not necessarily need to be severe for a perilymph fistula to develop, as cases have been reported in children who had mild head injuries.[15] Symptoms can include vertigo, tinnitus, aural fullness, and sensorineural hearing loss, which can be stable or fluctuating in nature.

Because the clinical presentation of perilymph fistula is similar to that of other otologic conditions, such as Meniere's disease or labyrinthine concussion, it can be challenging to diagnose based on symptoms alone. While there is no single test that is both highly sensitive and specific, there are several specialized tests that can be performed to help determine whether a fistula may be present. One is the fistula test, where pressure is applied to the ear by pressing on the tragus or using pneumatic otoscopy. A positive fistula test is when the patient exhibits nystagmus as pressure is applied to the ear. In the Tulio phenomenon, nystagmus or vertigo can be provoked with loud sounds. Imaging with CT or MRI can be helpful to look for signs suggestive of perilymph fistula, such as air in the cochlea, vestibule, or semicircular canals, or fluid in the round or oval windows.[14]

Treatment of symptomatic traumatic perilymph fistula is best accomplished with surgical exploration followed by plugging of the fistula with tissue, usually perichondrium or fascia. The oval and round windows are typically both treated when perilymph fistula is suspected if a visible injury is not observed. There is some literature to suggest that the blood patch procedure, where autologous blood is injected through the tympanic membrane, can be used to help both diagnose and treat a perilymph fistula. Patients are advised to avoid exposure to situations that may alter pressure in the inner ear, such as air travel, scuba diving, loud noises, or heavy

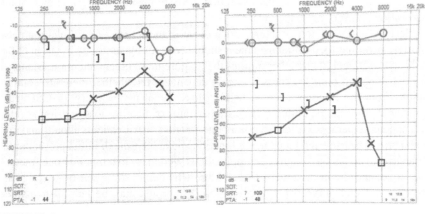

FIGURE 16.4

Audiogram of patient who had a perilymph fistula repaired with subsequent refistulation following loud noise exposure.

lifting. Fig. 16.4 shows audiograms after repair of perilymphatic fistula following traumatic stapes subluxation from Q-tip trauma with preservation of normal bone line (left) with subsequent refistulation after patient experienced acute onset vertigo while listening to very loud, bass-heavy music during his recovery period (right).

Temporal bone fracture

Trauma to the head can result in a temporal bone fracture, with children accounting for 8%−22% of all cases of temporal bone fracture.[15] These fractures have historically been classified as transverse or longitudinal relative to the direction of the injury to the petrous temporal bone. A third descriptor, an oblique fracture, was then introduced to describe fractures that cross the petrotympanic fissures. However, the utility of this classification system was lacking in categorizing fractures in a meaningful way that could both describe the nature of the fracture and serve as a predictor for clinical outcome. A newer classification system, where fractures are described as otic capsule violating and otic capsule sparing, has been shown to more closely correlate with clinical outcomes, such as sensorineural hearing loss.[16]

Temporal bone fractures are caused by high-impact trauma to the head. In children, fractures are usually caused by motor vehicle accidents or sports injuries. Given that significant blunt force is required to fracture the basilar skull, temporal bone fractures are often seen together with multiple injuries, and therefore, initial presentation is variable. A classic finding suggestive of temporal bone fracture is bruising over the mastoid bone, often called "Battle sign" or "Battle's sign." This can be accompanied by bruising over the eyes ("racoon eyes") or rhinorrhea due to CSF leak through the Eustachian tube. Patients may also present with hearing loss, facial nerve palsy, ear canal laceration, hemotympanum, tympanic membrane perforation, vertigo, or nystagmus.

Because temporal bone fractures often occur in the setting of multiple traumatic injuries, the initial focus of management should be hemodynamic stabilization of the child and treatment of any other injuries that require more urgent attention. Management of temporal bone fractures is largely dependent on whether there are complications from the fracture, such as hearing loss, facial nerve injury, or CSF leak. Compared with adults, children have higher rates of hearing loss and lower rates of facial nerve paralysis after temporal bone fracture.[17] All patients should undergo evaluation of hearing and facial nerve function and at the time of initial presentation. Patients who do not have signs of complications secondary to temporal bone fracture may be managed conservatively. For children who demonstrate sensorineural hearing loss or facial nerve palsy, a course of IV steroids may be helpful to reduce inflammation and may result in improved hearing and facial nerve function. Surgical exploration may be indicated for children who present with more serious complications, such as CSF leak or severe facial paralysis. There is a paucity of data comparing outcomes between surgical versus conservative treatment for acute facial paralysis in children who suffer temporal bone fracture. Many facial nerve injuries are recoverable and caused by neuropraxia, which often heal over time.[18] In some cases, the nerve may have been transected or crushed, which may result in unrecoverable function. Surgical exploration typically occurs when there is high suspicion that given the nature and location of the fracture, decompression of the facial nerve would result in improved function.

Conclusion

Many otologic injuries can be seen in the pediatric population. While most injuries are seen in the setting of accidental trauma, nonaccidental trauma must be ruled out. Further research exploring differences in prevalence of various otologic injuries and their complications in children compared with adults will help further refine management of pediatric ear injuries.

References

1. Burchhardt DM, David J, Eckert R, Robinette NL, Carron MA, Zuliani GF. Trauma patterns, symptoms, and complications associated with external auditory canal fractures. *Laryngoscope*. 2015;125(7):1579–1582. https://doi.org/10.1002/lary.25246.
2. Patel BC, Skidmore K, Hutchison J, et al. Cauliflower ear. Updated 2021 Nov 2. In: *StatPearls*. Treasure Island (FL): StatPearls Publishing; 2022 Jan-. Available from: https://www.ncbi.nlm.nih.gov/books/NBK470424/.
3. Williams CH, Sternard BT. Complex ear lacerations. Updated 2021 Aug 6. In: *StatPearls*. Treasure Island (FL): StatPearls Publishing; 2022 Jan-. Available from: https://www.ncbi.nlm.nih.gov/books/NBK525973/.

4. Delrue S, Verhaert N, Dinther JV, et al. Surgical management and hearing outcome of traumatic ossicular injuries. *J Int Adv Otol*. 2016;12(3):231−236. https://doi.org/10.5152/iao.2016.2868.

5. Steele BD, Brennan PO. A prospective survey of patients with presumed accidental ear injury presenting to a paediatric accident and emergency department. *Emerg Med J*. 2002;19(3):226−228. https://doi.org/10.1136/emj.19.3.226.

6. Ameen ZS, Chounthirath T, Smith GA, Jatana KR. Pediatric cotton-tip applicator-related ear injury treated in United States emergency departments, 1990-2010. *J Pediatr*. 2017; 186:124−130. https://doi.org/10.1016/j.jpeds.2017.03.049.

7. Mick P, Moxham P, Ludemann J. Penetrating and blast ear trauma: 7-year review of two pediatric practices. *J Otolaryngol Head Neck Surg*. 2008;37(6):774−776.

8. Remenschneider AK, Lookabaugh S, Aliphas A, et al. Otologic outcomes after blast injury: the Boston Marathon experience. *Otol Neurotol*. 2014;35(10):1825−1834. https://doi.org/10.1097/MAO.0000000000000616.

9. Dolhi N, Weimer AD. Tympanic membrane perforations. Updated 2021 Aug 11. In: *StatPearls*. Treasure Island (FL): StatPearls Publishing; 2022 Jan. Available from: https://www.ncbi.nlm.nih.gov/books/NBK557887/.

10. Indorewala S, Adedeji TO, Indorewala A, Nemade G. Tympanoplasty outcomes: a review of 789 cases. *Iran J Otorhinolaryngol*. 2015;27(79):101−108.

11. Guneri EA, Cakir Cetin A. Ossicular chain reconstruction: endoscopic or microscopic? *J Laryngol Otol*. 2020;134(12):1108−1114. https://doi.org/10.1017/S0022215120002728.

12. Campbell E, Tan NC. Ossicular-chain dislocation. Updated 2021 Aug 4. In: *StatPearls*. Treasure Island (FL): StatPearls Publishing; 2022 Jan. Available from: https://www-ncbi-nlm-nih-gov.dartmouth.idm.oclc.org/books/NBK560621/.

13. Sarna B, Abouzari M, Merna C, Jamshidi S, Saber T, Djalilian HR. Perilymphatic fistula: a review of classification, etiology, diagnosis, and treatment. *Front Neurol*. 2020;11: 1046. https://doi.org/10.3389/fneur.2020.01046. Published 2020 Sep. 15.

14. Johnson F, Semaan MT, Megerian CA. Temporal bone fracture: evaluation and management in the modern era. *Otolaryngol Clin*. 2008;41(3):597−618. https://doi.org/10.1016/j.otc.2008.01.006.

15. Little SC, Kesser BW. Radiographic classification of temporal bone fractures. *Arch Otolaryngol Head Neck Surg*. 2006;132:1300−1304.

16. Dunklebarger J, Branstetter 4th B, Lincoln A, et al. Pediatric temporal bone fractures: current trends and comparison of classification schemes. *Laryngoscope*. 2014;124(3): 781−784. https://doi.org/10.1002/lary.21891.

17. Patel A, Groppo E. Management of temporal bone trauma. *Craniomaxillofacial Trauma Reconstr*. 2010;3(2):105−113. https://doi.org/10.1055/s-0030-1254383.

18. Diaz RC, Cervenka B, Brodie HA. Treatment of temporal bone fractures. *J Neurol Surg B Skull Base*. 2016;77(5):419−429. https://doi.org/10.1055/s-0036-1584197.

Further reading

1 Krogmann RJ, Jamal Z, King KC. Auricular hematoma. Updated 2022 Jan 24. In: *StatPearls*. Treasure Island (FL): StatPearls Publishing; 2022 Jan. Available from: https://www-ncbi-nlm-nih-gov.dartmouth.idm.oclc.org/books/NBK531499/.

Pediatric vestibular dysfunction following head injury: Diagnosis and management

Graham Cochrane, PhD [1], Jacob R. Brodsky, MD, FACS, FAAP [2,3]

[1]*University of Alabama, School of Medicine, Birmingham, AL, United States;* [2]*Department of Otolaryngology and Communication Enhancement, Boston Children's Hospital, Boston, MA, United States;* [3]*Department of Otolaryngology, Harvard Medical School, Boston, MA, United States*

Introduction

The causes of vestibular symptoms after traumatic brain injury and concussion in children and adolescents are generally similar to those that impact adults. However, there are many unique considerations in the evaluation and management of children and adolescents with posttraumatic vestibular dysfunction relative to adults, which warrant special consideration. Posttraumatic dizziness and imbalance in the pediatric population are most commonly attributed to central causes at the level of the brain, as well as associated autonomic dysfunction. However, as many as 1 in 3 pediatric patients with posttraumatic vestibular symptoms have evidence of a causative peripheral vestibular condition.[1] It is important to note that such peripheral vestibular disorders can also occur concurrently with central vestibular dysfunction following a head injury, so they should not be treated as mutually exclusive.[2,3] Thus, this chapter is broken down into separate sections: (1) evaluation of pediatric posttraumatic dizziness, (2) posttraumatic peripheral vestibular disorders, and (3) posttraumatic central vestibular dysfunction and dysautonomia. A proposed algorithm for the evaluation and management of patients with posttraumatic dizziness is shown in Fig. 17.1.

Evaluation of pediatric posttraumatic dizziness

The history and physical examination are the highest yield components in the evaluation of pediatric patients with posttraumatic vestibular symptoms. Brief episodes of spinning vertigo that are triggered by specific rapid head movements, particularly when supine, should prompt the provider to evaluate for benign paroxysmal positional vertigo (BPPV) with diagnostic maneuvers, as summarized in further detail

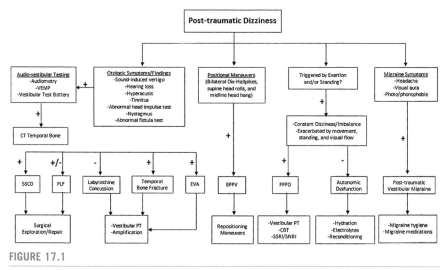

FIGURE 17.1

Algorithm for evaluation and management of pediatric patients with posttraumatic dizziness. Note that these diagnoses are not mutually exclusive and a single patient may have more than one of these conditions concurrently. Also note that central vestibulopathy is excluded from this algorithm, as it typically causes primarily balance impairment and not dizziness. *BPPV*, benign paroxysmal positional vertigo; *CBT*, cognitive behavioral therapy; *CT*, computed tomography; *EVA*, enlarged vestibular aqueduct; *PLF*, perilymphatic fistula; *PPPDs*, persistent postural perceptual dizziness; *PTs*, physical therapy; *SSCD*, superior semicircular canal dehiscence; *SSRI*, selective serotonin reuptake inhibitor; *SNRI*, serotonin norepinephrine reuptake inhibitor; *VEMP*, vestibular evoked myogenic potential.

in the section on BPPV in the following. Otologic symptoms, such as subjective hearing loss, unilateral tinnitus, ear pain, autophony, and/or conductive hyperacusis (described in further detail in the following), should prompt audiologic testing and evaluation by a vestibular specialist (otologist, oto-neurologist, and/or neurotologist). Dizziness that occurs specifically with standing and/or exertion suggests autonomic dysregulation. Dizziness that is constant with frequent flares and is exacerbated by visual triggers is suggestive of persistent postural–perceptual dizziness (PPPD). Physical examination findings that suggest a posttraumatic peripheral vestibular disorder include a positive diagnostic positional maneuver, corrective saccades on head impulse testing, direction-fixed horizontal/torsional nystagmus that is suppressed with fixation, diminished unilateral hearing, abnormal Rinne/Weber tuning fork testing, positive Hennebert's sign, and/or positive fistula test. In many cases, vestibular testing may also be warranted to further evaluate a patient for whom the suspicion of a posttraumatic peripheral vestibular condition is suspected. The examination techniques described before, as well as the role of different vestibular tests in diagnosing specific posttraumatic vestibular conditions, are discussed in further detail in the pertinent sections for individual conditions in the following, as well as in other relevant chapters in this book.

Vestibular testing may be more challenging to obtain in pediatric patients than in adults. Only a limited number of vestibular programs will test children and adolescents. Many younger children may not be able to tolerate or actively participate in some vestibular tests to a degree that will yield reliable results. In particular, caloric testing and dynamic subjective visual vertical testing can be very difficult for younger children to tolerate, while rotary chair, videonystagmography (without caloric testing), video head impulse testing (VHIT), vestibular evoked myogenic potential testing (VEMP), and static subjective visual vertical testing (SVV) are generally well tolerated. However, the testing audiologist or technician must be patient and reassuring, particularly in young children. The aid of an assistant is often essential in testing younger children, and the incorporation of light-up toys to help focus the child's attention can be very helpful. Children <7 years of age often have difficulty with understanding instructions adequately to provide reliable SVV results.[4] Similarly, children 4–7 years of age can typically provider reliable VHIT results in the horizontal canal plane, but not in the vertical planes.[5,6] VNG and VHIT goggles are generally too large to fit children <4 years of age, though most rotary chairs are equipped with a high-resolution infrared camera that allows for valuable, though limited, evaluation of the integrity of the vestibuloocular (VOR) reflex response and the presence of any nystagmus without the need for goggles in very young children. It is important that testing results be interpreted using age-specific norms, which can be obtained from the manufacturer and the medical literature, although ideally individual centers should obtain age-specific normative data for their own testing equipment, as results with different equipment can often vary to a significant degree.

Peripheral vestibular disorders

As many as 1 in 3 pediatric patients with dizziness after concussion have a contributing peripheral vestibular disorder, which may occur in isolation or concurrently with an additional central cause.[1–3,7] Fig. 17.2 shows a breakdown of the relative prevalence of individual peripheral vestibular conditions in children and adolescents with postconcussive dizziness based on data from a 2018 retrospective study of patients at the senior author's pediatric vestibular program and multidisciplinary concussion clinic.[1]

Benign paroxysmal positional vertigo

BPPV is a very common and easily treatable cause of posttraumatic vertigo, impacting as much as a third of children and adolescents with posttraumatic dizziness.[1–3,7–9] Unfortunately, it is frequently overlooked and vastly underdiagnosed, which is likely due primarily to the fact that most primary pediatric concussion providers (e.g., sports medicine providers, neurologists, and pediatricians) do not have significant experience in the evaluation and treatment of vestibular disorders. Similarly, most vestibular specialists do not routinely see patients with

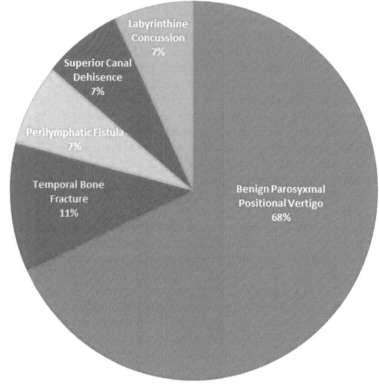

FIGURE 17.2

Relative percentage of peripheral vestibular disorders found in 28 patients diagnosed with peripheral vestibular dysfunction out of 109 pediatric patients evaluated for postconcussive dizziness in a pediatric vestibular program clinic.[1]

posttraumatic dizziness until they are several weeks, or even months out from their injury. One study found that the mean delay in diagnosis of BPPV in pediatric patients with postconcussive dizziness was approximately 4 months.[7] Thus, increasing awareness of the evaluation and management of BPPV among primary concussion providers may help to hasten recovery in many cases.

A more detailed discussion of BPPV is covered elsewhere in this book, so the focus of this section is on features of the condition that are specific to the posttraumatic pediatric population. Although BPPV is generally thought to be rare in children, it has actually been demonstrated in multiple recent studies to be much more common than previously supposed, particularly in the setting of concussion.[1–3,7–10] Although the posterior canal is most commonly involved in pediatric BPPV, as in adults, there is a much higher prevalence of horizontal and superior canal involvement in the pediatric age group. This difference is very pertinent to the history and the physical examination. The symptoms of horizontal and superior canal BPPV often differ significantly from those of posterior canal BPPV. Although posterior canal BPPV typically causes episodes of vertigo primarily when turning the head in bed, horizontal canal BPPV can also cause episodic vertigo when upright. Superior canal BPPV can also cause vertigo when supine but is particularly prone to causing symptoms when going from supine to upright, which may cause it to frequently be mistaken for the very common entity of posttraumatic hemodynamic intolerance (described elsewhere in this chapter). Patients with superior canal BPPV may even report symptoms with walking upright and particularly with bending over.

Diagnosis of suspected BPPV is confirmed with diagnostic positional maneuvers. Due to the higher incidence of horizontal and superior canal involvement in pediatric BPPV, it is ideal to use video goggles (VNG or Frenzel lenses) during the assessment and all six semicircular canals should be assessed. The latter is achieved by including not only bilateral Dix-Hallpike maneuvers in the examination (which evaluate both the posterior and superior canals), but also bilateral supine head roll maneuvers (horizontal canals), and a midline head-hang maneuver (superior canals). The presence of characteristic nystagmus and subjective vertigo with a given maneuver is diagnostic of BPPV in the tested canal. Posterior canal BPPV is associated with an upbeating torsional geotropic nystagmus with the Dix-Hallpike maneuver toward the affected side. Horizontal canal BPPV is associated with horizontal nystagmus that can be either geotropic or apogeotropic, with the affected side being that toward which the fast phase of nystagmus beats. Superior canal BPPV is associated with downbeating nystagmus with the Dix-Hallpike maneuver and midline head-hang maneuver, often with an accompanying torsional and/or horizontal component, which typically beats toward the affected ear. It should be noted that some children have difficulty tolerating the Dix-Hallpike maneuver in the presence of posterior or superior canal BPPV, because the movement of going from sitting directly to lying supine along with accompanying vertigo can induce a sense of falling and feel particularly vulnerable. In these children, we have found a partial Semont maneuver to be effective in evaluating for BPPV of the posterior canals. For this maneuver, the child is seating on the side of the examination table or on a parent's lap with their legs hanging of the side in front of them. Their head is turned 45° away from the side being testing, and then they are tipped sideways until they are lying on the shoulder of the side being tested with their head brought down into a hanging position with the head still angled upward. This achieves the same head movement and final head position as the Dix-Hallpike maneuver but can be less frightening and easier to achieve reliably in some younger children.

Treatment of BPPV consists of therapeutic canalith repositioning maneuvers, which are tailored to the affected canal(s). The posterior canal is typically treated with the Epley or Semont therapeutic maneuvers.[11,12] The horizontal canal is treated with a Lempert or Gufoni maneuver.[13,14] The superior canal can be treated effectively with a reverse Epley maneuver or with a standing inversion maneuver.[15] In the latter maneuver, the patient is bent over from a standing position until the head is pointed forward the floor and rotated away from the affected side. This position is held for 1 min, and then the patient is rapidly brought back up to the standing position by an assistant. Treatment-resistant cases of BPPV are uncommon, particularly following a head injury, but they may be somewhat more common in children than in adults.[8] Patients with treatment resistant BPPV may benefit from vitamin D supplementation.[16] In truly treatment resistant cases, surgical occlusion of the affected canal may be beneficial.[17]

Labyrinthine concussion

Labyrinthine concussion is a poorly understood entity that causes sudden loss of ipsilateral peripheral vestibular function and/or hearing following a head injury without grossly apparent violation of the labyrinth (e.g., fracture or fistula).[18] The pathophysiology of this phenomenon is unclear, partly due to its overall rarity. However, milder variations of this phenomenon may be more common than previously supposed, as evidenced by an increasing body of literature showing mild peripheral vestibular losses and/or hearing loss in a significant proportion of patients with concussion.[1,9] Diagnosis of labyrinthine concussion after a head injury should be suspected in the presence of sudden hearing loss, unilateral tinnitus, and/or vertigo exacerbated by rapid head movements. Examination findings that would support this diagnosis include a positive head impulse test on the affected side, contraversive direction-fixed nystagmus that is reduced with fixation, and tuning fork testing that is suggestive of a new sensorineural hearing loss (SNHL) in the affected ear. Diagnosis of labyrinthine concussion is confirmed by demonstrating evidence of a new unilateral SNHL on audiologic testing and/or unilateral vestibular loss on vestibular testing. Temporal bone imaging should be considered when the diagnosis is made, if not already done, to rule out a fracture. Treatment consists of vestibular rehabilitation and hearing amplification, if warranted. The role of steroids in the setting of posttraumatic sudden SNHL remains unclear and is covered elsewhere in this book. Classroom accommodations for children with a persistent hearing loss are important to recommend, ideally consisting of a minimum of preferential seating at the front of the classroom and an FM system, when available.

Temporal bone fracture

Diagnosis of temporal bone fracture in a child with a traumatic head injury is typically made on initial presentation, though occasionally it may be missed in the setting of a concussion where a scan was not performed. Most temporal bone fractures are essentially asymptomatic, but if the otic capsule or internal auditory canal is impacted, then resulting symptoms can include hearing loss, vertigo, imbalance, and/or facial nerve weakness. Exam findings are similar to those described for labyrinthine concussion before, though ipsilateral facial muscle weakness may be present. Ear pain and swelling may also be present. Audiologic testing may reveal an SNHL, conductive hearing loss (from ossicular chain disruption, hemotympanum, or tympanic membrane perforation), or a mixed hearing loss. Vestibular test findings may be similar to those described for labyrinthine concussion before, though they may also often be normal. Diagnosis is confirmed by computed tomography (CT) of the temporal bones. Hemotympanum will typically clear spontaneously, and traumatic tympanic membrane perforations may heal without intervention. Acute surgical intervention is rarely necessary, unless a bone fragment is noted to be compressing the cochlear, vestibular, and/or facial nerves, or if a cerebrospinal fluid leak is suspected. Nonurgent surgical management may be warranted for ossicular chain disruption or tympanic membrane perforations that do not heal spontaneously. The primary treatment for persistent vestibular symptoms from a temporal bone fracture is vestibular rehabilitation, if vestibular deficits/symptoms are present. The hearing loss can be managed with amplification, if surgical intervention is not warranted or does not adequately resolve the hearing loss. Classroom accommodations should also be provided when a significant hearing loss is present, as described before in the labyrinthine concussion section.

Superior canal dehiscence

Although not a traumatic peripheral vestibular disorder, per se, superior semicircular canal dehiscence (SSCD) can often become symptomatic after a head injury, so it warrants inclusion in the differential diagnosis of the child or adolescent with post-traumatic vertigo. The etiology of SSCD is thought to be primarily congenital with thinning of the bony roof of the superior semicircular canal that separates it from the dura of the middle cranial fossa; however, many cases may also be due to benign intracranial hypertension, leading to thinning of the bone over time.[19] A traumatic injury may cause a dehiscence of the already thinned bone, leading to the condition becoming symptomatic. The proposed mechanism of the disorder involves the so-called "third-window" effect, where the dehiscence leads to a third entry point into the otic capsule, in addition to the round and oval windows, resulting in conduction of sound pressure through the superior canal and adding an additional route for sound pressure to enter and exit the cochlea. Symptoms may include dysequilibrium, oscillopsia, sound-induced vertigo (Tullio's phenomenon), hearing loss, autophony, and conductive hyperacusis. Diagnosis is confirmed by a combination of audiometric findings, temporal bone CT (with thin, oblique cuts through the superior semicircular canal plane), and VEMP testing. VEMP results typically demonstrate a reduced threshold and increased amplitude in the affected ear. Treatment is most effectively achieved through surgical resurfacing or occlusion of the affected superior canal via a middle cranial fossa or a transmastoid approach. Transcanal round window occlusion is also sometimes effective at reducing the auditory and vestibular symptoms, though it does not resolve the associated hearing loss, and results with this approach are variable.[20] The overall prevalence of symptomatic SSCD in the pediatric population is unclear but appears to be relatively low.[1,2,21] It is an especially challenging diagnosis to confirm in children, since the roof of the superior canal is already thinner in younger children, in general.

Perilymphatic fistula

A perilymphatic fistula results from a traumatic violation of the round and/or oval window membrane. This will typically cause symptoms that are similar to those of SSCD, including hearing loss, tinnitus, dysequilibrium, sound-induced vertigo, autophony, and conductive hyperacusis. Examination may reveal a positive fistula sign, where tragal pumping of insufflation of the affected ear canal with a pneumatic bulb triggers vertigo and nystagmus; however, this test is not particularly sensitive or specific.[22] Audiometry may reveal a conductive, sensorineural, or mixed hearing loss. Vestibular testing may show unilateral vestibular loss and/or a third window pattern on VEMP testing, though it can also be normal. Temporal bone CT may show pneumolabyrinth, accumulation of fluid in the middle ear, and/or ossicular chain disruption, but also can often be normal. Diagnosis can only be confirmed definitively with surgical exploration of the middle ear, so a high degree of clinical suspicion is paramount. Repair is performed with tissue grafting (e.g., fat, perichondrium, fascia), often along with tissue glue, which is done at the time of middle ear exploration. This can typically be done via a transcanal approach and lends itself particularly well to the use of endoscopic techniques, except in the setting of a particularly brisk leak where a postauricular approach with a microscope may be preferable, particularly in younger children.[23]

Enlarged vestibular aqueduct

Enlarged vestibular aqueduct (EVA) is not a traumatic lesion but can become symptomatic following even very minor head injuries; thus, it warrants discussion in this chapter. EVA is the most common cause of congenital hearing loss that is grossly visible on temporal bone imaging. Children with EVA may have hearing loss at birth, but it can often be delayed in onset and fluctuates over time in many cases. It can be seen in the setting of mutations in the SLC26A4 gene, which is associated with Pendred syndrome when mutations are homozygous, but EVA can also be seen in conjunction with other hearing loss syndromes and often occurs as an isolated anomaly. Patients with EVA are often prone to sudden drops in hearing and/or vestibular function following impacts to the head that may be milder than that required to sustain a concussion or a major traumatic brain injury. Historically, patients with EVA were discouraged from sports activities, though this advice is no longer considered routine.[24] Audiologic testing in children with EVA typically shows a sensorineural or mixed hearing loss that may be unilateral or bilateral. Vestibular testing may show a third window pattern on VEMP testing and a unilateral or bilateral vestibular loss on other vestibular tests.[25,26] Diagnosis is confirmed by temporal bone CT, though very large vestibular aqueducts can sometimes be seen on MRI. There are multiple different diagnostic criteria for EVA, all of which are based on measurements of the vestibular aqueducts on temporal bone CT. The most commonly used criteria are the Cincinnati criteria, which indicate that EVA is confirmed by the presence of combined measurements of the aqueduct of

>0.9 mm at the midpoint and >1.9 mm at the operculum.[25] EVA is often also associated with an incomplete partition anomaly, type II (IP2), which was formerly known as a Mondini malformation. This anomaly also includes a shortened cochlear of only 1.5 turns, a deficient modiolus, and a deficient interscalar septum.[27] Treatment for EVA-induced vestibular dysfunction may include vestibular PT. Management of EVA-associated hearing loss may include amplification with hearing aids, classroom accommodations, or cochlear implantation. Many providers administer a course of corticosteroids to patients with EVA who have a sudden drop in hearing or vestibular function, particularly after a head injury, but evidence for the benefit of this approach is lacking.

Central vestibular dysfunction and autonomic dysfunction

Dizziness following head trauma in children frequently results from damage to central nervous system structures and tracts.[1] Rotational head trauma is hypothesized to impart mechanical stress onto neurons, disrupting axonal white matter integrity.[28,29] White matter microstructural changes and diffuse neurometabolic alterations resulting from that stress in turn impair the ability of neurons to propagate action potentials efficiently and induce neuroinflammatory changes, worsening clinical outcomes and lengthening recovery times.[28-30] While these changes are not identifiable on common imaging tools such as CT and basic MRI, tools such as diffusion tensor imaging have shown promise in identifying microstructural and functional changes in white matter following several types of pediatric head trauma.[31-34].

Damage to white matter tracts of the central vestibular system, i.e., brainstem neuronal tracts originating from the vestibular nuclei, therefore can manifest with symptoms of dizziness, imbalance, and disorientation in the absence of identifiable damage to the peripheral vestibular organs themselves.[35] Autonomic dysregulation may arise from similar damage to white matter tracts and neurometabolic changes of regions of cortex responsible for managing the autonomic nervous system, producing symptoms of dizziness in the case of hemodynamic intolerance.[36] Inflammatory responses to microstructural neuronal changes of central vestibular tracts and vascular structures are also likely responsible for induction of migraine-associated dizziness/vestibular migraine following head trauma.[37] Damage to these systems may result in maladaptive changes that lead to chronic debilitating dizziness in the form of persistent postural–perceptual dizziness even after the initial injury has resolved.[38] Proper identification of these conditions is vital to determine the proper treatment as, despite similar inciting processes and a shared symptom of dizziness, interventions for each differ greatly.

As dizziness from these central causes is due to diffuse metabolic and microstructural damage, treatment for these causes focuses on rehabilitation, lifestyle modifications, and medications rather than surgical intervention. It should be noted that both peripheral and central vestibular dysfunction can manifest following a single pediatric head injury or that several central processes may occur simultaneously;

in these cases, a combination of multiple treatment modalities is advised.[39] The following discussion will focus on cases of vestibular symptomatology in the absence of the causes of peripheral vestibular dysfunction discussed previously in this chapter and with a singular central diagnosis.

Central vestibulopathy

Imbalance and dizziness have been frequently cited as two of the most common symptoms following head trauma. These symptoms can be seen in both adults and children following head trauma without vestibular end-organ pathology such as impaired VOR or VEMP.[1,40–42] Imbalance and dizziness in these children may arise instead from disruption of white matter tracts of central vestibular sensory integration pathways.[43] Disturbances of these tracts impair the inability of the nervous system to properly utilize peripheral vestibular signals, even if those incoming signals are intact.

Central vestibular pathways can be probed clinically through higher-level vestibular testing that requires integration across multiple sensory modalities. The most commonly measured central sensory integration functions in clinic are static balance and gait due to their ease of administration, but other integrative measures such as subjective visual vertical and VOR cancellation tasks may also assess these processes.[41] Both measures of static balance and gait have been associated with DTI MRI changes following pediatric TBI, suggesting that loss of white matter integrity is related to impairments in the central sensory integration process and resulting balance impairments.[44,45] In addition, static balance and gait step variability—a function believed to be driven heavily by central vestibular processing and not peripheral vestibular functioning—have been correlated in children with TBI, further underscoring central vestibular and sensory integration as a pathophysiological mechanism for balance and gait impairments postinjury.[46,47] Even in children with severe TBI leading to changes in brain matter gray volume, gait abnormalities have best correlated with loss of volume in regions of the brain crucial for sensory integration like the superior parietal lobe.[48]

Assessment of static balance following TBI in children can be completed several ways and usually takes the form of measurement of postural sway and falls. Standalone balance assessments such as the BESS and BOT-2 allow for more standardized grading of balance ability than simple observation by the clinician and appear to be more sensitive to balance dysfunction than subjective self-reported balance status.[49] More comprehensive postinjury tools such as the SCAT include a standardized balance assessment as one of several composite measures. Each of these tools has been validated in children with and without TBI and is sensitive for detecting mild TBI, or concussion.[50–53] While these tools are most commonly utilized for concussion, some evidence suggests that concussion evaluation tools for balance may not be tolerable in more severe forms of TBI when physical disability impairs ability to perform the task.[54]

Computerized balance assessments of static posturography utilize force plate center-of-gravity sway to quantify balance function, such as the SOT or Wii Balance Board.[9,55] Wearable inertial sensors and smartphone accelerometer applications are in development and testing stages for more portable, real-life assessment of balance function.[56,57] These more sophisticated tools are believed to have higher sensitivity for detecting mild alterations in balance function that may persist, though require much more investment by the clinician both financially and in time needed for data processing and interpretation.[58,59] Even with sophisticated balance data, interpretation in children can be difficult. It has been well established that postural sway decreases as children age, but the exact mechanisms behind this maturation as well as age-specific expectations are unclear.[60] Several studies have suggested adult-like balance strategies are in place by age seven, while other studies still identify differences in preteen to teenage postural sway.[61–67] Therefore, interpretation of any type of balance data in a child should utilize individualized baseline data whenever possible and take into account normative data of the child's specific age and preinjury activity level.[68,69]

Gait function may be assessed through standardized observational grading, computerized walkways, and video analysis. Gait variables frequently included in postTBI analyses include step length, step variability, and sway during gait—sometimes referred to as "dynamic balance." Current evidence suggests that low-tech measures such as tandem gait speed and stability are reliable measures in children and can be as sensitive as computerized measures of balance function for detection of postconcussion deficits, especially when performed with a concurrent cognitive dual task.[70–75] Research on gait in children postconcussion has mainly focused on dynamic balance sway, but some studies have additionally identified deficits in gait parameters such as step length and walking speed.[72,76] Children with more severe TBI have more consistently demonstrated deficits in gait parameters such as step length and variability that also linger beyond resolution of other TBI symptoms.[77–79] Similar to balance data, gait data in children can be difficult to interpret across age ranges due to variable development and might not correlate well with self-perceived dizziness and imbalance.[80–82]

Vestibular rehabilitation has emerged as a promising tool for managing central vestibular dysfunction following head injuries in children, though there is a paucity of literature supporting its use.[83–85] Trials of vestibular rehabilitation in children have mainly focused on those with concussion and not more severe TBI. Protocols for such trials have been developed, and vestibular rehabilitation has been identified as a potential therapy for improving balance following such head injuries; however, these authors are unaware of a study that has specifically focused on vestibular rehabilitation of children following moderate-to-severe TBI.[86,87] The existing concussion literature does, however, indicate that imbalance improves following rehabilitation in both children and adults, suggesting that rehabilitation works through similar mechanisms to improve symptoms regardless of age.[83]

From the perspective of deficits in central vestibular processing, vestibular rehabilitation techniques such as balance training are hypothesized to work directly on rehabilitating central sensory integration pathways.[88-91] Vestibular rehabilitation exercises to improve balance and gait focus on training under different sensory conditions to alter the brain's reliance on specific sensory inputs. This can take the form of practicing balance with eyes closed to reduce the brain's weight of visual input, which has been shown to be increased following head injury.[92] Sensory reweighting therapies are of particular importance in younger children due to their underdeveloped somatosensory and visual systems for balance so that they do not develop maladaptive sensory processing strategies during critical sensory development periods.[93] Along with improving objective balance function, these exercises also appear to improve symptomatic dizziness in children, further supporting a link between disruption of central sensory processing pathways and dizziness.[83]

Autonomic dysregulation (dysautonomia)

Dizziness due to hemodynamic intolerance (HI) has been identified in children following both concussion and more severe head injury.[94-97] HI symptoms are driven by alterations in autonomic nervous system functioning such as decreases in cerebral perfusion and/or aberrant sympathetic nervous system responses to changes in position. This autonomic dysregulation is believed to precipitate symptoms such as dizziness, blurred vision, palpitations, lightheadedness, and fatigue.[36,98-100] A decrease in cerebral blood flow has been well documented in the TBI literature and associated with worse TBI symptoms and prognosis in both adolescents and young adults.[101-105] A decrease in cerebral blood flow further exacerbates the increase in neurometabolic demand of the brain following injury and simultaneously reduces blood flow to areas such as the insular cortex responsible for regulating the autonomic response.[28,36,104] Systemic reductions in neurotransmitter release and baroreceptor reflex sensitivity perpetuate this demand further and can result in presyncopal and syncopal symptoms upon changes in positioning.[36]

Two types of HI commonly diagnosed following head injury are orthostatic hypotension and postural orthostatic tachycardia syndrome (POTS). Orthostatic hypotension is defined as a reduction in systolic blood pressure or diastolic blood pressure of >20 mmHg or >10 mmHg, respectively, on standing or during head-up tilt (HUT) testing, whereas POTS is defined as an increase in heart rate of >40 bpm in children within 10 min of standing or during HUT without evidence of orthostatic hypotension.[106,107] Both of these physiologic responses represent abnormal autonomic responses to hemodynamic changes and may result in symptoms of dizziness know as hemodynamic orthostatic dizziness/vertigo.

Hemodynamic orthostatic dizziness/vertigo is defined by the Bárány Society as episodes of dizziness, unsteadiness, or vertigo that are triggered by postural changes in individuals who also meet the clinical criteria for orthostatic hypotension, postural orthostatic tachycardia syndrome, or syncope.[108] While these authors are unaware of a specific study utilizing this recent Bárány Society definition in children post-TBI, there are a number of studies investigating the incidence and management of both orthostatic hypotension and POTS in children post-TBI with symptoms suspicious for general HI.

Posttraumatic head injury HI has been identified in 8.7% of all children seen in a postconcussion clinic and has been shown to prolong recovery time but is not frequently assessed for properly if at all.[94,96,97] In a study of children with persistent postconcussion symptoms including lightheadedness, 70% demonstrated abnormal HUT results.[96] One retrospective study of new pediatric POTS diagnoses revealed that 11.2% of patients had sustained a head injury within the 3 months prior to their POTS diagnosis.[109] Despite the seemingly high prevalence of HI post-TBI, a major criticism of HI studies in head injury is that no study has prospectively assessed pre-injury orthostatic vital signs and HUT responses. As these are not routinely examined and the prevalence of HI symptoms in children is unknown, it is unclear how many children may have qualified for a diagnosis of orthostatic hypotension or POTS prior to their head injury.[110] Prospective studies evaluating the relationship between development of HI and TBI are needed to better understand this complex interaction and better define diagnostic criteria. Nevertheless, there has been an association with normalization of orthostatic vital signs and resolution of orthostatic symptoms in children with TBI.[96] As HI symptoms can play a major role in recovery, are easily assessed, and can potentially be managed through lifestyle changes and medications, they should be managed regardless of their true etiology.

Clinical suspicion of HI in a child with TBI should be raised when the child endorses symptoms of lightheadedness, palpitations, blurred vision, etc. that are associated with changes in position and/or abate upon laying down. The gold standard clinical examination to follow up such symptoms is an HUT; however, as multiple HUT protocols exist and are frequently being modified, specific clinic HUT should be requested to properly interpret results.[110] Furthermore, as HUT likely requires later referral to a specialty clinic, investigation of these symptoms can be completed in an initial clinic visit utilizing supine-to-standing orthostatic vital sign measurements. Like with HUT protocols, different supine-to-standing orthostatic protocols exist with regard to how long patients should remain supine prior to blood pressure and heart rate measurements standing and how long they should remain standing before checking vital signs again. Currently, supine-to-standing measurements are validated for the diagnosis of orthostatic hypotension in children after 3 minutes of standing, though delayed orthostatic hypotension may be missed.[106,110] A standing time of 10 minutes is required to rule out POTS; some published clinic protocols as long as 17 min, which may be more sensitive for diagnosis but is likely too long to be widely adopted.[111]

In addition to the difficulties in standardization and time requirements of these clinical examinations, there is growing research to suggest that specific orthostatic vital sign cutoffs are not good predictors of symptomatology or responsivity to treatment in children, both with idiopathic HI and post-TBI HI.[95,112,113] Initial treatment strategies for HI symptoms are low risk, consisting of graded exercise plans (already commonly incorporated into a post-TBI treatment plan), compression garments, and increasing fluid and salt intake.[114–116] Negative HUT or orthostatic vital signs therefore should not preclude attempting conservative management in a child with strong clinical suspicion for hemodynamic orthostatic dizziness based on their reported symptoms. Pharmacological treatment can be initiated if conservative management fails, typically with a very low dose of fludrocortisone or, if not tolerated, midodrine.[117,118] Beta-blockers, while useful for HI symptoms such as palpitations, are contraindicated in patients with dizziness/lightheadedness-predominant HI due to concerns of exacerbating those symptoms.[115] Future prospective studies should examine the effect these drugs have on HI in children as these treatment recommendations are based on prospective studies completed in adults, with some subjective efficacy reported in children.[94]

Vestibular migraine

Head injury is hypothesized to precipitate migraine-type headaches due to inflammation-mediated hyperexcitability of neuronal pathways and inflammatory vascular responses, most specifically in the trigeminovascular system.[119,120] Due to significant overlap between trigeminal and vestibular tracts both anatomically and biochemically, migraine-associated dizziness is hypothesized to occur due to simultaneous disruption of vestibular pathways.[121,122] These inflammatory responses are believed to be driven by axonal damage and the neurometabolic cascade theory described previously.[28] Currently, it is unknown whether chronic post-TBI migraine headaches differ significantly in pathogenesis when compared with idiopathic migraine that is also known to commonly present with vertiginous symptoms.[122–125] As both types of migraine respond similarly to antimigraine medications, some argue the delineation may not be clinically relevant for proper management.[37,119,126]

Though it has not received the same amount of research focus as post-TBI migraine pain, migraine-associated dizziness has been identified a potential cause of dizziness following TBI in at least two studies that included both adults and children.[127,128] As official diagnostic criteria for vestibular migraine (VM) were not available prior to one of these studies and not clearly utilized in the other, it is unclear whether these cases of migraine-associated dizziness in children post-TBI met formal criteria for VM.[127–130] However, as VM has been identified as one of the most common cause of episodic dizziness in both children, even using diagnostic criteria based off adults, it is reasonable to suggest that a portion of migraine-associated dizziness in children post-TBI would meet VM criteria.[122,131,132] Prospective studies evaluating this relationship in children using formalized criteria better suited for children are needed, as children with VM frequently present with few to no objective clinical vestibular deficits and are instead diagnosed based on descriptions of their dizziness and chronicity of migraine attacks.[131,132]

Management of VM in children has primarily focused on utilization of typical antimigraine medications and lifestyle modifications, based off treatment recommendations for adult VM.[131–133] Potential medications include either prophylactic or abortive regimens. Based on one retrospective study of VM in children, prophylactic medications such as amitriptyline and nortriptyline, cyproheptadine, and topiramate demonstrated the most efficacy and abortive triptan medications were tolerated with no obvious side effects.[131] Vestibular suppressants such as meclizine were also associated with minor improvements in symptoms, but not resolution. As with diagnostic criteria, more data are needed on medication regimens specifically targeted to children for management of VM.[132]

Medication regimens appear to be easier to adhere to when compared with lifestyle modifications such as dietary restrictions, which can be difficult to maintain in children.[131] Other lifestyle modifications studied in general pediatric migraine that may be easier to adhere to, such as improving sleep hygiene and ensuring adequate hydration, should be examined as supplemental therapies for VM in children.[134] In fact, many of these modifications are recommended for improvement of general postconcussion symptoms and should therefore be encouraged in children with any of the diagnoses described in this chapter.[135]

There is some evidence to suggest that vestibular rehabilitation may be efficacious in improving symptoms of both idiopathic TM and post-TBI VM.[131,136] Vestibular rehabilitation has been investigated for management of more general post-TBI headache and dizziness and has demonstrated a strong benefit.[137] However, these findings have been seen primarily in children with concurrent balance dysfunction along with their VM symptoms or in combined study samples of both children and adults without a clear diagnosis. Metanalyses suggest the overall data on vestibular rehabilitation in VM is not definitive; therefore, more high-quality, blinded studies need to be done to better characterize this intervention both in general and specifically in children.[133,138]

Persistent postural–perceptual dizziness

PPPD is a newly recognized unifying diagnosis for a chronic experience of dizziness, unsteadiness, or nonspinning vertigo. These symptoms can be preceded by vestibular diseases described previously in this chapter as well as other neurological, medical, or psychiatric disease.[38,139] The diagnostic criteria for PPPD were defined by the International Classification of Vestibular Disorders in 2017 (Tables 17.1) and incorporate elements of multiple functional dizziness disorders that were formerly classified by various names, including chronic subjective dizziness, space-motion discomfort, and phobic postural vertigo.[140] These symptoms can be notoriously difficult for patients to describe, especially pediatric patients, making proper diagnosis challenging.[141] It has been hypothesized that PPPD is primarily driven by maladaptive reorganization of vestibular pathways following some insult; unsurprisingly, then, PPPD can present alongside other vestibular diagnoses and is not a diagnosis of exclusion.[38,142] Comorbid vestibular deficits can further complicate the picture and delay proper treatment.[38]

Despite the recent establishment of official diagnostic criteria, several features commonly seen in patients with PPPD have been identified and studied in patients with TBI previously. Spatial disorientation has long been identified as a major cause of dizziness following head injury and shares similarities with the space-motion

Table 17.1 International classification of vestibular disorders consensus criteria for the diagnosis of persistent postural perceptual dizziness (PPPDs).[140] Patients must meet all five of criteria A through E.

Criteria	Additional details
A. One or more symptoms of dizziness, unsteadiness, or nonspinning vertigo are present on most days for 3 months or more.	**1.** Symptoms last for prolonged (hours-long) periods of time, but may wax and wane in severity. **2.** Symptoms need not be present continuously throughout the entire day.
B. Persistent symptoms occur without specific provocation, but are exacerbated by three factors:	**1.** Upright posture. **2.** Active or passive motion without regard to direction or position. **3.** Exposure to moving visual stimuli or complex visual patterns.
C. The disorder is precipitated by conditions that cause vertigo, unsteadiness, dizziness, or problems with balance including acute, episodic, or chronic vestibular syndromes, other neurologic or medical illnesses, or psychological distress.	**1.** When the precipitant is an acute or episodic condition, symptoms settle into the pattern of criterion a as the precipitant resolves, but they may occur intermittently at first, and then consolidate into a persistent course. **2.** When the precipitant is a chronic syndrome, symptoms may develop slowly at first and worsen gradually.
D. Symptoms cause significant distress or functional impairment.	
E. Symptoms are not better accounted for by another disease or disorder.	

discomfort aspect of PPPD.[127] Patients with PPPD commonly experience increased reliance on visual inputs for balance as well as severe visual hypersensitivity, where their vertigo worsens when exposed to environments with complex visual stimuli—two likely interrelated phenomena well described in concussion literature as well.[38,143,144] As future studies incorporate PPPD screening into TBI assessment, the relationship between symptom onset and head injury will become more clear.

While a new diagnosis in both adults and pediatric populations, PPPD has been rapidly researched in adults and may be a more unfamiliar diagnosis to pediatricians. The few studies on children have suggested that PPPD may be a common diagnosis in children with chronic dizziness, especially after head injury, with 11.2% of all children with dizziness seen at a specialty clinic meeting diagnostic criteria for PPPD and 15.1% of those cases experiencing a precipitating concussion.[2,145] Of comorbid vestibular diagnoses, BPPV and vestibular migraine were most common with over half of children with PPPD also meeting for either BPPV or vestibular migraine. However, while these children met criteria for multiple diagnoses at the time of their PPPD diagnosis, PPPD symptoms persisted in 86% of children whose

BPPV symptoms had resolved. Objective clinical vestibular testing did not reliably identify children with PPPD.[145]

In addition to its relationship with both peripheral and central vestibular disease, the diagnosis of PPPD and its predecessors is frequently made in individuals with comorbid anxiety disorders.[38,139,146] In children diagnosed with PPPD, 28.3% of children also had a diagnosis of anxiety, demonstrating a similarly common relationship.[145] While not fully understood, it is hypothesized that individuals prone to anxiety may have more difficulty shifting away from postinsult reliance on visual sensory input and cautious ambulation back to preinjury postural control mechanisms.[38] This relationship may share a similar mechanism to the relationship between postconcussion syndrome symptoms and anxiety disorders seen in both children and adults. Importantly, a preexisting anxiety disorder is not a prerequisite for diagnosis of either PPPD or postconcussion syndrome.[139,147,148] Clinicians treating patients with these types of chronic dizziness diagnoses should ensure they are holistically evaluating their patients and addressing underlying psychological factors if present.[3]

Symptoms of PPPD can be debilitating for children; 43% of patients reported missing school or work time due to the impact of their PPPD.[145] However, there is little published evidence to guide treatment in children. Due to the complex interaction of vestibular maladaptation and psychological factors contributing to PPPD, treatment plans generally consist of a combination of vestibular rehabilitation techniques, cognitive behavioral therapy (CBT), and SSRI management in both adults and children. Wang et al. reported these three methods as the most prescribed treatments in their sample, with a third of patients undergoing multiple treatment modalities.[145] While there were limited data to suggest a definitive treatment, almost half (n = 7, 39%) of the 18 pediatric patients who reported symptom resolution underwent treatment with all three modalities. More general pediatricians working with children with dizziness need to keep PPPD in mind as a potential diagnosis, especially in the setting of ongoing postconcussion syndrome and better elucidate the efficacy of different treatment modalities in the pediatric population.

Conclusion

In summary, dizziness and imbalance following head injuries are often multifactorial in children and adolescents. Both peripheral and central causes may be present, as well as autonomic dysfunction. BPPV should be considered when positional vertigo symptoms are present and providers should have a low threshold for performing diagnostic and/or therapeutic positional maneuvers, when appropriate. If otologic symptoms are present, particularly hearing loss and/or sound-induced vertigo, then third window lesions should be considered, such as perilymphatic fistula or superior semicircular canal dehiscence. Central vestibular dysfunction is common after concussion and is typically managed with vestibular physical therapy. Autonomic dysfunction is also frequently a factor, which is generally managed with reconditioning and optimizing hydration but may warrant additional medical workup when it is treatment-resistant. Lastly, PPPD is a relatively common, but often overlooked, cause of chronic dizziness in adolescents with concussion, which requires intensive multimodal treatment.

References

1. Brodsky JR, Shoshany TN, Lipson S, Zhou G. Peripheral vestibular disorders in children and adolescents with concussion. *Otolaryngol Head Neck Surg*. 2018;159(2):365−370. https://doi.org/10.1177/0194599818770618.
2. Wang A, Zhou G, Lipson S, Kawai K, Corcoran M, Brodsky JR. Multifactorial characteristics of pediatric dizziness and imbalance. *Laryngoscope*. 2021;131(4): E1308−e1314. https://doi.org/10.1002/lary.29024. In eng.
3. Shah AS, Raghuram A, Kaur K, et al. Specialty-specific diagnoses in pediatric patients with postconcussion syndrome: experience from a multidisciplinary concussion clinic. *Clin J Sport Med*. 2021. https://doi.org/10.1097/jsm.0000000000000891. In eng.
4. Brodsky JR, Cusick BA, Kenna MA, Zhou G. Subjective visual vertical testing in children and adolescents. *Laryngoscope*. 2016;126(3):727−731. https://doi.org/10.1002/lary.25389. In eng.
5. Hamilton SS, Zhou G, Brodsky JR. Video head impulse testing (VHIT) in the pediatric population. *Int J Pediatr Otorhinolaryngol*. 2015;79(8):1283−1287. https://doi.org/10.1016/j.ijporl.2015.05.033. In eng.
6. Zhou G, Goutos C, Lipson S, Brodsky J. Range of peak head velocity in video head impulse testing for pediatric patients. *Otol Neurotol*. 2018;39(5):e357−e361. https://doi.org/10.1097/mao.0000000000001793. In eng.
7. Wang A, Zhou G, Kawai K, O'Brien M, Shearer AE, Brodsky JR. Benign paroxysmal positional vertigo in children and adolescents with concussion. *Sport Health*. 2021; 13(4):380−386. https://doi.org/10.1177/1941738120970515. In eng.
8. Brodsky JR, Lipson S, Wilber J, Zhou G. Benign paroxysmal positional vertigo (BPPV) in children and adolescents: clinical features and response to therapy in 110 pediatric patients. *Otol Neurotol*. 2018;39(3):344−350. https://doi.org/10.1097/mao.0000000000001673. In eng.
9. Zhou G, Brodsky JR. Objective vestibular testing of children with dizziness and balance complaints following sports-related concussions. *Otolaryngol Head Neck Surg*. 2015; 152(6):1133−1139. https://doi.org/10.1177/0194599815576720. In eng.
10. Balzanelli C, Spataro D, Redaelli de Zinis LO. Benign positional paroxysmal vertigo in children. *Audiol Res*. 2021;11(1):47−54. https://doi.org/10.3390/audiolres11010006. In eng.
11. Epley JM. The canalith repositioning procedure: for treatment of benign paroxysmal positional vertigo. *Otolaryngol Head Neck Surg*. 1992;107(3):399−404. https://doi.org/10.1177/019459989210700310. In eng.
12. Semont A, Freyss G, Vitte E. Curing the BPPV with a liberatory maneuver. *Adv Oto-Rhino-Laryngol*. 1988;42:290−293. https://doi.org/10.1159/000416126. In eng.
13. Lempert T, Tiel-Wilck K. A positional maneuver for treatment of horizontal-canal benign positional vertigo. *Laryngoscope*. 1996;106(4):476−478. https://doi.org/10.1097/00005537-199604000-00015. In eng.

14. Gufoni M, Mastrosimone L, Di Nasso F. [Repositioning maneuver in benign paroxysmal vertigo of horizontal semicircular canal]. *Acta Otorhinolaryngol Ital*. 1998; 18(6):363−367. In ita.

15. Jackson LE, Morgan B, Fletcher Jr JC, Krueger WW. Anterior canal benign paroxysmal positional vertigo: an underappreciated entity. *Otol Neurotol*. 2007;28(2):218−222. https://doi.org/10.1097/01.mao.0000247825.90774.6b. In eng.

16. Abdelmaksoud AA, Fahim DFM, Bazeed SES, Alemam MF, Aref ZF. Relation between vitamin D deficiency and benign paroxysmal positional vertigo. *Sci Rep*. 2021;11(1): 16855. https://doi.org/10.1038/s41598-021-96445-x. In eng.

17. Beyea JA, Agrawal SK, Parnes LS. Transmastoid semicircular canal occlusion: a safe and highly effective treatment for benign paroxysmal positional vertigo and superior canal dehiscence. *Laryngoscope*. 2012;122(8):1862−1866. https://doi.org/10.1002/lary.23390. In eng.

18. Bartholomew RA, Lubner RJ, Knoll RM, et al. Labyrinthine concussion: historic otopathologic antecedents of a challenging diagnosis. *Laryngoscope Investig Otolaryngol*. 2020;5(2):267−277. https://doi.org/10.1002/lio2.360. In eng.

19. Steenerson KK, Crane BT, Minor LB. Superior semicircular canal dehiscence syndrome. *Semin Neurol*. 2020;40(1):151−159. https://doi.org/10.1055/s-0039-3402738. In eng.

20. Walsh EM. Current management of superior semicircular canal dehiscence syndrome. *Curr Opin Otolaryngol Head Neck Surg*. 2020;28(5):340−345. https://doi.org/10.1097/moo.0000000000000657. In eng.

21. Lee GS, Zhou G, Poe D, et al. Clinical experience in diagnosis and management of superior semicircular canal dehiscence in children. *Laryngoscope*. 2011;121(10): 2256−2261. https://doi.org/10.1002/lary.22134. In eng.

22. Hain TC, Ostrowski VB. Limits of normal for pressure sensitivity in the fistula test. *Audiol Neuro Otol*. 1997;2(6):384−390. https://doi.org/10.1159/000259263. In eng.

23. Rawal R, Z X, Lipson S, Brodsky JR. Endoscopic repair of traumatic perilymphatic fistula in children: a case series. *J Int Adv Otol*. 2021;17(2):182−185.

24. Brodsky JR, Choi SS. Should children with an enlarged vestibular aqueduct be restricted from playing contact sports? *Laryngoscope*. 2018;128(10):2219−2220. https://doi.org/10.1002/lary.27119.

25. Gopen Q, Zhou G, Whittemore K, Kenna M. Enlarged vestibular aqueduct: review of controversial aspects. *Laryngoscope*. 2011;121(9):1971−1978. https://doi.org/10.1002/lary.22083.

26. Zhou G, Gopen Q. Characteristics of vestibular evoked myogenic potentials in children with enlarged vestibular aqueduct. *Laryngoscope*. 2011;121(1):220−225. https://doi.org/10.1002/lary.21184.

27. Sennaroglu L. Cochlear implantation in inner ear malformations—a review article. *Cochlear Implants Int*. 2010;11(1):4−41. https://doi.org/10.1002/cii.416. In eng.

28. Giza CC, Hovda DA. The new neurometabolic cascade of concussion. *Neurosurgery*. 2014;75(Suppl. 4):S24−S33. https://doi.org/10.1227/NEU.0000000000000505.

29. MacFarlane MP, Glenn TC. Neurochemical cascade of concussion. *Brain Inj*. 2015; 29(2):139−153. https://doi.org/10.3109/02699052.2014.965208.

30. Wu YC, Harezlak J, Elsaid NMH, et al. Longitudinal white-matter abnormalities in sports-related concussion: a diffusion MRI study. *Neurology*. 2020;95(7):e781−e792. https://doi.org/10.1212/WNL.0000000000009930.

31. Imagawa KK, Hamilton A, Ceschin R, et al. Characterization of microstructural injury: a novel approach in infant abusive head trauma-initial experience. *J Neurotrauma.* 2014;31(19):1632−1638. https://doi.org/10.1089/neu.2013.3228.

32. Utsunomiya H. Diffusion MRI abnormalities in pediatric neurological disorders. *Brain Dev.* 2011;33(3):235−242. https://doi.org/10.1016/j.braindev.2010.08.015.

33. Watson CG, DeMaster D, Ewing-Cobbs L. Graph theory analysis of DTI tractography in children with traumatic injury. *Neuroimage Clin.* 2019;21:101673. https://doi.org/10.1016/j.nicl.2019.101673.

34. Dennis EL, Babikian T, Giza CC, Thompson PM, Asarnow RF. Neuroimaging of the injured pediatric brain: methods and new lessons. *Neuroscientist.* 2018;24(6):652−670. https://doi.org/10.1177/1073858418759489.

35. Alhilali LM, Yaeger K, Collins M, Fakhran S. Detection of central white matter injury underlying vestibulopathy after mild traumatic brain injury. *Radiology.* 2014;272(1):224−232. https://doi.org/10.1148/radiol.14132670. In eng.

36. La Fountaine MF. An anatomical and physiological basis for the cardiovascular autonomic nervous system consequences of sport-related brain injury. *Int J Psychophysiol.* 2018;132(Pt A):155−166. https://doi.org/10.1016/j.ijpsycho.2017.11.016.

37. Fife TD, Kalra D. Persistent vertigo and dizziness after mild traumatic brain injury. *Ann N Y Acad Sci.* 2015;1343:97−105. https://doi.org/10.1111/nyas.12678.

38. Popkirov S, Staab JP, Stone J. Persistent postural-perceptual dizziness (PPPD): a common, characteristic and treatable cause of chronic dizziness. *Practical Neurol.* 2018;18(1):5−13. https://doi.org/10.1136/practneurol-2017-001809.

39. O'Reilly RC, Greywoode J, Morlet T, et al. Comprehensive vestibular and balance testing in the dizzy pediatric population. *Otolaryngol Head Neck Surg.* 2011;144(2):142−148. https://doi.org/10.1177/0194599810393679.

40. Alkathiry AA, Kontos AP, Furman JM, Whitney SL, Anson ER, Sparto PJ. Vestibulo-ocular reflex function in adolescents with sport-related concussion: preliminary results. *Sport Health.* 2019;11(6):479−485. https://doi.org/10.1177/1941738119865262.

41. Christy JB, Cochrane GD, Almutairi A, Busettini C, Swanson MW, Weise KK. Peripheral vestibular and balance function in athletes with and without concussion. *J Neurol Phys Ther.* 2019;43(3):153−159. https://doi.org/10.1097/NPT.0000000000000280.

42. Campbell KR, Parrington L, Peterka RJ, et al. Exploring persistent complaints of imbalance after mTBI: oculomotor, peripheral vestibular and central sensory integration function. *J Vestib Res.* 2021. https://doi.org/10.3233/VES-201590.

43. Peterka RJ. Sensorimotor integration in human postural control. *J Neurophysiol.* 2002;88(3):1097−1118. https://doi.org/10.1152/jn.2002.88.3.1097.

44. Caeyenberghs K, Leemans A, Geurts M, et al. Brain-behavior relationships in young traumatic brain injury patients: DTI metrics are highly correlated with postural control. *Hum Brain Mapp.* 2010;31(7):992−1002. https://doi.org/10.1002/hbm.20911.

45. Caeyenberghs K, Leemans A, Geurts M, et al. Correlations between white matter integrity and motor function in traumatic brain injury patients. *Neurorehabilit Neural Repair.* 2011;25(6):492−502. https://doi.org/10.1177/1545968310394870.

46. Katz-Leurer M, Rotem H, Lewitus H, Keren O, Meyer S. Relationship between balance abilities and gait characteristics in children with post-traumatic brain injury. *Brain Inj.* 2008;22(2):153−159. https://doi.org/10.1080/02699050801895399.

47. Gimmon Y, Millar J, Pak R, Liu E, Schubert MC. Central not peripheral vestibular processing impairs gait coordination. *Exp Brain Res.* 2017;235(11):3345−3355. https://doi.org/10.1007/s00221-017-5061-x.

48. Drijkoningen D, Chalavi S, Sunaert S, Duysens J, Swinnen SP, Caeyenberghs K. Regional gray matter volume loss is associated with gait impairments in young brain-injured individuals. *J Neurotrauma*. 2017;34(5):1022−1034. https://doi.org/10.1089/neu.2016.4500.

49. Rochefort C, Walters-Stewart C, Aglipay M, Barrowman N, Zemek R, Sveistrup H. Self-reported balance status is not a reliable indicator of balance performance in adolescents at one-month post-concussion. *J Sci Med Sport*. 2017;20(11):970−975. https://doi.org/10.1016/j.jsams.2017.04.008.

50. Hansen C, Cushman D, Anderson N, et al. A normative dataset of the balance error scoring system in children aged between 5 and 14. *Clin J Sport Med*. 2016;26(6):497−501. https://doi.org/10.1097/JSM.0000000000000285.

51. Jirovec J, Musalek M, Mess F. Test of motor proficiency second edition (BOT-2): compatibility of the complete and short form and its usefulness for middle-age school children. *Front Pediatr*. 2019;7:153. https://doi.org/10.3389/fped.2019.00153.

52. Khanna NK, Baumgartner K, LaBella CR. Balance error scoring system performance in children and adolescents with no history of concussion. *Sport Health*. 2015;7(4):341−345. https://doi.org/10.1177/1941738115571508.

53. Babl FE, Dionisio D, Davenport L, et al. Accuracy of components of SCAT to identify children with concussion. *Pediatrics*. 2017;140(2). https://doi.org/10.1542/peds.2016-3258.

54. Kruse AJ, Nugent AS, Peterson AR. Using sideline concussion tests in the emergency department. *Open Access Emerg Med*. 2018;10:113−121. https://doi.org/10.2147/OAEM.S165995.

55. Clark RA, Bryant AL, Pua Y, McCrory P, Bennell K, Hunt M. Validity and reliability of the Nintendo Wii balance board for assessment of standing balance. *Gait Posture*. 2010;31(3):307−310. https://doi.org/10.1016/j.gaitpost.2009.11.012.

56. Brett BL, Zuckerman SL, Terry DP, Solomon GS, Iverson GL. Normative data for the sway balance system. *Clin J Sport Med*. 2020;30(5):458−464. https://doi.org/10.1097/JSM.0000000000000632.

57. Garcia-Soidan JL, Leiros-Rodriguez R, Romo-Perez V, Garcia-Lineira J. Accelerometric assessment of postural balance in children: a systematic review. *Diagnostics*. 2020;11(1). https://doi.org/10.3390/diagnostics11010008.

58. Ruhe A, Fejer R, Gansslen A, Klein W. Assessing postural stability in the concussed athlete: what to do, what to expect, and when. *Sport Health*. 2014;6(5):427−433. https://doi.org/10.1177/1941738114541238.

59. Rochefort C, Walters-Stewart C, Aglipay M, Barrowman N, Zemek R, Sveistrup H. Balance markers in adolescents at 1 Month postconcussion. *Orthop J Sports Med*. 2017;5(3). https://doi.org/10.1177/2325967117695507, 2325967117695507.

60. Verbecque E, Vereeck L, Hallemans A. Postural sway in children: a literature review. *Gait Posture*. 2016;49:402−410. https://doi.org/10.1016/j.gaitpost.2016.08.003.

61. Bourelle S, Dey N, Sifaki-Pistolla D, et al. Computerized static posturography and laterality in children. Influence of age. *Acta Bioeng Biomech*. 2017;19(2):129−139. https://www.ncbi.nlm.nih.gov/pubmed/28869624.

62. Shumway-Cook A, Woollacott MH. The growth of stability: postural control from a development perspective. *J Mot Behav*. 1985;17(2):131−147. https://doi.org/10.1080/00222895.1985.10735341.

63. Cochrane GD, Christy JB, Almutairi A, et al. Vestibular, oculomotor, and balance function in children with and without concussion. *J Head Trauma Rehabil*. 2021;36(4):264−273. https://doi.org/10.1097/HTR.0000000000000651.

64. Riach CL, Hayes KC. Maturation of postural sway in young children. *Dev Med Child Neurol*. 1987;29(5):650−658. https://doi.org/10.1111/j.1469-8749.1987.tb08507.x.

65. Olivier I, Cuisinier R, Vaugoyeau M, Nougier V, Assaiante C. Age-related differences in cognitive and postural dual-task performance. *Gait Posture*. 2010;32(4):494−499. https://doi.org/10.1016/j.gaitpost.2010.07.008.

66. Pierret J, Beyaert C, Paysant J, Caudron S. How do children aged 6 to 11 stabilize themselves on an unstable sitting device? The progressive development of axial segment control. *Hum Mov Sci*. 2020;71:102624. https://doi.org/10.1016/j.humov.2020.102624.

67. Rine RM, Rubish K, Feeney C. Measurement of sensory system effectiveness and maturational changes in postural control in young children. *Pediatr Phys Ther*. 1998;10(1):16−22. https://journals.lww.com/pedpt/Fulltext/1998/01010/Measurement_of_Sensory_System_Effectiveness_and.4.aspx.

68. Opala-Berdzik A, Glowacka M, Wilusz K, Kolacz P, Szydlo K, Juras G. Quiet standing postural sway of 10- to 13-year-old, national-level, female acrobatic gymnasts. *Acta Bioeng Biomech*. 2018;20(2):117−123. https://www.ncbi.nlm.nih.gov/pubmed/30220710.

69. Rogge AK, Hamacher D, Cappagli G, et al. Balance, gait, and navigation performance are related to physical exercise in blind and visually impaired children and adolescents. *Exp Brain Res*. 2021;239(4):1111−1123. https://doi.org/10.1007/s00221-021-06038-3.

70. Howell DR, Osternig LR, Chou LS. Adolescents demonstrate greater gait balance control deficits after concussion than young adults. *Am J Sports Med*. 2015;43(3):625−632. https://doi.org/10.1177/0363546514560994.

71. Howell DR, Osternig LR, Chou LS. Detection of acute and long-term effects of concussion: dual-task gait balance control versus computerized neurocognitive test. *Arch Phys Med Rehabil*. 2018;99(7):1318−1324. https://doi.org/10.1016/j.apmr.2018.01.025.

72. Sambasivan K, Grilli L, Gagnon I. Balance and mobility in clinically recovered children and adolescents after a mild traumatic brain injury. *J Pediatr Rehabil Med*. 2015;8(4):335−344. https://doi.org/10.3233/PRM-150351.

73. Van Deventer KA, Seehusen CN, Walker GA, Wilson JC, Howell DR. The diagnostic and prognostic utility of the dual-task tandem gait test for pediatric concussion. *J Sport Health Sci*. 2021;10(2):131−137. https://doi.org/10.1016/j.jshs.2020.08.005.

74. Howell DR, Brilliant AN, Meehan 3rd WP. Tandem gait test-retest reliability among healthy child and adolescent athletes. *J Athl Train*. 2019;54(12):1254−1259. https://doi.org/10.4085/1062-6050-525-18.

75. Howell DR, Osternig LR, Chou LS. Dual-task effect on gait balance control in adolescents with concussion. *Arch Phys Med Rehabil*. 2013;94(8):1513−1520. https://doi.org/10.1016/j.apmr.2013.04.015.

76. Howell DR, Lugade V, Potter MN, Walker G, Wilson JC. A multifaceted and clinically viable paradigm to quantify postural control impairments among adolescents with concussion. *Physiol Meas*. 2019;40(8):084006. https://doi.org/10.1088/1361-6579/ab3552.

77. Katz-Leurer M, Rotem H, Keren O, Meyer S. Balance abilities and gait characteristics in post-traumatic brain injury, cerebral palsy and typically developed children. *Dev Neurorehabil*. 2009;12(2):100−105. https://doi.org/10.1080/17518420902800928.

78. Katz-Leurer M, Rotem H, Keren O, Meyer S. Effect of concurrent cognitive tasks on gait features among children post-severe traumatic brain injury and typically-developed controls. *Brain Inj*. 2011;25(6):581−586. https://doi.org/10.3109/02699052.2011.572943.

79. Kuhtz-Buschbeck JP, Hoppe B, Golge M, Dreesmann M, Damm-Stunitz U, Ritz A. Sensorimotor recovery in children after traumatic brain injury: analyses of gait, gross motor, and fine motor skills. *Dev Med Child Neurol*. 2003;45(12):821−828. https://doi.org/10.1017/s001216220300152x.

80. Smulligan KL, Wingerson MJ, Seehusen CN, Magliato SN, Wilson JC, Howell DR. Patient perception of dizziness and imbalance does not correlate with gait measures in adolescent athletes post-concussion. *Gait Posture*. 2021;90:289−294. https://doi.org/10.1016/j.gaitpost.2021.09.184.

81. Bach MM, Daffertshofer A, Dominici N. The development of mature gait patterns in children during walking and running. *Eur J Appl Physiol*. 2021;121(4):1073−1085. https://doi.org/10.1007/s00421-020-04592-2.

82. Leban B, Cimolin V, Porta M, et al. Age-related changes in smoothness of gait of healthy children and early adolescents. *J Mot Behav*. 2020;52(6):694−702. https://doi.org/10.1080/00222895.2019.1680949.

83. Alsalaheen BA, Mucha A, Morris LO, et al. Vestibular rehabilitation for dizziness and balance disorders after concussion. *J Neurol Phys Ther*. 2010;34(2):87−93. https://doi.org/10.1097/NPT.0b013e3181dde568.

84. Storey EP, Wiebe DJ, D'Alonzo BA, et al. Vestibular rehabilitation is associated with visuovestibular improvement in pediatric concussion. *J Neurol Phys Ther*. 2018;42(3):134−141. https://doi.org/10.1097/NPT.0000000000000228.

85. Dobney DM, Miller MB, Tufts E. Non-pharmacological rehabilitation interventions for concussion in children: a scoping review. *Disabil Rehabil*. 2019;41(6):727−739. https://doi.org/10.1080/09638288.2017.1400595.

86. Sorek G, Katz-Leurer M, Gagnon I, et al. The development and the inter-rater agreement of a treatment protocol for vestibular/oculomotor rehabilitation in children and adolescents post-moderate-severe TBI. *Brain Inj*. 2021:1−10. https://doi.org/10.1080/02699052.2021.1972454.

87. Popernack ML, Gray N, Reuter-Rice K. Moderate-to-Severe traumatic brain injury in children: complications and rehabilitation strategies. *J Pediatr Health Care*. 2015;29(3):e1−e7. https://doi.org/10.1016/j.pedhc.2014.09.003.

88. Appiah-Kubi KO, Wright WG. Vestibular training promotes adaptation of multisensory integration in postural control. *Gait Posture*. 2019;73:215−220. https://doi.org/10.1016/j.gaitpost.2019.07.197.

89. Han BI, Song HS, Kim JS. Vestibular rehabilitation therapy: review of indications, mechanisms, and key exercises. *J Clin Neurol*. 2011;7(4):184−196. https://doi.org/10.3988/jcn.2011.7.4.184.

90. Herdman SJ. Role of vestibular adaptation in vestibular rehabilitation. *Otolaryngol Head Neck Surg*. 1998;119(1):49−54. https://doi.org/10.1016/S0194-5998(98)70195-0.

91. Whitney SL, Alghadir AH, Anwer S. Recent evidence about the effectiveness of vestibular rehabilitation. *Curr Treat Options Neurol*. 2016;18(3):13. https://doi.org/10.1007/s11940-016-0395-4.

92. Caccese JB, Santos FV, Yamaguchi FK, Buckley TA, Jeka JJ. Persistent visual and vestibular impairments for postural control following concussion: a cross-sectional study in university students. *Sports Med*. 2021;51(10):2209−2220. https://doi.org/10.1007/s40279-021-01472-3.

93. Rine RM. Vestibular rehabilitation for children. *Semin Hear*. 2018;39(3):334−344. https://doi.org/10.1055/s-0038-1666822.

94. Gould SJ, Cochrane GD, Johnson J, Hebson CL, Kazamel M. Orthostatic intolerance in post-concussion patients. *Phys Sportsmed*. 2021:1–6. https://doi.org/10.1080/00913847.2021.1953357.

95. Haider MN, Patel KS, Willer BS, et al. Symptoms upon postural change and orthostatic hypotension in adolescents with concussion. *Brain Inj*. 2021;35(2):226–232. https://doi.org/10.1080/02699052.2021.1871951.

96. Heyer GL, Fischer A, Wilson J, et al. Orthostatic intolerance and autonomic dysfunction in youth with persistent postconcussion symptoms: a head-upright tilt table study. *Clin J Sport Med*. 2016;26(1):40–45. https://doi.org/10.1097/JSM.0000000000000183.

97. Sorek G, Gagnon I, Schneider K, et al. The integrated functions of the cardiac autonomic and vestibular/oculomotor systems in adolescents following severe traumatic brain injury and typically developing controls. *Brain Inj*. 2020;34(11):1480–1488. https://doi.org/10.1080/02699052.2020.1807055.

98. Lanier JB, Mote MB, Clay EC. Evaluation and management of orthostatic hypotension. *Am Fam Physician*. 2011;84(5):527–536. https://www.ncbi.nlm.nih.gov/pubmed/21888303.

99. Nilsson D, Sutton R, Tas W, Burri P, Melander O, Fedorowski A. Orthostatic changes in hemodynamics and cardiovascular biomarkers in dysautonomic patients. *PLoS One*. 2015;10(6):e0128962. https://doi.org/10.1371/journal.pone.0128962.

100. Task Force for the D, Management of S, European Society of C, et al. Guidelines for the diagnosis and management of syncope (version 2009). *Eur Heart J*. 2009;30(21):2631–2671. https://doi.org/10.1093/eurheartj/ehp298.

101. Rostami E, Nilsson P, Enblad P. Cerebral blood flow measurement in healthy children and children suffering severe traumatic brain injury-what do we know? *Front Neurol*. 2020;11:274. https://doi.org/10.3389/fneur.2020.00274.

102. Udomphorn Y, Armstead WM, Vavilala MS. Cerebral blood flow and autoregulation after pediatric traumatic brain injury. *Pediatr Neurol*. 2008;38(4):225–234. https://doi.org/10.1016/j.pediatrneurol.2007.09.012.

103. Len TK, Neary JP, Asmundson GJ, Goodman DG, Bjornson B, Bhambhani YN. Cerebrovascular reactivity impairment after sport-induced concussion. *Med Sci Sports Exerc*. 2011;43(12):2241–2248. https://doi.org/10.1249/MSS.0b013e3182249539.

104. Meier TB, Bellgowan PS, Singh R, Kuplicki R, Polanski DW, Mayer AR. Recovery of cerebral blood flow following sports-related concussion. *JAMA Neurol*. 2015;72(5):530–538. https://doi.org/10.1001/jamaneurol.2014.4778.

105. Wang Y, Nelson LD, LaRoche AA, et al. Cerebral blood flow alterations in acute sport-related concussion. *J Neurotrauma*. 2016;33(13):1227–1236. https://doi.org/10.1089/neu.2015.4072.

106. Freeman R, Wieling W, Axelrod FB, et al. Consensus statement on the definition of orthostatic hypotension, neurally mediated syncope and the postural tachycardia syndrome. *Clin Auton Res*. 2011;21(2):69–72. https://doi.org/10.1007/s10286-011-0119-5.

107. Gibbons CH, Freeman R. Delayed orthostatic hypotension: a frequent cause of orthostatic intolerance. *Neurology*. 2006;67(1):28–32. https://doi.org/10.1212/01.wnl.0000223828.28215.0b.

108. Kim HA, Bisdorff A, Bronstein AM, et al. Hemodynamic orthostatic dizziness/vertigo: diagnostic criteria. *J Vestib Res*. 2019;29(2–3):45–56. https://doi.org/10.3233/VES-190655.

109. Boris JR, Bernadzikowski T. Demographics of a large paediatric postural orthostatic tachycardia syndrome program. *Cardiol Young.* 2018;28(5):668–674. https://doi.org/10.1017/S1047951117002888.

110. Stewart JM, Boris JR, Chelimsky G, et al. Pediatric disorders of orthostatic intolerance. *Pediatrics.* 2018;141(1). https://doi.org/10.1542/peds.2017-1673.

111. Kokorelis C, Slomine B, Rowe PC, Suskauer S. Screening for orthostatic intolerance in symptomatic children presenting for concussion care. *Clin Pediatr.* 2020;59(1):75–82. https://doi.org/10.1177/0009922819885656.

112. Boris JR, Huang J, Bernadzikowski T. Orthostatic heart rate does not predict symptomatic burden in pediatric patients with chronic orthostatic intolerance. *Clin Auton Res.* 2020;30(1):19–28. https://doi.org/10.1007/s10286-019-00622-y.

113. Singer W, Sletten DM, Opfer-Gehrking TL, Brands CK, Fischer PR, Low PA. Postural tachycardia in children and adolescents: what is abnormal? *J Pediatr.* 2012;160(2): 222–226. https://doi.org/10.1016/j.jpeds.2011.08.054.

114. Bruce BK, Harrison TE, Bee SM, et al. Improvement in functioning and psychological distress in adolescents with postural orthostatic tachycardia syndrome following interdisciplinary treatment. *Clin Pediatr.* 2016;55(14):1300–1304. https://doi.org/10.1177/0009922816638663.

115. Hebson CL, McConnell ME, Hannon DW. Pediatric dysautonomia: much-maligned, often overmedicated, but not as complex as you think. *Congenit Heart Dis.* 2019; 14(2):156–161. https://doi.org/10.1111/chd.12720.

116. Miranda NA, Boris JR, Kouvel KM, Stiles L. Activity and exercise intolerance after concussion: identification and management of postural orthostatic tachycardia syndrome. *J Neurol Phys Ther.* 2018;42(3):163–171. https://doi.org/10.1097/NPT.0000000000000231.

117. Sheldon R, Raj SR, Rose MS, et al. Fludrocortisone for the prevention of vasovagal syncope: a randomized, placebo-controlled trial. *J Am Coll Cardiol.* 2016;68(1):1–9. https://doi.org/10.1016/j.jacc.2016.04.030.

118. Izcovich A, Gonzalez Malla C, Manzotti M, Catalano HN, Guyatt G. Midodrine for orthostatic hypotension and recurrent reflex syncope: a systematic review. *Neurology.* 2014;83(13):1170–1177. https://doi.org/10.1212/WNL.0000000000000815.

119. Capi M, Pomes LM, Andolina G, Curto M, Martelletti P, Lionetto L. Persistent posttraumatic headache and migraine: pre-clinical comparisons. *Int J Environ Res Publ Health.* 2020;17(7). https://doi.org/10.3390/ijerph17072585.

120. Ruff RL, Blake K. Pathophysiological links between traumatic brain injury and post-traumatic headaches. *F1000Res.* 2016;5. https://doi.org/10.12688/f1000research.9017.1.

121. Balaban CD. Migraine, vertigo and migrainous vertigo: links between vestibular and pain mechanisms. *J Vestib Res.* 2011;21(6):315–321. https://doi.org/10.3233/VES-2011-0428.

122. Dieterich M, Obermann M, Celebisoy N. Vestibular migraine: the most frequent entity of episodic vertigo. *J Neurol.* 2016;263(Suppl 1):S82–S89. https://doi.org/10.1007/s00415-015-7905-2.

123. Beh SC. Vestibular migraine: how to sort it out and what to do about it. *J Neuro Ophthalmol.* 2019;39(2):208–219. https://doi.org/10.1097/WNO.0000000000000791.

124. Hilton DB, Shermetaro C. Migraine associated vertigo. Treasure Island (FL) *StatPearls.* 2021.

125. Versino M, Sances G, Anghileri E, et al. Dizziness and migraine: a causal relationship? *Funct Neurol.* 2003;18(2):97−101. https://www.ncbi.nlm.nih.gov/pubmed/12911141.

126. Haas DC. Chronic post-traumatic headaches classified and compared with natural headaches. *Cephalalgia.* 1996;16(7):486−493. https://doi.org/10.1046/j.1468-2982.1996.1607486.x.

127. Hoffer ME, Gottshall KR, Moore R, Balough BJ, Wester D. Characterizing and treating dizziness after mild head trauma. *Otol Neurotol.* 2004;25(2):135−138. http://www.ncbi.nlm.nih.gov/pubmed/15021772.

128. Marcus HJ, Paine H, Sargeant M, et al. Vestibular dysfunction in acute traumatic brain injury. *J Neurol.* 2019;266(10):2430−2433. https://doi.org/10.1007/s00415-019-09403-z.

129. Headache Classification Committee of the International Headache S. The international classification of headache disorders, 3rd edition (beta version). *Cephalalgia.* 2013; 33(9):629−808. https://doi.org/10.1177/0333102413485658.

130. Lempert T, Olesen J, Furman J, et al. Vestibular migraine: diagnostic criteria. *J Vestib Res.* 2012;22(4):167−172. https://doi.org/10.3233/VES-2012-0453.

131. Brodsky JR, Cusick BA, Zhou G. Evaluation and management of vestibular migraine in children: experience from a pediatric vestibular clinic. *Eur J Paediatr Neurol.* 2016; 20(1):85−92. https://doi.org/10.1016/j.ejpn.2015.09.011.

132. Langhagen T, Landgraf MN, Huppert D, Heinen F, Jahn K. Vestibular migraine in children and adolescents. *Curr Pain Headache Rep.* 2016;20(12):67. https://doi.org/10.1007/s11916-016-0600-x.

133. Lauritsen CG, Marmura MJ. Current treatment options: vestibular migraine. *Curr Treat Options Neurol.* 2017;19(11):38. https://doi.org/10.1007/s11940-017-0476-z.

134. Raucci U, Boni A, Evangelisti M, et al. Lifestyle modifications to help prevent headache at a developmental age. *Front Neurol.* 2020;11:618375. https://doi.org/10.3389/fneur.2020.618375.

135. Barlow KM. Postconcussion syndrome: a review. *J Child Neurol.* 2016;31(1):57−67. https://doi.org/10.1177/0883073814543305.

136. Gottshall KR, Moore RJ, Hoffer ME. Vestibular rehabilitation for migraine-associated dizziness. *Int Tinnitus J.* 2005;11(1):81−84. https://www.ncbi.nlm.nih.gov/pubmed/16419697.

137. Schneider KJ, Meeuwisse WH, Nettel-Aguirre A, et al. Cervicovestibular rehabilitation in sport-related concussion: a randomised controlled trial. *Br J Sports Med.* 2014; 48(17):1294−1298. https://doi.org/10.1136/bjsports-2013-093267.

138. Alghadir AH, Anwer S. Effects of vestibular rehabilitation in the management of a vestibular migraine: a review. *Front Neurol.* 2018;9:440. https://doi.org/10.3389/fneur.2018.00440.

139. Dieterich M, Staab JP. Functional dizziness: from phobic postural vertigo and chronic subjective dizziness to persistent postural-perceptual dizziness. *Curr Opin Neurol.* 2017;30(1):107−113. https://doi.org/10.1097/WCO.0000000000000417.

140. Staab JP, Eckhardt-Henn A, Horii A, et al. Diagnostic criteria for persistent postural-perceptual dizziness (PPPD): consensus document of the committee for the classification of vestibular disorders of the Barany society. *J Vestib Res.* 2017;27(4):191−208. https://doi.org/10.3233/VES-170622.

141. Jahn K, Langhagen T, Heinen F. Vertigo and dizziness in children. *Curr Opin Neurol.* 2015;28(1):78−82. https://doi.org/10.1097/WCO.0000000000000157.

142. Staab JP. Persistent postural-perceptual dizziness. *Semin Neurol*. 2020;40(1):130–137. https://doi.org/10.1055/s-0039-3402736.

143. Pavlou M, Whitney SL, Alkathiry AA, et al. Visually induced dizziness in children and validation of the pediatric visually induced dizziness questionnaire. *Front Neurol*. 2017; 8:656. https://doi.org/10.3389/fneur.2017.00656.

144. Broglio SP, Collins MW, Williams RM, Mucha A, Kontos AP. Current and emerging rehabilitation for concussion: a review of the evidence. *Clin Sports Med*. 2015;34(2): 213–231. https://doi.org/10.1016/j.csm.2014.12.005.

145. Wang A, Fleischman KM, Kawai K, Corcoran M, Brodsky JR. Persistent postural-perceptual dizziness in children and adolescents. *Otol Neurotol*. 2021;42(8): e1093–e1100. https://doi.org/10.1097/MAO.0000000000003212.

146. Staab JP. Chronic subjective dizziness. *Continuum*. 2012;18(5 Neuro-otology): 1118–1141. https://doi.org/10.1212/01.CON.0000421622.56525.58.

147. Goreth MB, Palokas M. Association between premorbid neuropsychological conditions and pediatric mild traumatic brain injury/concussion recovery time and symptom severity: a systematic review. *JBI Database Syst Rev Implement Rep*. 2019;17(7): 1464–1493. https://doi.org/10.11124/JBISRIR-2017-004008.

148. Martin AK, Petersen AJ, Sesma HW, et al. Concussion symptomology and recovery in children and adolescents with pre-existing anxiety. *J Neurol Neurosurg Psychiatry*. 2020;91(10):1060–1066. https://doi.org/10.1136/jnnp-2020-323137.

Index

'*Note*: Page numbers followed by "f " indicate figures and "t" indicate tables.'

9780323874823